Emergency Department Analgesia

An Evidence-Based Guide

Edited by
STEPHEN H. THOMAS

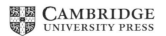
CAMBRIDGE
UNIVERSITY PRESS

CAMBRIDGE UNIVERSITY PRESS
Cambridge, New York, Melbourne, Madrid, Cape Town, Singapore, São Paulo, Delhi

Cambridge University Press
The Edinburgh Building, Cambridge CB2 8RU, UK

Published in the United States of America by Cambridge University Press, New York

www.cambridge.org
Information on this title: www.cambridge.org/9780521696012

First published 2008

Printed in the United States at Cambridge University Press, New York

A catalog record for this publication is available from the British Library

ISBN 978-0-521-69601-2 paperback

Contents

Contributors

Jeremy Ackerman, MD
Resident in Emergency Medicine, Stony Brook State University of New York and Medical Center, Stony Brook, NY, USA

Polly Bijur, PhD, MPH
Professor of Emergency Medicine, Albert Einstein College of Medicine, New York, USA

Hans Bradshaw, MD
Resident, Emergency Medicine/ Pediatrics, University of Arizona, Tucson, AZ, USA

Ciaran J. Browne, MB, BCh
Resident, Harvard Affiliated Emergency Medicine Residency, Brigham & Women's Hospital and Massachusetts General Hospital, Boston, MA, USA

John H. Burton, MD
Director of Emergency Medicine Residency, Albany Medical College/ Albany Medical Center, Albany, NY, USA

Lisa Calder, MD
Clinical Investigator, Ottawa Health Research Institute and Department of Emergency Medicine, University of Ottawa and Ottawa Hospital, Ottawa, ON, Canada

David Cline, MD
Associate Professor and Research Director, Department of Emergency Medicine, Wake Forest University Baptist Medical Center, Winston-Salem, NC, USA

Rita K. Cydulka, MD, MS
Associate Professor and Vice Chair, Department of Emergency Medicine, Case Western Reserve University School of Medicine and MetroHealth Medical Center, Cleveland, OH, USA

Deborah B. Diercks, MD
Associate Professor of Emergency Medicine, University of California Davis Medical Center, Sacramento, CA, USA

James Ducharme, MD
Professor and Clinical Director of Emergency Medicine Dalhousie University and Atlantic Health Sciences Corporation, St. John, NB, USA

Megan L. Fix, MD
Attending Physician, Maine Medical Center Department of Emergency Medicine, Portland, ME, USA

Michel Galinski, MD
Attending Physician, Service d'aide
medicale d'urgence de Seine Saint-
Denis, Avicenne Hospital, Bobigny,
France

Ula Hwang, MD, MPH
Assistant Professor of Emergency
Medicine, Mt. Sinai School of
Medicine, New York, USA

Jonathan S. Ilgen, MD
Resident, Harvard Affiliated
Emergency Medicine Residency,
Brigham & Women's Hospital and
Massachusetts General Hospital,
Boston, MA, USA

Andy Jagoda, MD
Professor and Emergency Medicine
Residency Site Director, Mt. Sinai
School of Medicine, New York, USA

Samuel Kim, MD, MDiv
Resident in Emergency Medicine,
Albany Medical College/Albany
Medical Center, Albany, NY, USA

Robert Knopp, MD
Professor and Assistant Emergency
Medicine Residency Director,
Regions Hospital and University of
Minnesota, St. Paul, MN, USA

Jason B. Lester, MD, MBA
Resident in Emergency Medicine,
St. Vincent Mercy Medical Center,
Toledo, OH, USA

Adam Levine, MD, MPH
Resident, Harvard Affiliated
Emergency Medicine Residency,
Brigham & Women's Hospital and
Massachusetts General Hospital,
Boston, MA, USA

Todd M. Listwa, MD
Resident, Harvard Affiliated
Emergency Medicine Residency,
Brigham & Women's Hospital and
Massachusetts General Hospital,
Boston, MA, USA

Frank LoVecchio, DO, MPH, ABMT
Professor of Emergency Medicine at
Arizona College of Osteopathic
Medicine and Research Director of the
Maricopa Medical Center Department
of Emergency Medicine, Phoenix,
AZ, USA

Sharon E. Mace, MD
Director of Observation Medicine and
Pediatric Education, Cleveland Clinic
Foundation/MetroHealth Medical
Center, Cleveland, OH, USA

Alan P. Marco, MD, MMM
Chairman and Residency Program
Director, Department of
Anesthesiology, University of Toledo
Medical Center,Toledo, OH, USA

Catherine A. Marco, MD
Clinical Professor of Emergency
Medicine, St. Vincent Mercy Medical
Center, Toledo, OH, USA

Chris McEachin, RN, EMTP
Paramedic, Wayne State University
and William Beaumont Hospital, Royal
Oak, MI, USA

James R. Miner, MD
Assistant Professor and Director of
Quality Assurance, University of
Minnesota and Hennepin County
Medical Center, New York, USA

Kalani Olmsted, MD
Resident in Emergency Medicine,
University of California Davis Medical
Center, Sacramento, CA, USA

Sohan Parekh, MD
Resident in Emergency Medicine,
Mt. Sinai School of Medicine, New
York, USA

Peter Rosen, MD
Visiting Lecturer, Harvard Medical
School and Beth Israel Deaconess
Medical Center, Boston, MA, USA

Michael S. Runyon, MD
Director of Medical Student
Education, Carolinas Medical Center,
Charlotte, NC, USA

Michael T. Schultz, MD
Resident in Emergency Medicine,
Carolinas Medical Center, Charlotte,
NC, USA

Adam J. Singer, MD
Professor and Vice Chair for Research,
Stony Brook State University of New
York and Medical Center, Stony Brook,
NY, USA

Robert A. Swor, DO
Clinical Associate Professor and EMS
Fellowship Director, Wayne State
University and William Beaumont
Hospital, Royal Oak, MI, USA

Joshua H. Tamayo-Sarver, MD, PhD
Resident in Emergency Medicine,
Harbor-UCLA Medical Center,
Torrance, CA, USA

Stephen H. Thomas, MD, MPH
Director of Academic Affairs at
Massachusetts General Hospital and
Associate Professor of Surgery at
Harvard Medical School, Boston,
MA, USA

Michael Turturro, MD
Clinical Professor and
Vice Chair and Director of Academic
Affairs, University of Pittsburgh and
The Mercy Hospital of Pittsburgh,
Pittsburgh, PA, USA

Michael Walta, MD
Resident, Harvard Affiliated
Emergency Medicine Residency,
Brigham & Women's Hospital and
Massachusetts General Hospital,
Boston, MA, USA

Benjamin A. White, MD
Resident, Harvard Affiliated
Emergency Medicine Residency,
Brigham & Women's Hospital and
Massachusetts General Hospital,
Boston, MA, USA

Beth Wicklund, MD
Resident in Emergency Medicine,
Regions Hospital and University of
Minnesota, St. Paul, MN, USA

Susan R. Wilcox, MD
Resident, Harvard Affiliated
Emergency Medicine Residency,
Brigham & Women's Hospital and
Massachusetts General Hospital,
Boston, MA, USA

Nathanael Wood, MD
Resident in Emergency Medicine,
Albany Medical College/Albany
Medical Center, Albany, NY, USA

Dale P. Woolridge, MD, PhD
Director of Emergency Medicine/
Pediatrics Residency Program and
Assistant Professor of Emergency
Medicine and Pediatrics, University of
Arizona, Tucson, AZ, USA

Andrew Worster, MD, MSc
Associate Professor of Medicine and
Clinical Epidemiology/Biostatistics
and Research Director, McMaster
University and Hamilton Health
Sciences, Cambridge, ON, USA

Janet Simmons Young, MD
Assistant Professor of Emergency
Medicine, University of North
Carolina, Chapel Hill, NC, USA

Kelly Young, MD
Associate Professor of Clinical
Medicine, Harbor-UCLA Medical
Center, Torrance, CA, USA

Foreword

There is a current fashion that I would label "arousal of emergency physician guilt." Far too many articles in our literature – and far too many hidden agendas – are addressed by declaring that the emergency physician must be aware of some rare entity, usually in an article that declares itself the first to report that entity in the emergency medicine literature. Moreover, there are many groups outside of emergency medicine that wish to blame the emergency physician for any error that is made. Such a one is the special interest group that has decided not to pay for care should we fail to draw a blood culture before treating a community-acquired pneumonia. The results of such culture might be of interest for the infectious disease specialists but cannot be shown to alter therapy, improve outcome, or lower the cost of medical care. We all profess belief in evidence-based medicine, but only if our own interests are served.

Nevertheless, there are areas of medicine in which our practice needs improvement, and it is part of the intellectual honesty of emergency medicine practitioners to obtain the evidence upon which an improved practice can be based. Pain management is certainly one such area. For too long the emergency physician has had a reputation for being very stoic about the patient's agony. That there is merit to this criticism is borne out by the reality that we often fail to treat painful musculoskeletal conditions, that we often underdose our analgesic therapy, and that for too long we perpetuate legends about pain that reinforce our unnecessary failure to treat pain adequately. For example, for years we were taught that infants did not perceive pain, and did not require analgesia. Another example is the often-present notion that if we give analgesia to patients with abdominal pain, we will mask their disease and prevent timely diagnosis and surgery.

The root cause of all of this is the reality that nowhere in medicine is the doctor as dependent upon the patient's history as in the presence of pain. If God had been a more helpful biomedical engineer, there would be a color code to light up the part of the body hurting in a brilliant color, the intensity of which would vary with the degree of pain. Unfortunately, there are no objective findings that define the presence of pain. A change in vital signs (e.g. tachycardia) does not mean that there is pain, and stable vital signs do not mean pain is absent. Moreover, the vital sign changes are often inconsistent; pain can simultaneously elevate blood pressure and decrease heart rate.

Furthermore, we are conditioned to worry about causing or contributing to addictive behaviors, although it is impossible to show that diseases (e.g. sickle cell) that cause significant episodes of pain lead to addiction. Because of these worries, we often underdose analgesic therapy, and formulate incorrect perceptions about patients when they are in-between pain crises. For example, if one sees a patient with renal colic, the perception of the patient's pain is quite different if the patient is viewed during stone movement rather than during the periods between movement.

This text is an effort to help to solve some of the dilemmas that exist in the recognition and management of a patient's pain. By reviewing the data that exist concerning the efficacy of various forms of pain relief in different conditions, we hope to assist the physician in forming intelligent judgment about which therapies are efficacious, what dosages to use, and what therapy does not work despite the legends that surround it.

The book cannot replace an empathetic and sensitive physician evaluation. There is no question that some patients cannot describe the nuances of their pain; they either do not have the language skills, or they are so focused upon their distress that they cannot talk about it. They know they are hurting, and whether the pain is throbbing, stabbing, radiating, or the worst they have ever felt is colored by their individual abilities to withstand discomfort, as well as their individual abilities to describe it. It requires experience and sympathy, as well as a willingness to trust the patient, to obtain an appreciation of how the patient feels. Many older patients appear stoic, but this may be because they cannot perceive or describe pain as readily as a younger patient, even though they are hurting. Some patients are so frightened of pain that any degree is enough to induce hysteria and even collapse. Some of this may be learned behavior, induced by the patient's historic and immediate culture. Some of this is variation on how patients tolerate discomfort. Some patients do not describe pain because they wish to deny the presence of a disease, such as a heart attack. Some do not describe pain because they do not want to appear demanding or cowardly. It is useful, therefore, for the physician to know what conditions produce pain, search to find the patients who possess it, and trust the answers that the patient gives. I personally am more concerned about relieving a patient's pain than I am about giving pain medicine to a patient who has a drug dependency rather than true pain.

There are many places in medicine where we are frustrated by not having adequate answers to solve problems, and pain management is one of these. There are certain kinds of pain for which we have no good answer (e.g. chronic back pain syndrome). The book has tried to find evidence to support practices that have utility, but there are many patients who remain in torment, and who also torment the medical staff because we cannot relieve their problems.

It is useful to recall that even when we do not possess good evidence from effective, well-executed prospective studies, which have been successfully blinded and have enough patients to avoid a type II error, we may still have a clinical problem to deal with. In those cases, we would recommend, as described appropriately in the book, a useful (even if not optimal) approach. Where there are no data for changing a practice, we would recommend using what your experience dictates. Historic anecdotal experience should not supersede good prospective evidence, but where there is no good evidence, it only makes sense to continue to do something that seems to work. There is no doubt there often is a placebo effect that can occur from a concerned physician who is trying to relieve discomfort. The fact that this may not be reproducible in a long clinical trial with multiple physicians does not negate some efficacy for a single physician.

It is also easy to fall into the trap of trusting anything that is written from a controlled study, even when it contradicts your own experience. For example, meperidine has fallen out of favor in some measure because of theoretical dangers. One can find rare examples of meperidine causing seizures when given in repeated doses, but it is inappropriate to deny a half-century's experience with millions of doses of the drug that produced analgesia without problem.

The authors of the book are aware of all these problems and try to make allowances for varying attitudes about evidence, as well as varying quality of the evidence. Upon reading many of the chapters concerning the difficult pain areas, I was often struck by the absence of a superior management, but overall, was left with a sense of comfort that, by drawing upon clinical experience, I would not be harming the patient.

In many chapters, one finds recommendations for how to avoid problems that the reader might otherwise not have considered, such as systemic absorption of ocular medications – therefore NSAID drops should not be used in pregnant patients. Most readers would probably know that the NSAIDs can prematurely close a ductus that needs to be patent in the fetus, but would they think of it in relationship to an ophthalmic drop?

This book is very useful for a wide group of readers with varying experience. Many students and residents will be commencing their clinical practice and attempting to learn appropriate dosages as well as which medications are preferable. For them, this book will provide an indispensable reference. It is probably best read in conjunction with caring for a given patient rather than trying to absorb the material by reading the book from cover to cover, which could be confusing and would certainly represent an unretainable amount of information.

The more experienced physician will also profit from the material in the book. There is always room to discover what your own individual style of practice is based upon, alter it where there is new information that you did not previously possess, or continue with your old style as you supplement the book evidence with your own clinical experience.

While the book is oriented towards the emergency physician and acute care provider, the material is broad enough that it would certainly also be useful for any office practice, as well as for many inpatient physicians in a variety of specialties.

The book has been very carefully edited to try to make the language, and the recommendations, uniform. In this respect, the book's broad subject matter and international scope render drug names a challenge. One thing I found particularly helpful is the tabulated lexicon of brand and generic names. While I understand the reason for using generic names, that is not the way most new agents are learned, and I am frequently lost as to what drug is being talked about when only the generic name is used.

While we have earned some of the opprobrium that is connected with pain management, it is quite clear that reading this book will alter the way one thinks about pain management and remind one to be more empathetic and generous. It will give the emergency physician good sound evidence upon which to base practice. I am sure that our patients will be grateful for this guidance to their improved care.

Peter Rosen MD
Boston

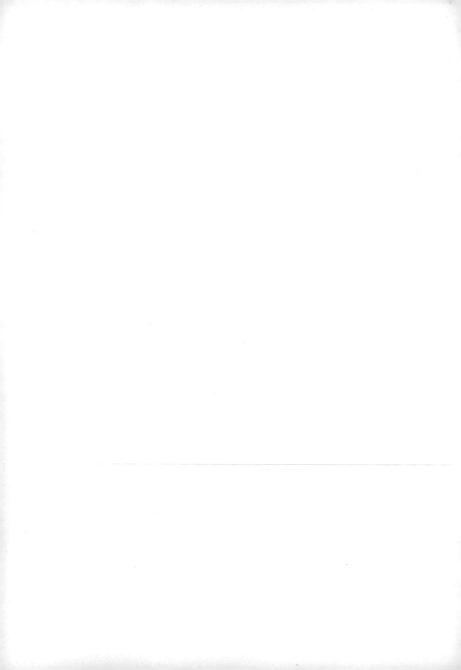

Preface

A typical shift in the Emergency Department (ED) finds the acute care provider making dozens of pain care decisions. How should discomfort be assessed? Which patients should be treated? What agent, administration route, and dosing interval should be chosen?

Busy ED clinicians answer the preceding and similar questions by calling on habit, educated guesswork, and – where available – evidence. This text's purpose is to present data-driven and experience-based recommendations, from research and clinical experts, that can be relied upon for guidance in treating pain in the ED.

Why a new text? The ED physician can already obtain detailed information on pain physiology and pharmacology. A number of excellent references exist, several written by chapter authors appearing in this text. While clinical chapters in major Emergency Medicine (EM) texts often provide cogent discussions of pain care, it is difficult for comprehensive texts to include fine detail on symptomatic relief. Analgesia may or may not be the most important part of an individual patient encounter, but it plays some role in the vast majority of ED visits. There is thus room for a reference that strives to provide highly focused, practical recommendations for ED pain care.

This text aims to combine a literature survey and consultation with a seasoned EM clinician. To facilitate this combination, chapter authors were given wide latitude to determine which evidence (*e.g.* data from non-ED settings) to include. Though clinical chapters follow a similar format, chapter lengths are uneven, due to varying levels of evidence addressing a given condition.

Treatment chapters begin with *Agents*, a listing of the drugs discussed. This listing may include analgesics or drug classes that are not recommended in the final analysis. The next section, *Evidence*, summarizes the available studies and applicable data. The *Evidence* section is subdivided for some conditions, particularly where there are many data. To aid clinicians seeking quick reference, pain-relief drug names are italicized (*morphine*) and analgesic drug classes are boldfaced (**opioids**).

Text users seeking quick reference may find that all they need are the *Summary and recommendations* sections of each chapter. These sections in the diagnosis-based chapters provide a *First-line* recommendation, the authors' opinion as to the best single choice for the condition. This choice may represent a clearly superior agent, or it may represent a selection of one drug among many with similar safety and efficacy.

Since clinicians treating pain have to select a single drug, this text's chapter authors were asked to do the same. The fact that more than one drug may be a "right" answer to a clinical situation is reflected in the authors' provision of *Reasonable* recommendations. The *Reasonable* classifications should be interpreted as just that – analgesic approaches that may or may not be as good as the *First-line* choice, but which are defensible as selections for the case at hand. The next sections in the *Summary and recommendations* provide advice for pregnant patients and for children; both safety and efficacy are considered. The clinical chapters conclude with mention of *Special circumstances* that may modify analgesia recommendations.

I hope that this text with its wisdom of many experienced authors proves useful to increasingly busy ED clinicians. Whether the reference confirms old habits as state-of-the-art, identifies new approaches that may be helpful, or even helps settle arguments (meperidine for biliary colic?), this book will be successful if you, the clinician, find that it assists your efforts to improve the comfort of your patients.

Acknowledgments

Many thanks to this text's chapter authors, who took on the time-consuming job of reviewing countless studies in order to define EM analgesia's state-of-the-art. Special appreciation is due Peter Rosen, whose invaluable mentorship included sagacious review and (characteristically blunt) commentary on each chapter of this text.

As an ED Attending at Massachusetts General Hospital, I've learned far more than my share from the MGH housestaff and Harvard medical students. I exhort these outstanding young clinicians to persist in asking "*Where's the data?*", while continuing to err on the side of the patient in cases where evidence is inconclusive.

The most important acknowledgments go to those from whom the most forbearance has been required, during the two years it has taken to prepare this book. To Cathrine, for her unwavering support and inevitable good humor, I owe the thanks of a lifetime. To Sarah Alice and Caroline, I will make good on the agreed-upon bribe (cookies), for tolerating long work hours and not causing (irreparable) damage to the manuscript.

Abbreviations

BID	twice daily
CNS	central nervous system
COX	cyclooxygenase
ED	emergency department
EM	emergency medicine
EMS	emergency medical services
FDA	US Food and Drug Administration
GI	gastrointestinal
HIV	human immunodeficiency virus
HS	at bedtime
ICP	intracranial pressure
IM	intramuscular
IN	intranasal
IU	international units
IV	intravenous
n	number of patients or study subjects
NSAID	nonsteroidal anti-inflammatory drug
OTM	oral transmucosal
PCA	patient-controlled analgesia
PO	oral
PR	rectal
q	every (e.g. q8 h = every 8h)
QD	(once) daily
QID	four times daily
RCT	randomized, controlled trial
SC	subcutaneous
SL	sublingual
SSRI	selective serotonin reuptake inhibitor
TD	transdermal
TID	three times daily
VAS	visual analog scale

General considerations

Introduction and general approach to pain

JAMES DUCHARME

■ Topics

- Becoming comfortable with treating pain
- General principles of pain assessment
- General principles of pain management

■ Introduction

Emergency physicians are frequently very busy at work. There is little time to make use of a standard reference text to find material that may be relevant to the patient in front of us. Many such texts, while invaluable at providing comprehensive evidence necessary to stay up to date, are not always user-friendly for immediate bedside care. This book hopes to provide a hands-on resource, by providing the clinician with practical information on pain management that can be used while working.

This book is intended to guide decision-making for the care of individual patients. Its main goal is to give an evidence-based set of recommendations – without implying they are the *only* "right" answers – for various painful conditions encountered in the acute care setting. The text also aims to over-view clinically relevant aspects of some general topics such as pain management in various populations.

Research and medical knowledge being the incomplete and evolving entities that they are, the available evidence may be of poor or even conflicting quality. The authors have been asked to wade through analgesia research, interpreting and incorporating the literature into their most reasonable practical recommendations for pain management. The intent of the authors is not to try and exhaustively critique the evidence. Rather, their goal is to present the best possible scientific basis for pain management decisions that must be made today, regardless of the quality of available data.

No text of the brevity and practicality envisioned for this book could be sufficiently comprehensive to cover all possibly acceptable approaches. By making specific recommendations when evidence may be poor, conflicting, or absent, authors will necessarily be somewhat subjective, and there will inevitably be room for disagreement. Finally, however, clinicians must make decisions about the patients in front of them. This book aims to help users to do just that.

■ Becoming comfortable with treating pain

Knowledge of analgesics should be a core area for our practice – up to 70% of ED patients register with a primary complaint of pain.[1] Unfortunately, pain education in medicine lags behind other areas. Many physicians graduate from medical school with almost no training in pain management or analgesic use. Attitudes such as opiophobia accompany us as we enter training and are often reinforced by the training we receive.[2] Lack of knowledge and, even more importantly, lack of understanding leave us unprepared. We often do not recognize how our own cultural and moral beliefs can negatively impact on patient pain management. For instance, when emergency physicians were surveyed about the incidence of addiction among sickle cell patients suffering from vaso-occlusive crises, 53% felt that more than 20% of patients were addicted, although the actual addiction rate is less than 2%.[3] Such beliefs can only be corrected if we learn how to differentiate drug-seeking behavior derived from oligoanalgesia – as is the case with sicklers – from similar, but not identical, behavior seen with addicts. It is only with such knowledge that our comfort level can improve, while our distrust of patients seemingly always in severe pain can diminish.

A nurse once said to me, "The patients always say their pain is 10/10, how can we believe them?" The answer is often so obvious as to be invisible: why come to an ED if pain is minimal? Every elderly patient we see in the ED is ill, but we do not infer that all elderly people are sick. Similarly, although a large portion of society suffers from chronic pain, most people do not. Our practice sees patients at their worst. They are in pain, afraid, and ill or injured. Let us not ever forget that as we apply the excellent advice seen in the following pages.

Since no physician consciously chooses to see a patient suffer, oligoanalgesia arises from unrecognized beliefs and attitudes.[2,4] For optimal application of the recommendations of this book, any such beliefs must be either unlearned or recognized and accounted for in day-to-day practice. If we do not believe the patient who says his pain is 10/10, then it does not matter how many times we document it: we still will not improve that patient's pain.[5] We must all come to accept that the vast majority of patients coming to an ED are in pain. Patients with true drug-seeking behavior create an emotionally charged atmosphere, thereby leaving the impression of being a large part of our practice. They, in fact, represent about 1% of our patient population.[6]

Pain management in EM has improved tremendously as we have become more aware of our past inadequacies. Excellent research, including many studies conducted by authors in this book, has allowed us to provide better care. It is now standard care to provide analgesia for patients with undifferentiated abdominal pain while performing necessary investigations.[7] New frontiers, such as nurse-initiated analgesics while the patient is in triage or with the use of delegated acts, are growing rapidly.[8-11] Patients in many EDs are now routinely provided topical or local anesthesia for simple (yet painful) procedures such as placement of intravenous catheters or nasogastric tubes.[12,13] It is hoped that, by providing practical information on analgesia, this book can further the goal of making all acute care providers comfortable treating pain.

■ General principles of pain assessment

The subject of ascertainment of pain levels is sufficiently important to warrant its own chapter in this text. Some general principles are outlined here. The Joint Commission on the Accreditation of Healthcare Organizations has mandated documentation of pain levels for patients in the ED.[14] That mandate cannot make us believe the patient, nor can it ensure that our assessment will agree with the report of pain by the patient. More than 15 years ago, Choiniere and colleagues reported that healthcare workers consistently scored pain at a different level to that scored by the patients.[15] Recent literature shows that even seasoned physicians inaccurately assess patients' pain levels. In fact, discrepancy between pain scores assigned by patients and physicians increases with provider experience.[16]

We have to remind ourselves constantly that the patient hasn't previously suffered a hundred broken tibias or episodes of trauma – the painful episode prompting the current ED visit may be the first ever of such intensity for that particular patient. Furthermore, patients (such as sicklers) with recurrent painful episodes may believe pain justification behavior is the only way they can convince us to appreciate the degree to which they are suffering. Finally, we must remember that fear and the impression of loss of control will further increase any pain sensation. Pain scores are uni-dimensional tools. They do not and cannot account for any of the above emotional overlay. Pain scores can be guides, but as with any guide they have to be believed to be followed.

The most important pain score is the first one. Scoring of pain at arrival should be used as part of a comprehensive triage tool to ascertain maximal times to physician assessment. Triage pain scores can also be used to initiate nurse-driven pain treatment protocols. After the initial pain score, further pain scoring (with few exceptions) should either not occur or play a minor role in determining need for further analgesia. The risk with longitudinal pain scoring lies in having pain management endpoints defined by an arbitrary number, rather than by the patient. As is the case with pain reporting, pain management endpoints should be patient driven. Healthcare workers should allow the patient to choose how much (or how little) pain they wish to continue to have. Patients rarely wish to have no pain; they wish to be comfortable and functional. Depending on home or work requirements, patients may be willing to have a higher degree of pain in order to avoid any adverse effects of medication. Instead of repeating pain score assessments, a patient's comfort needs may be better met by simply asking "do you want more pain medication?"

■ General principles of pain management

In many situations, expedited pain control can and should be achieved. Patients with any severe pain, especially those with renal colic, migraine headache, vaso-occlusive sickle crisis and breakthrough cancer pain should expect – and receive – rapid pain control. If an ED has prolonged waiting times or excessive delays, protocols that allow pain management prior to physician assessment should be considered for patients with such diagnoses. Other indications for advanced pain management directives could include obvious fractures, burns or amputations.

Clinicians should insure that, in cases where proffered analgesics are declined, the refusal is not caused by patients' own barriers to accepting clinically indicated medication. Providers should also keep in mind exceptions to the rule of patient self-determination of analgesia endpoints. Examples of situations in which complete pain relief should be sought include acute myocardial infarction, where no pain is acceptable, and migraine headaches, where discharge with pain is associated with increased chance of recurrent cephalalgia.[16,17]

Even when a physician sees a patient quickly, there may still be unacceptable delays to adequate pain management. Clinicians who routinely order titrated opioids for pain control may be unaware of intrinsic departmental barriers to rapid titration. Nursing workload may mean that an order for opioids "every 10 min as needed" results, operationally, in administration of medication at much longer intervals. Every ED should consider flow studies in order to identify specific barriers to the rapid delivery of titrated analgesics.

While initiation of analgesics is improving, we need to improve our rate of recurrent analgesic provision. In one study, only 15% of patients with polytrauma received more than one dose of analgesic.[18] We need to address our inability to treat pain adequately in specific subgroups: young children, the elderly, the cognitively impaired, and the polytrauma patient.[19] By applying standard approaches as described in this book, we can certainly further improve our pain management.

There is no such thing as "one drug fits all." Given genetic variation in relevant physiology (e.g. mu opioid receptors), it is important we know about many drugs in each class of analgesic.[20] It is more than likely clinicians will encounter patients who are unable to respond to certain analgesics. Before thinking "drug seeker," remember "genetic variability" it is entirely possible; that the patient being seen in ED cannot benefit from a specific medication that is known to be helpful (usually) for a given condition. It is equally important to remember that, for many types of severe pain (e.g. renal colic), combination therapy is superior to monotherapy.[21]

We can see that pain management is like any aspect of medicine: physician knowledge, physician experience, and patient expectation must all be combined to ensure optimal care. Too often our knowledge of pain management fails us – this book will certainly go a long way to correct that weakness. Failure to believe and include the patient is another reason for oligoanalgesia and patient dissatisfaction. Finally, we must all recognize that we each bring our own biases and experiences to the bedside ... it is up to us to determine if those biases and experiences aid rather than harm our patients.

References

1. Johnston CC, Gagnon AJ, Fullerton L, *et al.* One-week survey of pain intensity on admission to and discharge from the emergency department: a pilot study. *J Emerg Med.* 1998;**16**:377–382.

2. Weinstein SM, Laux LF, Thornby JI, *et al.* Medical students' attitudes toward pain and the use of opioid analgesics: implications for changing medical school curriculum. *South Med J.* 2000;**93**:472–478.

3. Shapiro BS, Benjamin LJ, Payne R, *et al.* Sickle cell-related pain: perceptions of medical practitioners. *J Pain Symptom Manage.* 1997;**14**:168–174.

4. Wilson JE, Pendleton JM. Oligoanalgesia in the emergency department. *Am J Emerg Med.* 1989;**7**:620–623.

5. Thomas S, Andruskiewicz L. Ongoing visual analog score display improves ED care. *J Emerg Med.* 2004;**26**:389–394.

6. Makower RM, Pennycook AG, Moulton C. Intravenous drug abusers attending an inner city accident and emergency department. *Arch Emerg Med.* 1992;**9**:32–39.

7. Thomas SH, Silen W. Effect on diagnostic efficiency of analgesia for undifferentiated abdominal pain. *Br J Surg.* 2003;**90**:5–9.

8. Kelly A, Brumby C, Barnes C. Nurse-initiated, titrated intravenous opioid analgesia reduces time to analgesia for selected painful conditions. *Can J Emerg Med.* 2005;**7**:149–154.

9. Meunier-Sham J, Ryan K. Reducing pediatric pain during ED procedures with a nurse-driven protocol: an urban pediatric emergency department's experience. *J Emerg Nurs.* 2003;**29**:127–132.

10. Fry M, Holdgate A. Nurse-initiated intravenous morphine in the emergency department: efficacy, rate of adverse events and impact on time to analgesia. *Emerg Med (Freemantle)*. 2002;**14**:249–254.

11. Fry M, Ryan J, Alexander N. A prospective study of nurse initiated panadeine forte: expanding pain management in the ED. *Accid Emerg Nurs*. 2004;**12**:136–140.

12. Singer AJ, Konia N. Comparison of topical anesthetics and vasoconstrictors vs lubricants prior to nasogastric intubation: a randomized, controlled trial. *Acad Emerg Med*. 1999;**6**:184–190.

13. Kleiber C, Sorenson M, Whiteside K, *et al*. Topical anesthetics for intravenous insertion in children: a randomized equivalency study. *Pediatrics*. 2002;**110**:758–761.

14. Gallagher RM. Physician variability in pain management: are the JCAHO standards enough? *Pain Med*. 2003;**4**:1–3.

15. Choiniere M, Melzack R, Girard N, *et al*. Comparisons between patients' and nurses' assessment of pain and medication efficacy in severe burn injuries. *Pain*. 1990;**40**:143–152.

16. Marquie L, Raufaste E, Lauque D, *et al*. Pain rating by patients and physicians: evidence of systematic pain miscalibration. *Pain*. 2003;**102**:289–296.

17. Ducharme J, Beveridge RC, Lee JS, *et al*. Emergency management of migraine: Is the headache really over? *Acad Emerg Med*. 1998;**5**:899–905.

18. Neighbor ML, Honner S, Kohn MA. Factors affecting emergency department opioid administration to severely injured patients. *Acad Emerg Med*. 2004;**11**:1290–1290.

19. Rupp T, Delaney KA. Inadequate analgesia in emergency medicine. *Ann Emerg Med*. 2004;**43**:494–503.

20. Wang H, Sun H, Della Penna K, *et al*. Chronic neuropathic pain is accompanied by global changes in gene expression and shares pathobiology with neurodegenerative diseases. *Neuroscience*. 2002;**114**:529–546.

21. Safdar B, Degutis L, Landry K, *et al*. Intravenous morphine plus ketorolac is superior to either drug alone for treatment of acute renal colic. *Ann Emerg Med*. 2006;**48**:173–181.

Assessment of pain

CATHERINE A. MARCO AND ALAN P. MARCO

■ Topics

- Necessity of pain quantification
- Principles of applying pain assessment mechanisms
- Specific pain assessment tools for various populations

■ Introduction

The Joint Commission on the Accreditation of Healthcare Organizations and various medical associations have endorsed the essential role of pain assessment in optimizing healthcare.[1,2] In fact, pain assessment plays an integral role in the ongoing efforts to improve overall pain management in the acute care setting; the use of pain scores in the ED setting increases rates of analgesia administration.[3–5] This chapter will overview the pain assessment process and outline some pain rating tools that have been useful in the acute care setting.

■ Is pain quantification necessary?

Because pain sensation is inherently subjective, it is typically assessed by patient self-report. Some form of explicit pain assessment is necessary, since studies in myriad patient populations have failed to identify consistently reliable surrogate markers for pain. Attempts to quantify pain using measurable behavioral and physiologic parameters (including vital signs) have been disappointing. Objective signs are neither consistent nor universal indicators of pain. Perhaps most importantly, the absence of such signs does not exclude the experience of pain.[6–10]

The very idea of quantifying pain is somewhat controversial. Germaine to the debate is a nineteenth century contention made by William Thomson (Lord Kelvin) that worthy knowledge should be quantifiable in the form of numbers. More recently, the "Curse of Kelvin," described as "the unthinking and inappropriate worship of quantifiable information in medicine," has been invoked by those concerned about objectification of information – such as pain – that is not amenable to direct quantification.[11,12]

For the clinician attending to a suffering patient, the philosophical debate about quantifying subjective sensation will usually be rendered moot by an institutional requirement for objective documentation of pain levels. Furthermore, the above-noted evidence does indicate that analgesia is improved by pain scoring – if for no other reason than focusing caregivers on pain assessment. Therefore, some form of this assessment needs to occur in the ED. As outlined in the initial chapter of this book, interpretation and application of pain score results requires clinical judgment. That said, the weight of available evidence supports performance of at least one objective pain rating for patients in ED.

■ Applying pain quantification tools

Pain self-ratings have long been known to be influenced by a range of clinical, psychological, and social factors. Patient pain ratings, and the reliability of available objective pain scales, have long been known to be affected by variables such as pain level, psychosocial factors, age, gender, ethnicity, cultural background, anxiety, and level of functional impairment.[13–17] More recently, investigators have demonstrated the importance of patient education regarding the use of the pain scale.[18] There is interpatient variation in terms of pain experiences, understanding of pain rating systems, and pain reporting and communication. For instance, a recent study at our institution demonstrated a breadth of pain scores in patients with similar injuries: scores ranged from 3 to 10 (on a 10-point scale) on the verbal numeric rating scale in patients with acute fractures.[19]

Despite pitfalls in self-reported pain scores, it is important for the objective pain rating to come from the patient. The necessity of pain self-report is supported by studies that consistently find clinicians' perception of patients' pain correlates poorly with self-reported pain levels.[20–23]

■ Pain assessment tools

In clinical practice, the most commonly used rating scale is the verbal numeric rating scale. Application of this scale simply entails asking the patient to rate pain level from 0 to 10, with 0 being no pain, and 10 being the worst pain imaginable. (Different approaches have been taken to the wording at the "top" end of pain scales; the most important *caveat* is that the pain descriptor be realistic.) The advantages of the verbal numeric rating scale include ease of administration and high agreement with the visual analog scales (illustrated) used in most clinical pain management studies in acute care.[24]

	Worst pain
No pain	imaginable

Typical instructions. Explain the line, which should be 10 cm in length, as representing the patient's current pain level ranging from "no pain" to "worst pain imaginable." Some versions of the scale have intermediate labels such as *slight*, *mild*, *moderate*, and *severe*, between the two end labels. Have the patient mark the point on the line corresponding to their pain. If repeat assessments are made, a new (unmarked) scale should be used.

Example of a visual analog scale.

Although the available literature leaves room for debate, it appears that in some cases basing therapy on a verbal pain descriptor (e.g. mild, moderate, severe), rather than a numerical rating, may suffice in the ED. Studies in both "healthy" patients and those being treated for pain find consistent corres pondence between pain categorization levels (i.e. no pain, mild pain, etc.) and ranges for 0–10 verbal numeric ratings.[25]

In some patient populations, the limitations of numeric scales necessitate the use of alternative approaches. Younger patients are one group for whom verbal numeric ratings scales perform suboptimally.[26] For children, visual tools such as the FACES scale, color scales, and visual pain "thermometers" or similar VASs have been used. Most of these tools have been found to

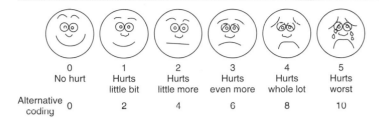

Brief word instructions. Point to each face using the words to describe the pain intensity. Ask the child to choose the face that best describes child's own pain and record the appropriate number.

Original instructions. Explain to the person that each face is for a person who feels happy because he has no pain (hurt) or sad because he has some or a lot of pain. **Face 0** is very happy because he doesn't hurt at all. **Face 1** hurts just a little bit. **Face 2** hurts a little more. **Face 3** hurts even more. **Face 4** hurts a whole lot. **Face 5** hurts as much as you can imagine, although you don't have to be crying to feel this bad. Ask the person to choose the face that best describes how he is feeling.

The Wong–Baker FACES Pain Rating Scale (for patients who are at least 3 years old). (With permission from Hockenberry MJ, Wilson D, Winkelstein ML. *Wong's Essentials of Pediatric Nursing*, 7th edn. St. Louis, MO: Mosby, 2005:1259. Copyright Mosby.)

have some potential clinical utility, although the value of some approaches (e.g. McGill Pain Questionnaire) lies mostly in clinical research.[27–33] Some tools have differing utility in various populations. Visual-based scales appear less reliable in the elderly, in whom spatial skills may deteriorate earlier than verbal skills.[34]

The Wong–Baker FACES Pain Rating Scale (FPRS), developed in the 1980s by clinicians working with children with burn, is an example of a valid and reliable pediatric pain assessment tool.[35,36] This scale is best used with children who are verbal, and who can follow the directions (as outlined in the figure) to indicate the depicted face that most represents their level of pain.

For the nonverbal child, several options exist. Although behavioral scales may not be ideal, some have been found to have clinical utility. The Faces, Legs, Activity, Cry, and Consolability (FLACC) behavioral pain assessment tool has good correlation with self-reported pain scores in both verbal and nonverbal children.[37,38] Furthermore, the FLACC has been validated in

The Face, Legs, Activity, Cry, Consolability (FLACC) Behavioral Assessment Tool[37]

Behavior	Description	Score
Face	No particular expression or smile	0
	Occasional grimace/frown, withdrawn or disinterested	1
	Frequent/constant quivering chin, clenched jaw	2
Legs	Normal position or relaxed	0
	Uneasy, restless, tense	1
	Kicking or legs drawn up	2
Activity	Lying quietly, normal position, moves easily	0
	Squirming, shifting back and forth, tense	1
	Arched, rigid or jerking	2
Cry	No cry	0
	Moans or whimpers, occasional complaint	1
	Crying steadily, screams or sobs, frequent complaints	2
Consolability	Content and relaxed	0
	Reassured by talking, occasional touching, or hugging	1
	Difficult to console or comfort	2

The Pain Assessment in Advanced Dementia (PAINAD) scale[43]

Behavior	Description	Score
Face	Smiling or inexpressive	0
	Sad – frightened – frown	1
	Facial grimacing	2
Breathing independent of vocalization	Normal	0
	Occasional labored breathing – short period of hyperventilation	1
	Noisy/labored – extended hyperventilation – Cheyne–Stokes respirations	2
Negative vocalization	None	0
	Occasional moan or groan – low level negative/disapproving speech	1
	Repeated troubled calling out – loud moaning or groaning – crying	2
Body language	Relaxed	0
	Tense – distressed pacing – fidgeting	1
	Rigid – fists clenched – knees up – pulling/pushing away – striking out	2
Consolability	No need to console	0
	Distracted or reassured by voice or touch	1
	Unable to console, distract, or reassure	2

children who are cognitively impaired.[39] Other behavioral scales for children include the COMFORT scale and the Toddler-Preschooler Postoperative Pain Scale (TPPS).[40,41]

In older adults who are cognitively intact, numerical rating scales or simple verbal reports of pain categories are preferred. Compared with visual rating scales, the more straightforward verbal rating approach is associated with more favorable error rates, easier use, and greater patient preference.[34] However, in the cognitively impaired adult, verbal descriptor scales may be combined with a "pain thermometer" form of vertical visual analog scale (with intermediate labels along the scale); in this setting the modified FACES scale was found to have weak correlation with other scales.[42] In advanced dementia, a tool similar to the FLACC scale (the Pain Assessment in Advanced Dementia [PAINAD]) scale has been developed and appears potentially useful for assessing pain in noncommunicative elderly patients.[43]

■ Summary and recommendations

First line: verbal numeric rating scale (0 to 10)

Reasonable: verbal reports of pain categories (none, mild, moderate, severe)

Pediatric: FACES scale (for verbal children)

Special cases:
■ *nonverbal pediatric patient*: FLACC
■ *adult with mild-moderate cognitive impairment*: verbal rating or labeled VAS
■ *nonverbal adult*: PAINAD

References

1. Phillips D. JCAHO pain management standards are unveiled. *JAMA*. 2000; **284**:428–429.
2. Anonymous. American Pain Society Quality of Care Committee: quality improvement guidelines for the treatment of acute pain and cancer pain. *JAMA*. 1995;**274**:1874–1880.

3. Silka P, Roth M, Moreno G. Pain scores improve analgesic administration patterns for trauma patients in the emergency department. *Acad Emerg Med.* 2004;**11**:264–270.

4. Nelson B, Cohen D, Lander O. Mandated pain scales improve frequency of ED analgesic administration. *Am J Emerg Med.* 2004;**22**:582–585.

5. Thomas S, Andruskiewicz L. Ongoing visual analog score display improves ED care. *J Emerg Med.* 2004;**26**:389–394.

6. Taksande A, Vilhekar K, Jain M, *et al.* Pain response of neonates to venipuncture. *Indian J Pediatr.* 2005;**72**:751–753.

7. Anonymous. Prevention and management of pain and stress in the neonate. American Academy of Pediatrics and Canadian Pediatric Society. *Pediatrics.* 2000;**105**:454–461.

8. Marco CA, Plewa MC, Buderer N, *et al.* Self-reported pain scores in the emergency department: lack of association with vital signs. *Acad Emerg Med.* 2006;**13**:974–979.

9. Craig K, Whitfield M, Grunau R, *et al.* Pain in the preterm neonate: behavioral and physiological indices. *Pain.* 1993;**52**:287–299.

10. Payen J, Bru O, Bosson J, *et al.* Assessing pain in critically ill sedated patients by using a behavioral pain scale. *Crit Care Med.* 2001;**29**:2258–2263.

11. Wears R. Patient satisfaction and the curse of Kelvin. *Ann Emerg Med.* 2005;**46**:11–12.

12. Feinstein A. On exorcising the ghost of Gauss and the curse of Kelvin. In Feinstein A (ed.) *Clinical Biostatistics.* St. Louis: CV Mosby, 1977:235.

13. Campbell T, Hughes J, Girder S. Relationship of ethnicity, gender, and ambulatory blood pressure to pain sensitivity: effects of individualized pain rating scales. *J Pain.* 2004;**5**:183–191.

14. Logan H, Gedney J, Sheffield D. Stress influences the level of negative affectivity after forehead cold pressor pain. *J Pain.* 2003;**4**:520–529.

15. Saastamoinen P, Leino-Arjas P, Laaksonen M, *et al.* Socio-economic differences in the prevalence of acute, chronic and disabling chronic pain among ageing employees. *Pain.* 2005;**114**:364–371.

16. Rosseland L, Stubhaug A. Gender is a confounding factor in pain trials: women report more pain than men after arthroscopic surgery. *Pain.* 2004;**112**:248–253.

17. Hobara M. Beliefs about appropriate pain behavior: cross-cultural and sex differences between Japanese and Euro-Americans. *Eur J Pain.* 2005;**9**:389–393.

18. Marco C, Marco A, Plewa M, *et al.* The Verbal Numeric Pain Scale: effects of patient education on self-reports of pain. *Acad Emerg Med.* 2006;**13**:853–859.

19. Marco CA, Plewa MC, Buderer N, *et al.* Comparison of oxycodone and hydrocodone for the treatment of acute pain associated with fractures: a double-blind, randomized, controlled trial. *Acad Emerg Med.* 2005;**12**:282–288.

20. Thomas SH, Borczuk P, Shackelford J, *et al.* Patient and physician agreement on abdominal pain severity and need for opioid analgesia. *Am J Emerg Med.* 1999;**17**:586–590.

21. Singer A, Richman P, Kowalska A. Comparison of patient and practitioner assessmsents of pain for commonly performed emergency department procedures. *Ann Emerg Med.* 1999;**33**:652–658.

22. Singer A, Gulla J, Thode H. Parents and practitioners are poor judges of young children's pain severity. *Acad Emerg Med.* 2002;**9**:609–612.

23. Labus J, Keefe F, Jensen M. Self-reports of pain intensity and direct observations of pain behavior: When are they correlated? *Pain.* 2003;**102**:109–124.

24. Bijur PE, Latimer CT, Gallagher EJ. Validation of a verbally administered numerical rating scale of acute pain for use in the emergency department. *Acad Emerg Med.* 2003,**10**.390–392.

25. Palos G, Mendoza T, Mobley B. Asking the community about cutpoints used to describe mild, moderate, and severe pain. *J Pain.* 2006;**7**:49–56.

26. Bailey B, Bergeron S, Gravel J, *et al.* Comparison of four pain scales in children with acute abdominal pain in a pediatric emergency department. *Ann Emerg Med.* 2007;**50**:379–383, 383, e371–372.

27. Gordon M, Greenfield E, Marvin J, *et al.* Use of pain assessment tools: is there a preference? *J Burn Care Rehabil.* 1998;**19**:451–454.

28. Choiniere M, Auger F, Latarjet J. Visual analogue thermometer: a valid and useful instrument for measuring pain in burned patients. *Burns.* 1994;**20**:229–235.

29. Boureau F, Doubrere J, Luu M. Study of verbal description in neuropathic pain. *Pain.* 1990;**42**:145–152.

30. Maio R, Garrison H, Spaite D, *et al.* Emergency Medical Services Outcomes Project (EMSOP) IV: pain assessment in out-of-hospital outcomes research. *Ann Emerg Med.* 2002;**40**:172–179.

31. Garron D, Leavitt F. Psychological and social correlates of the back pain classification scale. *J Pers Assess.* 1983;**47**:60–65.

32. Tammaro S, Berggren U, Bergenholtz G. Representation of verbal pain descriptors on a visual analogue scale by dental patients and dental students. *Eur J Oral Sci.* 1997;**105**:207–212.

33. Melzack R. The McGill Pain Questionnaire: major properties and scoring methods. *Pain*. 1975;**1**:277–299.

34. Gagliese L, Weizblit W, Chan V. The measurement of postoperative pain: a comparison of intensity scales in younger and older surgical patients. *Pain*. 2005;**117**:412–420.

35. Bieri D. The Faces Pain Scale for the self-assessment of the severity of pain experienced by children: development, initial validation, and preliminary investigation for the ratio scale properties. *Pain*. 1990;**41**:139–150.

36. Wong D, Baker C. Pain in children: comparison of assessment scales. *Pediatr Nurs*. 1988;**14**:901–907.

37. Voepel-Lewis SMT, Shayevitz J, Malviya S. The FLACC: a behavioral scale for scoring postoperative pain in young children. *Pediatr Nurs*. 1997;**23**:293–297.

38. Willis M, Merkel S, Voepel-Lewis T, *et al.* FLACC behavioral pain assessment scale: a comparison with the child's self-report. *Pediatr Nurs*. 2003;**29**:195–198.

39. Voelpel-Lewis T, Merkel S, Tait A. The reliability and validity of the FLACC observational tool as a measure of pain in children with cognitive impairment. *Anesth Analg*. 2002;**95**:1224–1229.

40. Ambuel B, Hamlett K, Marx C, *et al.* Assessing distress in pediatric intensive care environments: the COMFORT scale. *J Pediatr Psychol*. 1992;**17**:95–109.

41. Tarbell S, Cohen I, Marsh J. The Toddler–Preschooler Postoperative Pain Scale: an observational scale for measuring postoperative pain in children aged 1–5. *Pain*. 1992;**50**:273–280.

42. Taylor L, Harris J, Epps C, *et al.* Psychometric evaluation of selected pain intensity scales for use with cognitively impaired and cognitively intact older adults. *Rehab Nurs*. 2005;**30**:55–61.

43. Warden V, Hurley A, Volicer L. Development and psychometric evaluation of the Pain Assessment in Advanced Dementia (PAINAD) Scale. *JAMDA*. 2003: **4**(1) 9–15.

Prehospital analgesia

CHRIS McEACHIN AND ROBERT A. SWOR

■ Topics

- Importance of analgesia in prehospital care
- Barriers to prehospital pain relief
- Specific medications

■ Introduction

The use of analgesia in the prehospital setting has garnered increasing attention over the past several years. The added focus on prehospital pain relief has generated a body of literature that, while continuing to grow, sheds sufficient light to allow some conclusions about out-of-hospital analgesia. The importance of nonpharmacological approaches to pain relief (e.g. burn dressings) is acknowledged, but these approaches are not discussed since they lie outside the scope of this book.

While more studies are needed, there are definitely sufficient data to support some conclusions about pain relief in the out-of-hospital setting. This chapter intends to overview the importance of analgesia as an important endpoint (and one in need of improvement) in prehospital care. The discussion also aims to highlight potential barriers to administration of analgesics by EMS providers. The chapter concludes with outlining analgesic approaches that are addressed in the prehospital literature.

■ Importance of analgesia in prehospital care

One of the most important points about prehospital analgesia is that, in many settings, it is inadequate – the hospital's oligoanalgesia problems extend to the world of EMS.[1] As is the case in the ED setting, multifaceted barriers to adequate prehospital pain relief are not easily overcome even with education and protocol changes.[2] Consequently, the arena of prehospital analgesia should be one of keen interest for those wishing to improve EMS care in what has been denoted one of its most important endpoints: pain relief.[1–4]

Analgesia's importance is magnified by the frequency with which EMS providers interact with injured patients in significant pain. Moderate or severe pain is present in nearly a third of all-diagnosis cases, and at least four out of five patients with extremity fractures.[5,6] Provision of analgesia thus represents an area where prehospital providers can positively make an important impact upon a large number of patients.[3,6]

In everyday practice, ED delays in analgesia administration magnify the beneficial impact of prehospital analgesia. Even if the transport time is only 10 min, a patient who will experience a 30-minute delay before receiving analgesia in the ED benefits from EMS analgesia administration. Thus, the time benefits of EMS analgesic administration exceed the prehospital transport time.[1,7,8]

The general issue of ED oligoanalgesia is addressed elsewhere in this text, but some studies deserve mention in the context of an EMS discussion. For instance, a helicopter EMS study of patients with extremity fractures who received prehospital *fentanyl* found a median delay to ED analgesia of 45 min, well beyond the expected clinical half-life of the prehospital **opioid**.[7] Another study, focusing on the same types of injury but in patients transported by ground EMS found a median time to analgesia of nearly 3 h.[9] While some of these patients could have had adequate pain control (e.g. from splinting), it seems unlikely that an average delay of 3 h in administering fracture analgesia is appropriate.

This chapter focuses on prehospital medication administration, with the understanding that not all medications will be available in all EMS systems. We also acknowledge that the needs of varying EMS systems will differ depending on factors such as transport distances and patient and provider characteristics. However, just as the problem of prehospital oligoanalgesia stretches across national boundaries and different crew configurations (including those in which a physician is on board the ambulance), some basic solutions will also likely be shared across multiple EMS system types.[4,9]

■ Barriers to prehospital pain relief

There are myriad reasons for suboptimal prehospital analgesia administration. Most are amenable to remedy, with the proper preparation and education. The issue of improving prehospital analgesia is reviewed in detail in the acute care literature, but some points warrant highlighting.[4]

The first perceived problem with out-of-hospital analgesia administration is that the drugs incur risk of hemodynamic or respiratory compromise. These concerns are mainly directed toward the **opioids**, which constitute the main (if not the only) analgesic available to most EMS providers.[10] Fortunately, a growing body of prehospital data demonstrates the rarity of any **opioid**-associated complications. Recent review of the available data overviews the substantial evidence, comprising thousands of prehospital **opioid** administrations (usually *morphine* or *fentanyl*), and concludes complications are extremely rare.[4,11-20]

In addition to concerns about potential hemodynamic and respiratory depression, the other major barrier to prehospital analgesia administration is the question of the drugs' effect on the clinical evaluation. Unfortunately, compared with the issues surrounding depression of vital signs, the impact of analgesics on patient assessment is relatively unstudied in the prehospital setting.

In the case of head injury, there is legitimate argument that mental status-altering drugs adversely impact subsequent ED assessment. The National Association of EMS Physicians (NAEMSP), for instance, recognizes head injury as a relative contraindication to analgesia.[21] The practical application of these concerns is problematic, because of the high prevalence of potential head injury in EMS patients. Universal withholding of analgesics for any patient for whom there may be head injury is an untenable approach, since such practice risks unnecessary suffering as well as intracranial pressure elevation associated with untreated pain.[10,21,22] We believe that clinical judgment and use of short-acting agents (e.g. *fentanyl*) will enable safe provision of field pain relief in nearly all cases.

Examination-related issues other than the neurological evaluation are also prominent reasons for physicians not to administer (or not to authorize) prehospital analgesia.[23] These concerns, which include the age-old issue of clouding of the abdominal examination, have been contradicted in cases other than trauma and are equally baseless in the injured patient.[24–26]

Even if analgesia is authorized and administered, inadequate dosing remains a common obstacle to effective pain relief. In children, for example, EMS studies suggest that analgesic underdosing occurs in most cases.[27] In adults as well, prehospital underdosing and inadequate pain relief occur more often than not.[6,28] Reviewers of the pain literature in EMS acknowledge the futility of administering 2 mg *morphine* to a healthy adult, and note the importance of EMS providers (and their protocols) allowing for administration of appropriate analgesic dosages.[12]

One remediable barrier to rapid prehospital pain relief is the unnecessary delay incurred by requiring medical control authorization prior to administering analgesics.[1,12,29] While protocols should include guidance as to when medical control should be consulted (e.g. patients with borderline vital signs), in the majority of instances initial analgesic doses should be provided before medical control discussions.

MEDICATIONS

The medications used for prehospital pain relief depend upon both the diagnosis and analgesic, availability (which, are in turn dictated by regional practice and EMS provider credentials). The diagnosis-specific alternatives are far fewer for the prehospital setting, given the limited number of agents carried by most EMS units. Other than nonpharmacological interventions (e.g. splinting), the main example of diagnosis-specific EMS pain relief is in cardiac events, where *oxygen*, *nitroglycerin*, and *aspirin* (although not for its analgesic effects) are administered. The remainder of this chapter addresses general analgesics that can be used in a variety of patients, with and without trauma, encountered in the field.

In austere settings, oral agents such as *acetaminophen* (*paracetamol*) and **NSAIDs** are useful.[30] However, it is unlikely that oral agents with such mild potency will be of use in most EMS situations. Furthermore, the side effects of **NSAIDs** (including the more controversial ones such as impairment of fracture healing) combine with their longer onset times to render this class inferior to **opioids** for prehospital use.

The **opioids** are the primary analgesic approach available to most EMS services. The need for patient acuity prehospital and the desire for rapid-onset, titrateable analgesia translate into preference for IV administration. While there may be occasional roles for IM or SC routes (e.g. in patients in whom there is no IV access), the ED factors that make the IV route best are also applicable out of hospital. For patients with significant pain and sufficient acuity to require IV access for reasons besides analgesia, the intraosseous route of **opioid** administration is effective.[31]

The prototypical **opioid** for use in prehospital care is *morphine*, which is consistently demonstrated to be useful for a variety of adult and pediatric conditions encountered in EMS.[10,13,21,27,28,29-35] The literature is not without shortcomings, but the conclusion of *morphine*'s utility in EMS is indisputable. In the EMS literature, generally recommended adult doses for *morphine* call for 2–5 mg portions titrated up to 10 mg per dose. Pediatric *morphine* dosing endorsed by the EMS for Children (EMS-C) initiative is 0.1 mg/kg (maximum dose 10 mg).

Compared with *morphine, fentanyl* is at least as effective and is easier to titrate.[7,10,12,14-18,22,28,31-33,35,36] The pharmacologic (in particular, hemodynamic) advantages of *fentanyl* make it particularly attractive for prehospital use,[19,20] Trauma anesthesia literature suggests that *fentanyl* is the preferred analgesic in patients with potential head injury.[22] *Fentanyl* is reported safe and effective (for both adults and children) when administered by either physician-staffed or nonphysician-staffed EMS systems.[7,14,15,18,31] Reports in the past few years have established *fentanyl*'s safe use in thousands of prehospital administrations by both ground and air EMS providers.[11,17] An example study finds no sequelae from *fentanyl* use in over 2000 patients (only one of whom required naloxone for respiratory depression).[17]

Intranasal *fentanyl* (given as a total dose of 1.5 μg/kg), having been found useful in a pediatric ED setting, is a promising avenue for prehospital pain relief, but further evidence of its logistical practicality is required before this can be recommended for routine use.[36] Similar conclusions are drawn about the OTM route for *fentanyl* delivery. The OTM route, familiar to many acute care providers as an adjunct for procedural sedation and analgesia, may have prehospital utility in some settings, but more data are required before its EMS use can be endorsed.[38]

Alfentanil is similar to *fentanyl* and is demonstrated comparable to *morphine* when used by physician-staffed (Finnish) EMS in cardiac patients.[39] There are no available data describing its effectiveness in other prehospital populations, and it is premature to recommend adoption of *alfentanil* for routine prehospital use.

Two other **opioids**, with agonist–antagonist activity, have also been studied for use in the field. *Nalbuphine* has been in use for decades in the USA and is also employed in the UK. Those who use the agent report favorably on its performance, but more robust data are needed before its widespread deployment in EMS can be recommended.[40,41] *Butorphanol* has the advantage that it can be administered by the intranasal route (i.e. when IV access is lacking). Despite this potential niche for prehospital use, there is insufficient evidence or experience to recommend *butorphanol*'s inclusion in the prehospital pharmacopoeia.[30]

The mixed-mechanism agent *tramadol* is used commonly in some (non-USA) venues. The drug has its roles in acute care medicine (see other chapters), but relative lack of trial data and high incidence (30%) of nausea figure prominently in assessments of *tramadol*'s role in prehospital care.[12] *Tramadol*'s **opioid** characteristics require medical and logistic (e.g. drug storage) attention, and the drug can also precipitate serotonin syndrome if used in patients taking monoamine oxidase inhibitors or other serotoninergic antidepressants.[42] While *tramadol* is probably effective for EMS use in some settings, there is little reason to select this agent over *morphine*.

The use of nonopioids in the out-of-hospital environment remains atypical, but emerging data seem likely to indicate some role for these agents. The main non-opioid analgesics discussed in the prehospital analgesia literature are *nitrous oxide*, *ketamine*, and **local anesthetic** injection for regional block. These agents are considered next, with the understanding that their availability may be limited to only a few EMS systems.

Nitrous oxide is the only inhaled agent available for prehospital use in the USA (other inhalational anesthetics are in use in other countries). *Nitrous oxide* has been used in the field for over three decades.[12] It appears safe, is moderately effective (> 80% rates of pain relief in the prehospital setting), and is recommended in prehospital reviews of analgesic methods for adults and children.[12,21,34,35] There are some patient-based disadvantages. *Nitrous oxide* use requires precautions (e.g. pneumothorax) attendant to administration of any gas, and there is vomiting (and thus aspiration risk) in 10–15% of patients.[32] It is the disadvantage of occupational risk (to ambulance providers) that is the main barrier to more widespread EMS use of *nitrous oxide*. Sufficient ventilation to keep *nitrous oxide* concentrations below acceptable levels is difficult to achieve in the enclosed ambulance compartment.

In some settings (with physician-staffed EMS), *ketamine* is found useful as a pain control adjunct for splinting, extrication, and transport of trauma victims.[35,43] Particularly in areas outside the USA, *ketamine* has been useful when given IV, IM, or intraosseously for a broad mix of patients including those in shock; clinical series and discussions of its use are consistently positive.[44–50] *Ketamine*'s near-100% efficacy is not surprising, given long ED experience with the drug's use in procedural sedation and analgesia. The experience in acute care teaches another lesson: *ketamine* use requires close familiarity with the agent's pharmacology and adverse effect profile. The problem is not vital signs depression, although there is some risk of apnea with rapid IV administration.[51] Instead, hesitance to embrace *ketamine* is related to other concerns (e.g. laryngospasm, hypersalivation, emergence phenomena) that, while not unique to *ketamine*, are noted more frequently with the dissociative agent than with alternatives such as the **opioids**. Another (controversial) question is that of *ketamine*-mediated (sympathomimetic) increases in intracranial pressure. The decades-old assumption that *ketamine*'s sympathomimetic effects can exacerbate ICP increases in head injury have been called into question, with recent reviews of the evidence noting that data are mixed.[52] Detailed discussion of these issues lies outside the scope of this chapter, but it is noteworthy that theorized dangers of *ketamine* in head injury do not appear to materialize in studies (including prospective trials in patients with ICP monitoring) of the drug's use in neurotrauma.[52–55] Clinical trials data are sparse for *ketamine*. There are no data demonstrating *ketamine*'s risks, but there are also no methodologically rigorous studies evaluating its risk-to-benefit profile in the

EMS setting. We do not believe that *ketamine*'s issues translate into a lack of any possible role for the drug's prehospital use.

Regional nerve blocks with **local anesthetic** injection are efficacious for field use in settings where physician prehospital providers are available. European studies demonstrate utility of this approach for patients with hip and femur fractures.[35] Nerve blocks appear unlikely to be widely adopted for EMS use by nonphysician crews, such as are the rule in the USA, but this approach does have appeal for physician crews.[30]

■ Summary and recommendations

First line:

■ morphine (initial dose 4–6 mg IV, then titrate)
■ fentanyl (initial dose 50–100 μg IV, then titrate)

Reasonable:

■ other opioid (e.g. hydromorphone initial dose 1 mg IV, then titrate)

Pregnancy:

■ morphine (initial dose 4–6 mg IV, then titrate) or fentanyl (initial dose 50–100 μg IV, then titrate); lower doses if delivery is imminent

Pediatrics:

■ morphine (initial dose 0.05–0.1 mg/kg IV, then titrate; maximum 10 mg/ dose) or fentanyl (initial dose 1–2 μg/kg, then titrate; maximum 100 μg/dose)

Special cases:

■ *EMS services operating with extended transport times*: protocols for these services should allow for adequate analgesia re-dosing

References

1. Turturro M. Pain, priorities, and prehospital care. *Prehosp Emerg Care.* 2002;**6**:486–488.
2. Fairbanks R, Kolstee K, Martin H, *et al.* Prehospital pain management is not adequate. *Prehosp Emerg Care.* 2007;**11**:134.

3. McEachin C, McDermott J, Swor R. Few EMS patients with lower-extremity fractures receive prehospital analgesia. *Prehosp Emerg Care.* 2002;**6**:406–410.

4. Thomas S, Shewakramani S. Prehospital analgesia. *J Emerg Med.* 2007; e17997072.

5. McLean S, Domeier R, DeVore H, *et al.* The feasibility of pain assessment in the prehospital setting. *Prehosp Emerg Care.* 2004;**8**:155–161.

6. McEachin C, Swor R, Seguin D, *et al.* EMS analgesia: the patient's perspective. *Prehosp Emerg Care.* 2004;**8**:103.

7. DeVellis P, Thomas SH, Wedel SK. Prehospital and emergency department analgesia for air-transported patients with fractures. *Prehosp Emerg Care.* 1998;**2**:293–296.

8. Abbuhl F, Reed D. Time to analgesia for patients with painful extremity injuries transported to the emergency department by ambulance. *Prehosp Emerg Care.* 2003;**7**:445–447.

9. Vassiliadis J, Hitos K, Hill C. Factors influencing prehospital and emergency department analgesia administration to patients with femoral neck fractures. *Emerg Med (Freemantle).* 2002;**14**:261–266.

10. Barber J, White N, Luria J. Controversies in pediatric emergency medicine: pediatric trauma. *Pediatr Emerg Care.* 2004;**20**:412–417.

11. Krauss B, Shah S, Thomas S. Fentanyl analgesia in the out-of-hospital setting: variables associated with hypotension in 1091 administrations among 500 consecutive patients. *Acad Emerg Med.* 2007; **14**(5, Suppl 1);S115.

12. McManus J, Sallee D. Pain management in the prehospital environment. *Emerg Med Clin North Am.* 2005;**23**:415–431.

13. Galinski M, Pommerie F, Ruscev M. Emergency ambulance management of acute pain in children: a national survey. *Presse Medicale.* 2005;**34**:1126–1128.

14. DeVellis P, Thomas S, Wedel S, *et al.* Prehospital fentanyl analgesia in air-transported pediatric trauma patients. *Pediatr Emerg Care.* 1998;**14**:321–323.

15. Thomas S, Rago O, Harrison T, *et al.* Fentanyl trauma analgesia use in air medical scene transports. *J Emerg Med.* 2005;**29**:179–185.

16. Galinski M, Ruscev M, Pommerie F. National survey of emergency management of acute pain in the prehospital setting. *Ann Fr Anesth Reanim.* 2004;**23**:1149–1154.

17. Kanowitz A, Dunn TM, Kanowitz EM, *et al.* Safety and effectiveness of fentanyl administration for prehospital pain management. *Prehosp Emerg Care.* 2006;**10**:1–7.

18. Kurtz T. Safety of IV fentanyl in adults requiring analgesia during ground interfacility transports by a critical care transport team. *Prehosp Emerg Care.* 2006;**10**:140.

19. Thomas S. Fentanyl in the prehospital setting. *Am J Emerg Med.* 2007;**25** (7):842–843.

20. Braude D, Richards M. Appeal for fentanyl prehospital use. *Prehosp Emerg Care.* 2004;**8**:441–442.

21. Mulligan-Smith D, O'Connor R, Markenson D. EMSC partnership for children: NAEMSP model pediatric protocols. *Prehosp Emerg Care.* 2000;**4**:111–128.

22. Tentillier E, Ammirati C. Prehospital management of patients with severe head injuries. *Ann Fr Anesth Reanim.* 2000;**19**:275–281.

23. Zohar Z, Eitan A, Halperin P, *et al.* Pain relief in major trauma patients: an Israeli perspective. *J Trauma.* 2001;**51**:767–772.

24. Thomas S, Silen W, Cheema F. Effects of morphine analgesia on diagnostic accuracy in emergency department patients with abdominal pain: a prospective, randomized trial. *J Am Coll Surg.* 2003;**196**:18–31.

25. Thomas SH, Silen W. Effect on diagnostic efficiency of analgesia for undifferentiated abdominal pain. *Br J Surg.* 2003;**90**:5–9.

26. Gallagher EJ, Esses D, Lee C, *et al.* Randomized clinical trial of morphine in acute abdominal pain. *Ann Emerg Med.* 2006;**48**:150–160.

27. Moller J, Ballnus S, Kohl M, *et al.* Evaluation of the performance of general emergency physicians in pediatric emergencies. *Pediatr Emerg Care.* 2002;**18**:424–428.

28. Ricard-Hibon A, Chollet C, Saada S, *et al.* A quality control program for acute pain management in out-of-hospital critical care medicine. *Ann Emerg Med.* 1999;**34**:738–744.

29. Fullerton-Gleason L, Crandall C, Sklar D. Prehospital administration of morphine for isolated extremity fractures: a change in protocol reduces time to medication. *Prehosp Emerg Care.* 2002;**6**:411–416.

30. Wedmore I, Johnson T, Czarnik J, *et al.* Pain management in the wilderness and operational setting. *Emerg Med Clin North Am.* 2005;**23**:585–601.

31. Helm M, Breschinski W, Lampl L, *et al.* Intraosseous puncture in preclinical emergency medicine: experiences of an air rescue service. *Anaesthetist.* 1996;**45**:1196–1202.

32. Alonso-Serra H, Wesley K. Prehospital pain management. *Prehosp Emerg Care.* 2003;**7**:482–488.

33. Ricard-Hibon A, Chollet C, Belpomme V, *et al.* Epidemiology of adverse effects of prehospital sedation analgesia. *Am J Emerg Med.* 2003;**21**:461–466.

34. Allison K, Porter K. Consensus on the prehospital approach to burns patient management. *Emerg Med J.* 2004;**21**:112–114.

35. Lee C, Porter K. Prehospital management of lower limb fractures. *Emerg Med J.* 2005;**22**:660–663.

36. Thomas S, Benevelli W, Brown D, *et al.* Safety of fentanyl for analgesia in adults undergoing air medical transport from trauma scenes. *Air Med J.* 1996;**15**:57–59.

37. Borland M, Jacobs I, Geelhoed G. Intranasal fentanyl reduces acute pain in children in the emergency department: a safety and efficacy study. *Emerg Med (Freemantle).* 2002;**14**:275–280.

38. Kotwal RS, O'Connor KC, Johnson TR, *et al.* A novel pain management strategy for combat casualty care. *Ann Emerg Med.* 2004;**44**:121–127.

39. Silfvast T, Saarnivaara L. Comparison of alfentanil and morphine in the prehospital treatment of patients with acute ischemic-type pain. *Euro J Emerg Med.* 2001;**8**:275–278.

40. Hyland-McGuire P, Guly H. Effects on patient care of introducing prehospital intravenous nalbuphine hydrochloride *J Accid Emerg Med.* 1998;**15**:99–101.

41. Houlihan KP, Mitchell RG, Flapan AD, *et al.* Excessive morphine requirements after pre-hospital nalbuphine analgesia. *J Accid Emerg Med.* 1999;**16**:29–31.

42. Kitson R, Carr B. Tramadol and severe serotonin syndrome. *Anaesthesia.* 2005;**60**:934–935.

43. Porter K. Ketamine in prehospital care. *Emerg Med J.* 2004;**21**:351–354.

44. Kuznetsova O, Marusanov VE, Biderman FM, *et al.* [Ketalar anesthesia in the first-aid stage with the victims of severe injury and traumatic shock.] *Vestn Khir Im I I Grek.* 1984;**132**:88–91.

45. Danilevich E, Kostiuchenko AL, Kuznetsova O, *et al.* [Combined anesthesia based on the use of ketamine in the prehospital stage in victims of severe trauma and shock.] *Anesteziol Reanimatol.* 1987(5):46–50.

46. Danilevich E, Gal'tseva IV, Kuznetsova O, *et al.* [Effect of ketamine anesthesia on patients with severe trauma at the pre-hospital stage on the course and outcome of shock.] *Vestn Khir Im I I Grek.* 1990;**145**:104–107.

47. Beliakov VA, Sinitsyn LN, Maksimov GA, *et al.* [Analgesia and anesthesia in the prehospital stage of mechanical trauma.] *Anesteziol Reanimatol.* 1993 (5):24–32.

48. Helm M, Breschinski W, Lampl L, *et al.* [Intraosseous puncture in preclincal emergency medicine. Experiences of an air rescue service.] *Anaesthesist.* 1996;**45**:1196–1202.

49. Roberts K, Bleetman A. An email audit of prehospital doctor activity in an area of the West Midlands. *Emerg Med J.* 2002;**19**:341–344.

50. Porter K. Ketamine in prehospital care. *Emerg Med J.* 2004;**21**:351–354.

51. Green SM, Clark R, Hostetler MA, *et al.* Inadvertent ketamine overdose in children: clinical manifestations and outcome. *Ann Emerg Med.* 1999;**34**:492–497.

52. Sehdev RS, Symmons DA, Kindl K. Ketamine for rapid sequence induction in patients with head injury in the emergency department. *Emerg Med Australas.* 2006;**18**:37–44.

53. Shapira Y, Artru AA, Lam AM. Ketamine decreases cerebral infarct volume and improves neurological outcome following experimental head trauma in rats. *J Neurosurg Anesthesiol.* 1992;**4**:231–240.

54. Albanese J, Garnier F, Bourgoin A, *et al.* [The agents used for sedation in neurointensive care unit.] *Ann Fr Anesth Reanim.* 2004;**23**:528–534.

55. Bar-Joseph G, Guilbord Y, Arzomarov T, *et al.* Ketamine (Ketalar) decreases intracranial pressure in children with intracranial hypertension In *Proceedings of the 5th International Conference on Pediatric Critical Care Medicine*, Geneva, June 2007.

Epidemiologic overview of pain treatment in the emergency department

POLLY BIJUR

■ Topics

- Trends in ED analgesia provision over time
- Heterogeneity in ED analgesia provision across demographic groups

■ Introduction

The study of epidemiology includes assessment of the distribution (or maldistribution) of healthcare resources to different segments of the population. This chapter considers the healthcare resource of pain treatment, with focus on findings relevant to acute care analgesia provision. The chapter discusses the evolution of ED analgesia provision over time and overviews the clinically relevant lessons of research into disparities in pain medication administration. The data are primarily from the USA, but the overarching messages have broader relevance.

■ Incidence

The most comprehensive view of acute care pain treatment in the USA is provided by the National Hospital Ambulatory Medical Care Survey (NHAMCS), which reports a representative sample of all ED visits. For the year 2004, the estimated number of ED visits was 18 162 million for mild pain, 26 074 million for moderate pain, and 16 617 million for severe pain. An estimated 71 829 million analgesic medications were administered in the ED. Using the NHAMCS terminology, 44% were narcotics, 35% NSAIDs, and 21% non-narcotic analgesics.[1]

■ Analgesia provision over time

The proportion of patients in acute pain who receive analgesics has increased over time. Two studies, carried out in 1987 and 1988, revealed extremely low rates of analgesia in two academic centers. One analysis reported only 44% of patients admitted to the hospital from one ED with painful disorders received any analgesia.[2] The second study found analgesics were administered to only 37% of patients with lower extremity fractures.[3] In contrast, an analysis of NHAMCS data collected from 1997 to 2000, showed that 64% of all patients with long-bone and clavicle fractures receive analgesics, and 73% of the patients with moderate to severe pain were treated for that pain.[4] This same level of treatment is observed in a recent prospective multisite study finding that 60% of patients with severe pain receive analgesics.[5]

If the data clearly indicate a favorable trend with respect to the proportion of suffering patients receiving analgesia, it is less certain that this increase in *analgesia provision* is translating into improved *pain relief*. One problem is the limitations of the relevant literature (e.g. lack of prospective analyses of the question of adequacy of pain management). Overall, compared with the quality of data addressing analgesia administration rates, information on pain treatment adequacy is less conclusive. The available studies do allow for some inferences.

Several recent prospective studies indicate that pain is not adequately controlled. In a single-center study of 1663 ED patients with painful disorders, investigators found that patients' average pain at discharge was 54 on a 0–100 mm VAS; under a third of patients reported a 50% decrease in pain intensity over the course of the visit.[6] Another ED group found that only 50% of patients had numeric pain scores reduced at least 2 points (on a 0–10 scale). In this study, three-quarters of patients were discharged with moderate or severe pain.[5] It is unrealistic to expect that all pain will be alleviated in all patients, but the finding is suggestive of room for improvement.

Thus, as assessed by either pain score reduction during an ED visit, or residual pain at discharge, current acute care analgesia practices fall short of the ideal. Further concerns are identified when investigators focus on another parameter: time to first analgesia administration. One study of severely injured and hospitalized patients had a mean average time lapse, between initial evaluation and analgesia administration, of 40 min.[7] Another group reported an average delay almost twice as long (78 min), and a third study found a median time to treatment of 90 min.[5,6] In fact, the problem of intractable delays in ED analgesia provision, even for those patients with obviously painful injuries, has been invoked as an important reason for the importance of prehospital pain care.[8] (The matter of prehospital pain care is addressed in a separate chapter.)

■ Distribution of pain treatment by demographic characteristics of patients

RACE AND ETHNICITY

In 1993, Todd *et al.* published a finding that Hispanic patients were only half as likely as whites to receive analgesia for long-bone fractures.[9] Since that time, many studies have shed light on the question of disparities in analgesia provision (particularly for predictably painful conditions such as long-bone fractures). Despite the early findings of unequal treatment in different racial and ethnic groups, the evidence that Hispanic and African-American patients receive less adequate pain management than white patients is not consistent.

The table summarizes nine ED investigations examining racial or ethnic analgesia disparities. Most of the studies failed to identify disparities in administration of "any analgesia" or "opioid analgesia." However, data from the largest available dataset, that of the NHAMCS, suggested a different conclusion, at least for some diagnoses.[4]

Distribution of pain treatment by race and ethnicity				
Author (year data collected)	Condition	Patient type (*n*)	Received any analgesics (%)	Received opioids (%)
Todd[9] (1990–1)	Long-bone fracture	White (108) Hispanic (31)	72 45	68 45
Karpman[18] (1992)	Long-bone fracture	White (55) Hispanic (29)	56 55	NR
Todd[19] (1992–5)	Long-bone fracture	White (90) African-American (127)	74 57	64 44

Distribution of pain treatment by race and ethnicity (cont.)

Author (year data collected)	Condition	Patient type (n)	Received any analgesics (%)	Received opioids (%)
Quintans-Rodriquez[13] (1998–9)	Long-bone fracture	White (181)	80	70
		African-American (58)	83	66
		Hispanic (46)	78	63
Tamayo-Sarver[4] (1997–9)	Long-bone fracture	White (602)	67	36
		African-American (80)	72	42
		Hispanic (71)	63	25
	Back problems	White (912)	80	43
		African-American (273)	70	21
		Hispanic (126)	77	35
	Migraine	White (471)	84	61
		African-American (92)	72	33
		Hispanic (43)	89	50
Neighbor[7] (1999)	Severe injuries resulting in hospitalization	White (179)	NR	53
		African-American (104)	NR	51
		Hispanic (103)	NR	43
Bijur (2000–2) unpublished	Long-bone fracture	White (81)	74	65
		African-American (133)	69	59
		Hispanic (235)	77	66
Miner[6] (2003–4)	Painful disorders	White (642)	73	NR
		African-American (749)	71	
		Hispanic (105)	73	
		Other (145)	72	
Heins[20] (2004)	Musculoskeletal pain	White (249)	NR	Odds ratio whites: African-Americans = 1.8
		African-American (603)	NR	

NR, not reported.

As is the case with many of the other studies of patients with fracture, NHAMCS data do not reveal an association between race/ethnicity and analgesia provision. For white, African-American, and Hispanic patients with extremity or clavicle fractures, analgesia was provided at statistically similar rates of 67%, 72%, and 63%, respectively. For low-back pain and migraines, however, analysis of NHAMCS identifies heterogeneous treatment. For these diagnoses, analgesia likelihood for African-American and Hispanic patients was lower than the corresponding likelihood for whites, and the difference remained significant even after adjustment for potential confounders.

AGE

Age-related heterogeneity in analgesia provision is a well-known issue. The treatment of pain in older adults can be impacted by age bias. Analgesia provision in geriatric patients is also affected by myriad issues relating to drug interactions and side effects. Geriatric analgesia is, therefore, addressed in detail in another chapter, which covers both the problems and potential solutions to underanalgesia in older patients. This chapter's discussion focuses on contrasts between treatment of children and of adults less than 70 years.

Results from five studies that addressed age and pain treatment are summarized in the table. Some studies were limited by small sample sizes, so the estimates about treatment should be interpreted with caution. With that limitation in mind, useful inferences can be drawn from the existing data.

NHAMCS information from 1997 to 2000 has been used to examine the relationship between age and analgesic practice in 2828 patients with long-bone or clavicle fractures.[10] One of the findings is that, compared with patients younger than 16 years of age, patients aged 16 to 69 are twice as likely to receive opioid analgesics. A similar trend to more analgesia is seen when analysis is restricted to patients with moderate to severe pain; compared with children, adults are approximately 40% more likely to receive analgesics.[11]

Author (year data collected) age group (years)	Condition	Sample size	Received any analgesics (%)	Received opioids (%)
Brown[10] *(1997–2000)*				
<16	All patients with	818	60	26
16–69	clavicle or long-bone fracture	1553	68	49
<16	Patients in moderate/	263	68	43
16–69	severe pain from clavicle or long-bone fracture	529	78	61
Selbst[3] *(1988)*				
<19	Sickle cell crisis	27	74	NR
19–65		26	100	NR
<19	Lower extremity	24	33	NR
19–65	fracture	139	31	NR
<19	Second, third-degree	106	15	NR
19–65	burn	23	65	NR
Neighbor[7] *(1999)*				
<11	Patients with severe	25	NR	49
11–64	injuries and hospitalized	188	NR	46
Alexander[12] *(1999–2000)*				
0.5–2	Long-bone fracture	96	35	15
6–10	and burns	84	52	43
Petrack[11] *(1993–4)*				
0–15	Long-bone fracture	120	53	43
16–65		120	73	45

NR, not reported.

If younger patients are at risk for lower analgesia rates, the risk for oligo-analgesia is even more pronounced in the youngest children. In a study of long-bone fractures and burns, Alexander *et al.* found analgesia rates of 35% of children between 6 and 24 months of age, compared with 52% analgesia rates in children aged 6 to 10 years.[12] In another study, characterized by low overall rates of analgesia, Selbst *et al.* found that 12% of children less than 24 months received analgesics, compared with 38% of children aged 2 to 18 years.[3]

SEX

Two retrospective studies suggest that women receive significantly more analgesics than men.[13,14] However, the preponderance of evidence argues against gender-related pain treatment. The differing conclusions in available studies may result from methodology. In a rigorous prospective study, univariate analysis showed that women were more likely to receive pain medication than men but this finding was nullified with use of multivariate correction for factors such as patient and physician perception of pain severity.[15] Several other studies also fail to find an association between patient gender and pain treatment.[7,14,16]

■ Discussion: lessons for the acute care provider

It is heartening that, over the past few decades, the approximate proportion of adult patients in pain receiving analgesics has increased from 40% to 70%. While it is true that over a fourth of patients in pain still do not receive any pain medication, it is not clear that "adequate pain treatment" means that all patients in pain should receive analgesics. There are patients who do not want pain medication, and instances in which the use of analgesics is ill-advised. However, nearly half of patients who do not receive analgesia indicate they do want treatment, and the modest 18% increase in analgesia use over 1997–2001 (based upon NHAMCS data) suggests that we are only beginning to move in the right direction.

There are grounds for optimism in the data, which suggests that racial/ethnic disparities in analgesia provision are diminishing with the passage of time. The literature should be interpreted with the *caveat* that most of the studies deal with extremity fractures. The long-bone fracture model is attractive for analgesia studies because the pain from fractures is thought to be of similar intensity; the situation approximates an experimental paradigm in which all subjects are exposed to the same pain stimulus. However, it has been suggested that the long-bone fracture model may fail to identify race/ethnicity-based differences in treatment of pain from conditions that are less objective and verifiable.[4] This concern is supported by the NHAMCS analysis finding of racial and ethnic disparities in treatment of migraines and back pain. Patients with conditions that rely more heavily on patient–doctor communication may be more vulnerable to disparate treatment. The evidence continues to be mixed on this subject. Two large studies of patients with varied painful conditions, comprising a mix of subjective and objective complaints, failed to find racial/ethnic disparities in pain management.[6,7] As investigation of this area continues, clinicians must remember the potential for significant inter-patient variation in pain experiences (even with similar diagnoses), pain reporting, and attitude toward medication use. The goal for acute care physicians should be to assess pain as objectively as possible, preventing provider characteristics (e.g. race, sex, stereotyping) from affecting the decision to treat patients in pain.

Age-related disparities in pain treatment represent another problem. Younger patients are clearly at risk for receiving insufficient analgesia – the younger the patient, the higher the risk. The reasons for pediatric oligoanalgesia can include concerns over adverse events, difficulty in communication (particularly with young children), and discounting of pain. Some of the same concerns are in effect in the geriatric population; these issues are discussed in a separate chapter. Like geriatric oligoanalgesia, the undertreatment of pain in children is an area of serious concern. The problem of age-related disparities in pain treatment warrants close attention in order to elucidate further the reasons for oligoanalgesia, and to identify strategies to improve pain management in vulnerable populations.

In contrast to the situations with race, ethnicity, and age, it appears that gender is not a major determinant of analgesia administration. Although there are some conflicting data, high-quality evidence suggests that the initial pain report and physician assessment of pain level account for apparent gender-related differences in treatment.[15]

In conclusion, the available evidence on pain treatment shows that the acute care community has improved in the delivery of pain relief, but that more improvement is still desirable. Issues regarding class of analgesic, dose, and adequacy of pain relief as reported by patients must be more fully explored. Evidence of long waiting times to treatment, suboptimal pain relief, and high levels of pain on discharge indicate that we are only beginning to address oligoanalgesia in the ED.

It is not clear that all pain must be relieved, or that the goal of good medical practice is not reached if some patients indicate incomplete analgesia upon ED discharge. Even though evolving literature is resolving some debates about withholding of analgesia (e.g. in patients with abdominal pain), there remain cases (e.g. hypotensive or head-injured patients) in which adminis-tration of pain medication may incur significant disadvantage. The results of studies mentioned herein should not be used to brand emergency physicians as less caring than other healthcare providers. Indeed, the specialty deserves kudos for focusing a self-reflective (and often critical) eye on ED pain care practices.

Although it seems hardly likely that any problems with oligoanalgesia are limited to the ED, emergency physicians are well advised to consider the components to improving acute care pain relief, as outlined by Todd.[17] In order to maintain and improve trends in equitable pain relief for all patients in the ED, leaders and practitioners in EM should advocate for increased federal funding, integration of acute care providers into the FDA analgesia review system, and inclusion of pain management curricula in medical school and residency programs.

References

1. McCaig LF, Nawar EW. National Hospital Ambulatory Medical Care Survey: 2004 emergency department summary. *Adv Data*. 2006(372):1–29.
2. Wilson JE, Pendleton JM. Oligoanalgesia in the emergency department. *Am J Emerg Med*. 1989;**7**:620–623.
3. Selbst S, Clark M. Analgesia use in the emergency department. *Ann Emerg Med*. 1990;**19**:1010–1013.

4. Tamayo-Sarver JH, Hinze SW, Cydulka RK, *et al.* Racial and ethnic disparities in emergency department analgesic prescription. *Am J Public Health.* 2003;**93**:2067–2073.

5. Hewitt DJ, Todd KH, Xiang J, *et al.* Tramadol/acetaminophen or hydrocodone/ acetaminophen for the treatment of ankle sprain: a randomized, placebo-controlled trial. *Ann Emerg Med.* 2007;**49**:468–480, 480, e461–462.

6. Burton JH, Miner JR, Shipley ER, *et al.* Propofol for emergency department procedural sedation and analgesia: a tale of three centers. *Acad Emerg Med.* 2006;**13**:24–30.

7. Neighbor ML, Honner S, Kohn MA. Factors affecting emergency department opioid administration to severely injured patients. *Acad Emerg Med.* 2004;**11**:1290–1296.

8. Thomas S, Shewakramani S. Prehospital analgesia. *J Emerg Med.* 2007; e17997072.

9. Todd K, Samaroo N, Hoffman J. Ethnicity as a risk factor for inadequate emergency department analgesia. *JAMA.* 1993;**269**:1537–1539.

10. Brown J, Klein E, Lewis C, *et al.* Emergency department analgesia for fracture pain. *Ann Emerg Med.* 2003;**42**:197–205.

11. Petrack EM, Christopher NC, Kriwinsky J. Pain management in the emergency department: patterns of analgesic utilization. *Pediatrics.* 1997;**99**:711–714.

12. Ray JG, Deniz S, Olivieri A, *et al.* Increased blood product use among coronary artery bypass patients prescribed preoperative aspirin and clopidogrel. *BMC Cardiovasc Disord.* 2003;**3**:3.

13. Quintans-Rodriquez A, Turegano-Fuentes F, Hernandez-Granados P, *et al.* Survival after prehospital advanced life support in severe trauma. *Eur J Emerg Med.* 1995;**2**:224–226.

14. Hostetler MA, Auinger P, Szilagyi PG. Parenteral analgesic and sedative use among ED patients in the United States: combined results from the National Hospital Ambulatory Medical Care Survey (NHAMCS) 1992–1997. *Am J Emerg Med.* 2002;**20**:139–143. [Erratum appears in *Am J Emerg Med* 2002 **20**:496.]

15. Raftery KA, Smith-Coggins R, Chen AH. Gender-associated differences in emergency department pain management. *Ann Emerg Med.* 1995;**26**:414–421.

16. Lewis L, Lasater L, Brooks C. Are emergency physicians too stingy with analgesics? *South Med J.* 1994;**87**:7–9.

17. Todd KH. Emergency medicine and pain: a topography of influence. *Ann Emerg Med.* 2004;**43**:504–506.

18. Karpman RR, Del Mar N, Bay C. Analgesia for emergency centers' orthopaedic patients: does an ethnic bias exist? *Clin Orthopaed Related Res.* 1997;**334**:270–275.

19. Todd KH, Deaton C, D'Adamo AP, *et al.* Ethnicity and analgesic practice. *Ann Emerg Med.* 2000;**35**:11–16.

20. Heins JK, Heins A, Grammas M, *et al.* Disparities in analgesia and opioid prescribing practices for patients with musculoskeletal pain in the emergency department. *J Emerg Nurs.* 2006;**32**:219–224.

Geriatric analgesia

ULA HWANG AND ANDY JAGODA

■ Topics

- Oligoanalgesia
- Loss of physiologic reserve
- Polypharmacy and adverse drug events
- Beers criteria
- Acetaminophen, NSAIDS, and opioids

■ Introduction

Analgesia care in geriatric patients requires consideration of several age-specific aspects of pain assessment and treatment. Perhaps most importantly, the elderly tend to have a more complex medical history and much comorbidity compared with younger adults. There is, therefore, higher potential for analgesia complications, as well as polypharmacy-related untoward drug effects. Older patients may suffer from physical and cognitive impairments that add to the challenge of pain evaluation and management. Some of the challenges of geriatric pain assessment, as well as recommended tools for pain evaluation in the elderly, are outlined in this chapter on pain assessment.

In geriatrics, some analgesic therapies have disease-specific utility (e.g. *calcitonin* for vertebral compression fractures) or particular concerns (e.g. **triptans**). Use of these agents is addressed in relevant chapters of this text. This chapter focuses more upon general principles of pain relief in older patients.

The well-recognized increased risk of adverse drug reactions in older adults has *not* been shown to be associated with age itself but is related rather to characteristics prevalent in older adults: polypharmacy, comorbidities, higher illness acuity, smaller body size, and changes in hepatorenal drug handling.[1] Regardless of the root cause of analgesia's risk in older patients, safe and effective geriatric pain care requires that the acute care provider maintains vigilance with regard to a variety of patient factors. Equally important is provider awareness of and avoidance of biases and legends, which produce poor pain care in the elderly.

■ Oligoanalgesia

Despite the fact that they experience acute and chronic pain as frequently as younger patients, older adults often receive significantly less analgesia for comparable conditions.[2] The disparity may be secondary to patients' medical complexities and the related fear of drug complications. Another potential cause of oligoanalgesia is underreporting of pain levels to providers. Older adults may have cognitive impairment, or they may be reticent (owing to self-doubt) to describe sensations as painful. Even when pain sensation is conveyed to providers, discomfort of medical staff and misguided beliefs about older adults' pain treatment can lead to inadequate treatment.[3,4]

Geriatric oligoanalgesia is well known to occur in the acute care setting, and the problem has serious ramifications.[2,5] Just as effective pain management improves patient outcomes and reduces length of stay and resource use, untreated pain prolongs functional impairment and increases risk of delirium.[6–9]

■ Decreased physiologic reserve: pharmacological implications

Aging changes the physiology of drug absorption, distribution, metabolism, and elimination.[1] Age-associated physiologic changes vary from patient to patient, in both degree and directionality (e.g. increased or decreased sensitivity). Even the directionality of some effects (e.g. increased or decreased drug sensitivity) may differ, both between patients and within an individual (i.e. varying effects at different receptor sites).

As adults pass their third decade, progressive loss of organ system functional reserve alters both pharmacokinetics (drug distribution and elimination) and pharmacodynamics (i.e. drug action at receptor sites).[10] These physiologic and pharmacologic changes have direct clinical implications for the safe and effective provision of analgesia to older patients.

Opioid therapy provides an illustrative example of how altered elderly pharmacology dictates a conservative approach to analgesia titration. Drug administration regimens must allow for longer circulation times. Lower **opioid** dosing is also necessitated by increased drug sensitivity, and by decreased renal and hepatic drug clearance owing to diminished organ cell mass and blood flow to the kidneys and liver.[11] In addition to hepatic and renal clearance changes, pharmacokinetics are also altered by the increased proportion of fatty tissue in older patients, and by decreases in lean body mass and total body water.

Given the between-patient variability in physiology of aging and its pharmacologic effects, there can be no "standard recommendation" that will precisely adjust medication dosing as needed. Rather, it is recommended that caution and awareness of the altered physiology inform decisions about choice and dosing of analgesics. In approaching pain medication prescription to older adults, the traditional dictum *primum non nocere* ("first do no harm") should be appended with an admonition to "start slow and go low." In geriatric patients in particular, the keys to safe and efficacious pain relief are conservative dosing, vigilant reassessment, and judicious titration.

To avoid hypoanalgesia, it is prudent to start with a lower dose but repeat it if the patient sustains inadequate relief. As repeated doses are given, it is critical to monitor the patient closely, not only to observe if pain relief has occurred but also to prevent a cumulative side effect of drug that might lead to confusion or respiratory or circulatory failure.

■ Polypharmacy and adverse drug events

Since 90% of elderly patients take at least one medication, with the average geriatric patient taking four drugs, it is no great surprise that adverse drug events are common in this population.[12,13]

An example is provided by warfarin, one of the most often-implicated drugs in adverse interactions in general.[14,15] One of warfarin's more important interactions entails potentiation of anticoagulation when the drug is combined with **NSAIDs** such as *ibuprofen*.[16] The **NSAIDs** are not the only analgesic implicated in warfarin–analgesia interaction: there is debate over whether warfarin's effects are potentiated by *acetaminophen (paracetamol)*.[17] Since it is impossible to remember every potential drug–drug interaction involving analgesics, it is prudent not only to be cautious with starting dosages of analgesia, but also to ask pharmacists to assist with recommendations on both dosage and on how to avoid potential or real drug interactions.

An adverse drug event is any complication stemming from the use of a medication. This umbrella, therefore includes expected drug side effects as well as drug sequelae occurring owing to inappropriate dosing or administration. Adverse drug events are a major problem, constituting the most common type of adverse event in the overall hospital population; older patients are much more likely than younger adults to suffer such adverse drug events.[18,19]

Education and awareness of the issues are useful steps, but ultimately the reduction of error in geriatric analgesia usage requires both system and personnel contributions including decision support-aided computerized physician order entry, unit dose drug distribution, ED pharmacist availability, patient counseling, and protocols for the use of high-risk drugs.[20]

■ Beers criteria: a practical tool to enhance safety in geriatric analgesia

To help in avoiding error, the Beers criteria were developed. These evidence-based guidelines, generated by a multispecialty panel using a modified Delphi approach, were initially developed to enhance safe prescribing of medications to nursing home patients.[21] The Beers criteria have been adopted by many healthcare authorities, including the Centers for Medicare and Medicaid Services, and are now the most often-used consensus criteria guiding medication use in older adults.[22,23]

There are no geriatric drug use guidelines designed expressly for the acute care setting. Consequently, the widespread acceptance and demonstrated utility of the Beers criteria in a variety of healthcare settings (i.e. in addition to nursing homes) constitute reasonable basis for their application to geriatric ED patients.[23,24] Selected recommendations are presented in the table.[24]

Analgesic approaches associated with risk in geriatric patients[24]	
Drug	Concerns with use in older patients
Opioids	
Meperidine	Confusion; disadvantages compared with other opioids
Pentazocine	Compared with other opioids, higher incidence of CNS side effects
Propoxyphene	Incurs opioid risks, with minimal (if any) analgesic benefit over acetaminophen monotherapy
NSAIDs	
General concerns	GI ulcers; asymptomatic/unknown renal disease (prevalent in elderly)
Indomethacin	More CNS adverse effects than other NSAIDs
Benzodiazepines	
Longer-acting agents (e.g. diazepam)	Extended half-life (days); prolonged sedation and fall/fracture risk
Shorter-acting agents (e.g. lorazepam)	High sensitivity to these agents; syncope/fall risk; impaired psychomotor function; efficacy and safety optimized by use of smaller doses
Non-benzodiazepine muscle relaxants (e.g. cyclobenzaprine)	Anticholinergic effects, sedation, and weakness

■ First-line analgesia: acetaminophen and NSAIDs

In geriatric patients as in other populations, first-line analgesia for mild-to-moderate pain should usually entail non-opioids. For the elderly, *acetaminophen* is the drug of first choice. *Acetaminophen*'s potential amplification of warfarin's anticoagulant effects has been mentioned, but even this is subject to debate, and there are no other major drug interactions of concern with *acetaminophen*.[25] Although *acetaminophen* should be used with caution in patients with hepatic disease, the overall safety profile of the drug is preferable to that of the main alternative, **NSAIDs**.

NSAIDs are widely prescribed, and frequently efficacious, in the acute care setting. **NSAIDs** are particularly effective in ameliorating pain from a variety of inflammatory conditions, including rheumatologic disorders often encountered in the elderly. However, it is well known that **NSAID** use, even in healthy younger adults, risks renal and gastrointestinal side effects. Older patients' physiology and associated alterations in drug pharmacokinetics and pharmacodynamics compound **NSAID**-associated risks.

Though the reasons for **NSAID** risk in geriatric patients are myriad, major contributing risks include concomitant use of steroids or anticoagulants. The combination of **NSAIDs** with either of these medication classes substantially increases the chance of peptic ulcer disease complications, including bleeding.[13] Older age also increases the risk of **NSAID**-related renal disease.[26]

NSAID-mediated sodium retention is a particular concern in elder patients, as hypertension and congestive heart failure exacerbation can result. In fact, use of **NSAIDs** (*indomethacin* and *piroxicam* in particular) appears to result in a systolic blood pressure elevation of approximately 5 mmHg in geriatric patients.[27] **NSAID**-related congestive heart failure risk from renal impairment and sodium retention is further increased by water retention, increased peripheral vascular resistance, and antagonism of beta-blocker effects.[28]

Whereas **NSAIDs** are characterized by a ceiling analgesic effect, risks of adverse effects continue to rise as doses are increased.[29] Therefore, especially for severe pain, increasing the **NSAID** dose beyond recommended levels serves only to increase adverse effect risk without improving analgesic benefit. For those instances where **NSAIDs** are used in the elderly, the lowest possible dose should be administered for the shortest reasonable duration, and vigilance for complications must be assured both in the ED and upon follow-up.

■ Opioids

Opioid selections for moderate (e.g. *hydrocodone*) or severe (e.g. *morphine*) pain in the elderly are generally similar to those for younger adults. As a guiding principle, "start low and go slow," is a prudent approach to prescribing **opioids** to the elderly. As long as appropriate pain reassessment is performed, instituting **opioid** therapy with low doses optimizes both safety and efficacy.

The common error with this approach, however, is to conclude that the low dose is the safe dose, and the adequate dose, and that more than the low dose is contraindicated. This is one of the legends that leads to hypoanalgesia. The patient must be carefully and frequently monitored so that more analgesia can be given soon enough to relieve pain, while the patient is being carefully observed for the development of undesirable side effects.

There are some **opioids** that should be avoided in geriatric patients. Specifically, clinicians should try to avoid *propoxyphene*, *codeine*, and *meperidine* (*pethidine*).[30-33] The analgesic benefit of these agents fails to counter the associated risks, which include impaired mental performance, delirium, falls (and hip fractures), ED visits and hospitalizations, and death.

Side effects of **opioids** are a reasonable source of concern. The most important are respiratory depression and constipation. In general, however, the risk of these negative effects with opioids is outweighed by the benefits of analgesia.

The clinical impact of **opioid**-related respiratory depression can be minimized by drug titration and observation for development of side effects. For patients in the ED, serious respiratory depression from parenteral **opioids** is best "treated" by prevention, but hypoventilation can be addressed with ventilatory support. When necessary, *naloxone* can be given, but administration of an **opioid** reversal agent usually translates into difficulty with subsequent pain management.

One of the most common adverse effects with **opioids** is constipation. Fortunately, constipation is relatively easily prevented with combination short-term therapy with *both* a stool softener (e.g. docusate) and a gentle laxative (e.g. senna). Stimulant laxatives (e.g. bisacodyl, cascara sagrada), while listed as "inappropriate" by Beers criteria, are occasionally indicated for short-term use with **opioid** analgesia.[32]

■ Summary and recommendations

First line:

- acetaminophen for mild pain (650 mg PO QID)
- hydrocodone for moderate pain (2.5–5 mg PO q4–6 h)
- morphine for severe pain (initial dose 0.05 mg/kg IV, then titrate)

Reasonable: other opioids (*not recommended*: codeine, meperidine, pentazocine, or propoxyphene)

Special cases:

■ if NSAIDs are used, ibuprofen is a reasonable choice (there is some evidence basis for avoiding indomethacin); safety is maximized by short-term use of the lowest effective dose (e.g. 200–400 mg PO TID–QID)

References

1. Beyth R, Shorr R. Medication use. In Duthie E, Katz P (eds.) *Duthie: Practice of Geriatrics*, 3rd edn. Philadelphia, PA: WB Saunders, 1998:38–47.

2. Jones J, Johnson K, McNinch M. Age as a risk factor for inadequate emergency department analgesia. *Am J Emerg Med*. 1996;**14**:157–160.

3. Gloth F. Geriatric pain: factors that limit pain relief and increase complications. *Geriatrics*. 2000;**55**:12–17.

4. Helme R, Meliala A, Gibson S. Methodologic factors which contribute to variations in experimental pain threshold reported for older people. *Neurosci Lett*. 2004;**361**:144–146.

5. Brown J, Klein E, Lewis C, *et al*. Emergency department analgesia for fracture pain. *Ann Emerg Med*. 2003;**42**:197–205.

6. Dubbleby W, Lander J. Cognitive status and postoperative pain: older adults *J Pain Symptom Manage*. 1994;**19**:19–27.

7. Hoenig H, Rubenstein L, Sloane R, *et al*. What is the role of timing in the surgical and rehabilitative care of community-dwelling older persons with acute hip fracture? *Arch Intern Med*. 1997;**157**:513–520.

8. Morrison R, Magaziner J, McLaughlin M. The impact of postoperative pain on outcomes following hip fracture. *Pain*. 2003;**103**:303–311.

9. Morrison R, Gilbert JMM. Relationship between pain and opioid analgesics on the development of delirium following hip fracture. *J Gerontol*. 2003;**58**:76–81.

10. Evans R, Ireland G, Morely J. Pharmacology and aging. In Sanders A (ed.) *Emergency Care of the Older Person*. St. Louis, MO: Beverly Cracom, 1996:29–42.

11. Wu C. Acute postoperative pain. In Miller R, ed. *Miller's Anesthesia*. 6 ed. Philadelphia, PA: Elsevier; 2005:2729–2762.

12. Hohl C, Dankoff J, Colacone A, *et al.* Polypharmacy, adverse drug-related events, and potential adverse drug interactions in elderly patients presenting to an emergency department. *Ann Emerg Med.* 2001;**38**:666–671.

13. Terrell KM, Heard K, Miller DK. Prescribing to older ED patients. *Am J Emerg Med.* 2006;**24**:468–478.

14. Gaddis G, Holt T, Woods M. Drug interactions in at-risk emergency department patients. *Acad Emerg Med.* 2002;**9**:1162–1167.

15. Cobaugh D, Krenzelok E. Adverse drug reactions and therapeutic errors in older adults: a hazard factor analysis. *Am J Health Syst Pharm.* 2006;**63**:2228–2234.

16. Schulman S, Henriksson K. Interaction of ibuprofen and warfarin on primary haemostasis. *Br J Rheumaol.* 1989;**28**:46–49.

17. Mahe I, Caulin C, Bergmann J. Does paracetamol potentiate the effects of oral anticoagulants: a literature review. *Drug Saf.* 2004;**27**:325–333.

18. Leape L, Brennan T, Laird N. The nature of adverse events in hospitalized patients. *N Engl J Med.* 1991;**324**:377–384.

19. Beers M, Storrie M, Lee G. Potential adverse drug interactions in the emergency room: an issue of quality of care. *Ann Intern Med.* 1990;**112**:61–64.

20. Kelly W, Rucker T. Compelling features of a safe medication-use system. *Am J Health Syst Pharm.* 2006;**63**:1461–1468.

21. Beers M, Ouslander J, Rollingher J, *et al.* Explicit criteria for determining inappropriate medication use in nursing home residents. *Arch Intern Med.* 1991;**151**:1825–1832.

22. Beers M. Explicit criteria for determining potentially inappropriate medication use by the elderly: an update. *Arch Intern Med.* 1997;**157**:1531–1536.

23. Fick D, Waller J, Maclean J. Potentially inappropriate medication use in a Medicare managed care population: association with higher costs and utilization. *J Managed Care Pharm.* 2001;**7**:401–413.

24. Fick D, Cooper J, Wade W, *et al.* Updating the Beers criteria for potentially inappropriate medication use in older adults: results of a U.S. consensus panel of experts. *Arch Intern Med.* 2003;**163**:2716–2724.

25. Toes M, Jones A, Prescott L. Drug interactions with paracetamol. *Am J Ther.* 2005;**12**:56–66.

26. Griffin M, Yared A, Ray W. Nonsteroidal anti-inflammatory drugs and acute renal failure in elderly persons. *Am J Epidemiol.* 2000;**151**:488–496.

27. Johnson A. NSAIDs and blood pressure: clinical importance for older patients. *Drugs Aging.* 1998;**12**:17–27.

28. Buffum M, Buffum J. Nonsteroidal anti-inflammatory drugs in the elderly. *Pain Manage Nurs.* 2000;**1**:40 50.

29. Ferrell B. Pain management. In Hazzard W, Blass J, Ettigner W (eds.) *Principles of Geriatric Medicine and Gerontology*, 4th edn. New York: McGraw-Hill, 1999:413–433.

30. Kamal-Bahl SJ, Stuart BC, Beers MH. Propoxyphene use and risk for hip fractures in older adults. *Am J Geriatr Pharmacother.* 2006;**4**:219–226.

31. Turturro MA, Paris PM, Yealy DM, *et al.* Hydrocodone versus codeine in acute musculoskeletal pain. *Ann Emerg Med.* 1991;**20**:1100–1103.

32. Perri M, 3rd, Menon AM, Deshpande AD, *et al.* Adverse outcomes associated with inappropriate drug use in nursing homes. *Ann Pharmacother.* 2005;**39**:405–411.

33. Fong HK, Sands LP, Leung JM. The role of postoperative analgesia in delirium and cognitive decline in elderly patients: a systematic review. *Anesth Analg.* 2006;**102**:1255–1266.

Chronic pain

DAVID CLINE AND STEPHEN H. THOMAS

■ Topics

- General approach and the chronic pain history
- Analgesic selections in chronic pain
- Pain medication contracts
- Chronic pain and drug-seeking behavior

■ Introduction

Chronic pain, by definition, has been present for three months or more. It should be considered as being distinct from acute pain, from both diagnostic and treatment perspectives. This chapter is intended to provide information for the acute care provider tasked with addressing chronic pain conditions. Much of the discussion in this chapter is closely related to pain syndromes (e.g. fibromyalgia, neck and back strain) considered in specific chapters in this book. Since many chronic pain issues (e.g. drug-seeking behavior) are pertinent across myriad diagnoses, this chapter's purpose is to introduce some concepts with broad relevance to acute care of the patient with chronic pain. Although "drug-seeking" behavior can occur with acute pain conditions (e.g. renal colic), symptom recurrence and chronicity are common, so this chapter also considers the ED approach to the patient making multiple visits.

■ General approach and the chronic pain history

The approach to the patient with chronic pain should indeed be different to that for a patient with acute pain. For instance, in injury-related chronic pain, the patient's discomfort persists long after the healing process is complete. This persistence of pain has impact on therapeutic decision-making. While rest, immobilization, compression, and elevation are cornerstones of the treatment of acute injury, these interventions tend to exacerbate chronic pain and associated disability. In fact, patients with chronic pain can benefit from an active progressive exercise program. This principle is illustrated by considering low-back pain, for which "chronic" but not "acute" sufferers reap benefit from exercise.[1]

With variable prevalence, long-standing pain is accompanied by a wide range of psychosocial issues that either precede or result from the chronic pain condition. Examples of such issues include depression, dependence, dysfunction, disability, dramatization, drug addiction, and doctor-shopping. These conditions render the acute evaluation job a difficult one for the ED care provider. To optimize the care of this patient population, emergency physicians should collect a *chronic pain history* that includes chronic pain conditions, a detailed listing of medication use and effectiveness, and any suspicious allergy listings. The patient should be directly queried, without taking a pejorative tone, about substance abuse problems. The chronic pain history is frequently aided by consultation of prior records when this information is available.

While the underlying diagnosis is typically in hand when a patient with chronic pain presents to the ED, the chronic pain history should include assessment for any changes associated with the current presentation, compared with previous episodes. This component of the history is critical, in order to minimize chances of missing a new life- or limb-threatening process (e.g. a cauda equina syndrome that has developed in a patient with chronic back pain).

If an emergent or urgent condition is not present, the next concern should be in selecting a treatment that does not exacerbate the presenting condition. When used inappropriately in chronic pain, some agents that are useful for acute conditions are not only ineffective but also associated with increased frequency of undesired effects.

Ultimately, the patient with chronic pain needs a regular doctor (and perhaps a pain specialist) to facilitate optimal management. Such longitudinal care is essential when certain medications (e.g. **opioids**) are used over an extended period. If the patient fails to follow through with longitudinal care providers, it may be reasonable to refuse medications such as **opioids** until a stable doctor–patient relationship is established. One of the most important tools for long-term pain care provision is the "pain contract." Acute care providers should seek to determine whether such a contract has been arranged for the patient presenting to the ED, and the terms of these contracts should be respected. In the rare instances when "out-of-contract" analgesia will be provided by the ED physician, contact with the longitudinal care provider is critical. In the occasionally inevitable instances for which the ED becomes the patient's de facto primary care clinic, the acute care provider may need to develop (and document for future providers' reference) a pain contract (see below).

■ Analgesic selections in chronic pain

Patients with chronic pain conditions tend to take analgesics for far longer than the few days or weeks that suffice for acute pain. Consequently, the prescribing clinician must be particularly cognizant of the risks of side effects associated with longer-term use of the medications. Consideration of the risks may impact medication selection (as risk-to-benefit calculations are weighed). Alternatively, side effects may prompt the addition of adjunctive drugs (e.g. stool softeners, anti-dyspeptics) to improve tolerance of pain relievers.

The fact that an agent or class is used frequently for a given condition should not lead to an assumption of efficacy. For instance, meta-analysis of **opioid** use for chronic low-back pain reveals that this oft-prescribed approach has only marginal efficacy and incurs a significant risk of addiction.[2] Similarly, despite their frequent prescription for neuropathic syndromes, **NSAIDs** – which are associated with well-described adverse effects – are generally unhelpful for neuropathy. Even for low-back pain, a condition in which there is some role for **NSAID** use in acute care, the chronic use of these analgesics may have unfavorable risk-to-benefit ratio. Besides well-publicized ulcer, renal, and cardiovascular risk (see the Arthritis chapter, p. 94), long-term **NSAID** use risks abdominal pain, diarrhea, edema, dry mouth, rash, dizziness, headache, and tiredness.[3] In the past, some experts have recommended **NSAIDs** for chronic low-back pain; these recommendations were modified by the reviewers' subsequent clarification that the supporting evidence came from studies of six (or fewer) weeks of **NSAID** use.[4,5]

The side effect problems of **NSAIDs** in chronic use may be ameliorated by use of agents with COX2 specificity. However, this practice brings with it another set of potential problems with cardiovascular disease. Some authors recommend avoiding the potential cardiovascular risk of **COX2-selective NSAIDs** by prescribing dual therapy with a nonselective **NSAID** plus a **proton pump inhibitor**.[6] This decision is not an easy one and should be informed by case-specific variables such as cost and gastrointestinal and cardiovascular risk profiles; some relevant risk-to-benefit information is presented in the Arthritis chapter (p. 94).

Therefore, **opioids** and **NSAIDs**, which are the mainstays of acute care analgesia, are often ineffective or contraindicated for chronic pain conditions. The ED provider is left with some medication selections that are quite out of the mainstream of acute care use. Effective analgesia in chronic pain may be gained by use of **antidepressants** or **anticonvulsants** – in patients who lack depressive symptoms or seizures. *Pregabalin*, *calcitonin*, and **bisphosphonates** are understandably not at the forefront of ED provider's minds when the term "analgesia" is mentioned. Nonetheless, these medications, used in conjunction with appropriate longitudinal follow-up care, may be particularly helpful in some chronic pain conditions.

The approach of the ED provider toward the unique pharmacopoeia of chronic pain should balance enthusiasm with caution. Care must be taken to incorporate available evidence as wisely as possible. The various chapters in this text outline specific evidence, but some examples are worth highlighting. In the various neuropathic pain syndromes, for instance, there is clinically significant (and diagnosis-dependent) variability even within drug classes such as **SSRIs** and **cyclic antidepressants**. Furthermore, while the **tricyclic antidepressants** are, generally speaking, the best drug class for neuropathic pain, they have little benefit in some commonly encountered neuropathic conditions (e.g. HIV-related neuropathy). The differences in chronic versus acute pain medication use extend to the **opioids**. *Tramadol*, as a rule, has a limited evidentiary role for most acute pain conditions – but the agent's monoamine uptake inhibition seems to render it useful for some chronic pain diagnoses. The bipartite lesson for the acute care provider is to maintain both an open mind and open communication (i.e. with physicians more experienced in use of these "non-ED" agents).

Regardless of the medication selected, the ED provider should be straightforward with patients about the expected course of pain relief. Prescribing *morphine* and *ketorolac* for acute renal colic is expected to yield results in minutes. Using *pregabalin* for diabetic neuropathy can reap rewards, but pain reduction takes at least a week and does not peak until the fourth week of treatment.[7] With rare exception, the ED provider, who is used to achieving near-complete analgesia for acute care conditions, will need to be content with a lesser degree of success in the setting of chronic pain. In many cases, the most important ED interventions are instituting a new prescription and arranging for follow-up – with the latter intervention being the most critical.

■ Pain medication contracts

The pain contract will uncommonly be instituted by the acute care provider. However, many ED patients will have pain contracts, and the acute care provider is well advised to have some familiarity with these agreements as they may be a source of very useful information.[2] Although further study of the utility of pain contracts in the acute care setting is needed, in some areas these agreements are used to minimize drug (usually **opioid**) abuse in the ED setting.[2]

There are many forms of pain contract, but the common element to all is an agreement (between patient and provider) on a plan for managing chronic pain. Intrinsic to most pain contracts is the patient's acknowledgment that, while the agreed-upon regimen may not completely alleviate pain, medications "outside the contract" will not be sought without knowledge of the patient's main provider.

Other elements of the pain contract include the listing of medication names and doses. Patients agree not to increase dosages without preapproval of the healthcare provider. The most useful contracts include requirements for patients to seek refills of analgesics at the prescribed interval only, and only during business hours (during which the primary provider is reachable for confirmation).

The pain contract usually specifies that patients are to pledge that they will not try and go outside the contracting provider to obtain extra pain medications. Furthermore, if patients do present to other providers with pain, they are to inform them of the agreed-upon medication regimen.

One of the most important (and ED-relevant) components of a pain contract is the patient's pledge to safekeep their medicines. Lost or stolen medications are often the chief complaint of many patients presenting to the ED for exacerbation of chronic pain. These patients make up some of the most challenging for the acute care provider. Lost and stolen drugs actually *are* occurring to some of the scores of patients who are taking long-term pain medications – especially considering the social situations often seen in this group. However, this is precisely the kind of unconfirmable history that places patients and acute care providers in a difficult position. Though it may seem draconian, the pain contract exists for the good of the patient; it is not the place of the acute care provider to ignore a nonreplacement clause of the pain contract.

Other clauses of the pain contract may deal with patients' promises to avoid illegal drugs, and to undergo drug screening. Furthermore, patients should be directed to keep follow up appointments with the chronic care provider.

If a patient has a pain contract, the contract should be viewed if available. If the contract is unavailable, or the ED physician suspects there may be a contract (but the patient is not reporting one), the patient's physician may be available for clarification. The guiding tenet is that when a pain contract is available, ED should be consistent with its terms.

In conditions anywhere near ideal, it is not the place of the ED physician to generate a pain contract. Furthermore, in the situation in which the acute care provider must institute a pain contract (hopefully in communication with the patient's follow-up physician), some of the previously outlined issues may be worth incorporating in a rudimentary, temporizing pain medication contract. If the ED pain contract *is* generated, then the document will be in the ED record, and it should be adhered to with the same vigor as any other pain contract (thus reinforcing the importance of generating a realistic, reasonable contract).

■ Chronic pain and drug-seeking behavior

Perhaps the most important point to make about drug-seeking behavior is that no physician's judgment is flawless and EM specialists with particular interest in pain note two complementary points: (1) virtually all acute care providers have been successfully misled by patients who are inappropriately seeking drugs, and (2) the inappropriate *denial* of analgesia to the apparent "drug-seeker" is a particularly concerning occupational hazard in the ED.[8] As a corollary to the preceding rules, the ED provider should understand that time spent arguing with patients or their families about pain medication prescription is time poorly spent for all involved. When patients' sincerity is questionable, but not clearly false, we believe that ED providers' clinical obligations outweigh any assumed responsibilities in the realm of policing society's drug misbehavior.

As outlined in this text's introductory sections, patients ought to receive the benefit of the doubt. Furthermore, clinicians should be aware that sometimes patients with legitimate pain are relegated to "drug-seeking" behavior in order to achieve the pain relief to which they are entitled. Through the discussions on how to handle potentially inappropriate drug-seeking behavior runs the thread that the acute care provider's initial assumption should be that patient requests for analgesia are valid.[8]

There are physicians who seem better versed in identifying faked pain than they are in relieving real pain. The successful ED provider must keep in mind the twin imperatives to minimize reinforcing inappropriate drug-seeking behavior while effectively managing the risk of denying analgesia where appropriate. There are some interventions that should be nonthreatening and yet can be very helpful in managing the patient with chronic pain with due diligence. Phoning the patient's physician and assessing the patient's pain contract are obvious examples. In some settings, contacting the patient's pharmacy will provide useful information (many pharmacy chains maintain computerized records, increasing this option's potential utility). Other interventions designed to minimize abuse of the ED are on shakier ground. Maintaining ED "frequent visitor" lists is an example of a commonly used approach that stirs discomfort in both ethicists and EM specialists.[9] In our opinion, these "habitual offender" lists are inconsistently applied and potentially problematic from a legal perspective. Considering that such lists should not be shared within a regions' EDs, they carry risks that are not incurred by simply documenting the same information in the medical record – which can be legitimately consulted by any future care provider.[8] The answer may be to develop statewide monitoring systems, appropriately governed and regulated with respect for ethical and privacy concerns, that are modeled along those that are already in place in much of the USA.[8] Until then, the ED provider dealing with the patient with chronic pain who may be inappropriately seeking analgesics must base decisions on an amalgamation of common sense, reasonable investigative effort, and willingness to give patients the benefit of the doubt.

References

1. Hayden JA, van Tulder MW, Malmivaara AV, *et al.* Meta-analysis: exercise therapy for nonspecific low back pain.*Ann Intern Med.* 2005;**142**(9):765–775.

2. Martell BA, O'Connor PG, Kerns RD, *et al.* Systematic review: opioid treatment for chronic back pain: prevalence, efficacy, and association with addiction. *Ann Intern Med.* 2007;**146**(2):116–127.

3. Koes BW, Scholten RJ, Mens JM, *et al.* Efficacy of non-steroidal anti-inflammatory drugs for low back pain: a systematic review of randomised clinical trials. *Ann Rheum Dis.* 1997;**56**(4):214–223.

4. van Tulder MW, Koes BW, Bouter LM. Conservative treatment of acute and chronic nonspecific low back pain. A systematic review of randomized controlled trials of the most common interventions. *Spine.* 1997;**22**(18):2128–2156.

5. van Tulder MW, Scholten RJ, Koes BW, *et al.* Nonsteroidal anti-inflammatory drugs for low back pain: a systematic review within the framework of the Cochrane Collaboration Back Review Group. *Spine.* 2000;**25**(19):2501–2513.

6. Hur C, Chan AT, Tramontano AC, *et al.* Coxibs versus combination NSAID and PPI therapy for chronic pain: an exploration of the risks, benefits, and costs. *Ann Pharmacother.* 2006;**40**(6):1052–1063.

7. Freynhagen R, Busche P, Konrad C, *et al.* [Effectiveness and time to onset of pregabalin in patients with neuropathic pain.] *Schmerz.* 2006;**20**(4):285–288, 290–282.

8. Millard WB. Grounding frequent flyers, not abandoning them: drug seekers in the ED. *Ann Emerg Med.* 2007;**49**(4):481–486.

9. Marco JMC, Larkin G. From Hippocrates to HIPAA: privacy and confidentiality in emergency medicine. *Ann Emerg Med.* 2005;**45**(1):53–67.

NSAIDs and opioids

BENJAMIN A. WHITE AND STEPHEN H. THOMAS

■ Topics covered

- NSAIDs
- Opioids

■ Introduction

The **NSAIDs** and **opioids** figure prominently in the daily practice of EM. Along with *acetaminophen* (*paracetamol*), these drugs constitute the primary methods of providing nonspecific pain relief in the acute care setting. The information in this chapter is intended to provide general reference for clinicians needing information about the two most commonly used analgesic classes.

■ NSAIDs

Information relevant to the **NSAIDs** is provided in the table on p. 399. Given varying drug availabilities in different countries, not every **NSAID** is covered.

In examining the evidence in this book on acute care use of **NSAIDs**, some common themes about this class emerge. First, for many disease processes, a **NSAID** is all the analgesic that is needed. Particularly when pain is mild or moderate, and related to acute injury or inflammation, an agent such as *ibuprofen* compares favorably with either *acetaminophen* or a weak **opioid**. In children with musculoskeletal injuries, for instance, well-executed trial data demonstrate that patients receiving *ibuprofen* do significantly better than those given either *acetaminophen* or *codeine*.[1] Although the ED physician should not reflexively prescribe **NSAIDs**, this class is not a bad place to start for many patients and acute care conditions.

Once a decision is made to use a **NSAID**, there is scarce efficacy evidence to support selecting one agent over another. When nonselective **NSAIDs** (i.e. not **COX-2 selective NSAIDs**) are similarly dosed, there are few (if any) broadly applicable safety or efficacy differences to guide drug choice. *Ibuprofen* initially appears to be associated with lower risk of GI side effects, but meta-analysis of over 10 studies concludes that the apparent safety advantage of *ibuprofen* is related primarily to lower relative dosage.[2]

Because of genetic variability or other factors, an individual patient may consistently respond better to, or have fewer side effects from, a given **NSAID**. However, there is scant evidence basis for selection of one drug or **NSAID** subclass over another. This general equivalence includes comparison of parenteral **NSAIDs** with their oral counterparts. There may be reasons to use a parenteral **NSAID** in some patients, but the available evidence does not support an assumption of improvements in analgesia with the IV or IM approach compared with PO dosing.[3,4] (In some settings, there may be differential **NSAID** effects with respect to blood pressure elevation in older patients; this is discussed in the chapter on geriatric analgesia, p. 42.)

The previous statements with regard to general **NSAID** safety and efficacy equivalence must be qualified by noting that they apply to nonselective **NSAIDs**. In terms of safety, the **COX-2 selective NSAIDs** should be considered in a different light. The decision-making surrounding use of these agents in the ED is potentially vexing. Acute care providers' suboptimal knowledge of patients' medical histories hinders performance of the risk-to-benefit calculations that should accompany consideration of prescribing **COX-2 selective NSAIDs**. Review of the literature emphasizes the importance of such risk-to-benefit calculations, given the need to weigh GI and cardiovascular risk profiles.

A Cochrane review in favor of the **COX-2 selective NSAIDs**, on the one hand, concluded that these agents are effective for short-term pain relief, and that the GI protection offered by drugs in this class allows their use in patients unable to tolerate nonselective **NSAIDs**.[5,6] On the other hand, cardiovascular risks of **COX-2 selective NSAIDs** are well publicized, and it is important to remember that GI advantages of this class may be completely offset by the low-dose aspirin many patients take for cardiovascular prophylaxis.

Though the data are premature, it appears possible that the newer, more-specific agents such as *lumaricoxib*, or the non-coxib (but still COX-2 selective) agent *nimesulide*, may be characterized by better safety profile than other **COX-2 selective NSAIDs**.[7–9]

For now, with a few possible exceptions such as arthritis pain (see p. 00), we recommend ED providers avoid use of the **COX-2 selective NSAIDs**. This general recommendation is subject to modification in particular clinical circumstances, as outlined in other chapters of this text. Further data will undoubtedly clarify the role of **COX-2 selective NSAIDs** for acute (and chronic) analgesia.

If the side effects of the **COX-2 selective NSAIDs** require further elucidation, there is much less uncertainty about risks associated with nonselective **NSAIDs**. Among the issues to consider are GI bleeding, renal insufficiency, and impaired fracture healing. These complications, which are less likely with a few days' use than with longer **NSAID** prescription, should inform – but not dominate – emergency physicians' drug decision-making.[10] Despite the well-characterized **NSAID** risks, this class is still often the best choice for ED patients. One reason is that the usual alternatives include agents with known adverse effects of their own (e.g. **opioids**), or drugs with lesser analgesic efficacy (e.g. *acetaminophen*).

The gastrointestinal risks of **NSAIDs** are reduced by co-administration of gastroprotective therapy such as *misoprostol* or, preferably, **proton pump inhibitors**.[11,12] Commentators supporting the use of **proton pump inhibitors** in patients receiving **NSAIDs** cite data showing that, compared with **NSAID** monotherapy, the dual-therapy approach reduces GI bleed incidence by over 80%.[13] Pharmaco-economic analysis suggests that, for short-course therapy prescribed from the ED, the combination will usually be more cost effective than **COX-2 selective NSAID** monotherapy.[14]

Perhaps surprisingly for many conditions described in this text, the combination of **NSAIDs** and **opioids** fails to accrue additive (or synergistic) analgesic results. The point is illustrated by recent data from a study of children with suspected fractures. The authors of the study found that children with mild-to-moderate pain responded equally well to *ibuprofen* (10 mg/kg PO), *oxycodone* (0.1 mg/kg PO), or the combination of the two, and preferred monotherapy for reasons of safety and simplicity.[15] The message for the ED physician is that single-drug therapy may be best. Do not assume that **NSAID**-associated risks – however small in an individual patient – are outweighed by analgesic benefit in a patient who is already going to be taking **opioids**.

We believe that the systemic use of **NSAIDs** in pregnant patients is not associated with favorable risk-to-benefit ratio. Most **NSAIDs** are FDA Pregnancy Category C, although the category changes to D toward the end of pregnancy. Even for topical applications (e.g. corneal abrasion), there are alternatives, even **opioids**, that are preferable. The risk of systemic and fetal effects, including those on the ductus arteriosus, is simply too high for **NSAID** administration to gravida. We also believe that, although the evidence of harm is not irrefutable, **NSAIDs** are best avoided in breastfeeding mothers.

NSAIDs (and *acetaminophen*) will always claim one advantage over **opioids**: antipyresis. Given the improvement in comfort that is inevitably achieved with defervescence, treatment of pain accompanied by fever should include either an **NSAID** or *acetaminophen*.

■ Opioids

In reviewing the recommendations and evidence from this text, it is clear that the **opioids** remain the most important class for the ED provider dealing with acute pain of moderate to high severity. Information relevant to the **opioids** is presented in the table on p. 402.

For most patients, the potential problems with **opioids** have little to do with efficacy in relieving pain. In fact, one of the causes for concern related to **opioids** is that these agents relieve pain so effectively that the ED physician fails to provide nonpharmacologic pain relief (e.g. splinting). More problematic is the potential that the acute care provider, falsely reassured by **opioid**-mediated pain relief, prematurely ceases the diagnostic search for the condition that caused the pain.

Perhaps the lengthy history of **opioids**' effectiveness is responsible for the relatively few rigorous analyses of their risks and benefits – either compared with each other or compared with non-opioid analgesics. There is abundant data on **opioid** use in the ED, however, and some common threads from this chapter are noteworthy.

First, equipotent doses of pure **opioid** agonists tend to be equally effective. There remains potential that an individual patient will respond better to one agent or another (perhaps from genetic variability), but the general equivalence of the **opioids** is demonstrated by a wealth of data.

One caveat to the general rule of **opioid** equivalence is that mixed agonist-antagonist agents have clinical characteristics that differ from those of the pure mu receptor agonists. The agonist–antagonists can be associated with more dysphoria and may precipitate withdrawal symptoms in patients who are not **opioid** naïve. Unless there is a specific reason, we prefer use of traditional pure mu agonists (e.g. *morphine*). (As a related point, the ED provider should be wary of administration of *naloxone* to patients in whom **opioids** may be necessary for analgesia; subsequent pain control can be complicated by the difficulty of overcoming **opioid** reversal agents.)

The second caveat to considering **opioid** deals with the imprecision of "**opioid** potency equivalence tables." The case of *hydromorphone*, which can be illustrated with high-quality data, serves well as an illustration of the difficulty of arriving at an evidence-based level of "equipotency" compared with *morphine*. A recent ED study found a dose of 0.015 mg/kg *hydromorphone* to be equally efficacious to 0.1 mg/kg *morphine*.[16] The resulting ratio of 15:1 markedly differs from what pain experts denote as the accepted standard: 7:1.[17] The situation is further obfuscated by trial evidence suggesting that, for PCA dosing, the *hydromorphone:morphine* potency ratio is roughly 3:1.[17] Confusion can be compounded when considering pediatric studies, which demonstrate risk for *hydromorphone* underdosing when adult equipotency data are applied in younger patients.[18] We do not recommend wholesale distrust or abandonment of equianalgesia tables, but we do suggest that acute care providers should not be dogmatic about applying such data.

The equianalgesia tables do provide an important **opioid** dosing starting point, the utility of which is underlined by another tenet we wish to emphasize. An **opioid**, like any other drug, ought to be given a fair trial in an individual patient before concluding that it is not efficacious. All too frequently, a few small doses of an **opioid** are given, then clinicians switch to a second **opioid** because of "failure" of the initial agent. This practice represents unnecessary polypharmacy. In the case of *morphine*, we have seen countless instances where providers wish to switch to a second **opioid** because of continuing pain after 10 mg (or less) – this switch despite the well-demonstrated fact that higher *morphine* doses are *usually* required for ED pain control.[19] In fact, data demonstrate that for children and adults, with a variety of medical and surgical conditions, 0.1 mg/kg IV *morphine* is unlikely to constitute adequate analgesia.[19,20] Ceiling doses of **opioids** will vary by drug and patient, so a specific "abandonment point" cannot be delineated. Rather, we advise the ED clinician to keep in mind that safety, efficacy, and ease of titration are optimized by giving one **opioid** a fair trial before switching to another.

On a related point, even when *morphine* is written in a correct initial dosage (i.e. in a range 0.1–0.15 mg/kg), well-intentioned providers often mistakenly administer the drug in staggered fashion, giving multiple (near-homeopathic) 1–2 mg injections over an extended time period. Such caution is encouraged when **opioids** are given to patients particularly likely to experience side effects, but the vast majority of ED patients in severe pain can easily tolerate a 4–6 mg initial *morphine* dose. In fact, savvy ED clinicians discussing *hydromorphone*'s advantages have noted that the drug's apparent incremental efficacy over *morphine* is simply a function of it being administered as ordered (i.e. in a single 1 mg dose), rather than split into aliquots as *morphine* often is.[16]

While a few doses of **opioids** given in generally recommended ranges are unlikely to cause serious side effects, it is our experience that nausea and vomiting are common, especially with aggressive **opioid** dosing such as advocated for many conditions in this text. We do not believe that prophylactic administration of **antiemetics** should be routine, but we do advocate early administration of such medications in patients who have a history of **opioid**-associated nausea. The ED provider should also be observant for, and quickly treat, nausea and vomiting that occur after **opioid** administration. Otherwise, many patients will find the side effects of the analgesia as unpleasant as, or worse than, the pain itself.

We believe that the systemic use of **opioids** in pregnant patients is often associated with favorable risk-to-benefit ratio. Most **opioids** are FDA Pregnancy Category C, although there are some exceptions such as *oxycodone* and *nalbuphine* which are Category B. Long-term use of **opioids**, especially during the peripartum period, increases the risk of **opioid** use during pregnancy. For short-term use as prescribed from the ED, the analgesic benefits of the **opioids** will counterbalance the risks for most pregnant patients with pain uncontrollable by other means. Since most **opioids** are excreted to some degree in breast milk, **opioids** are best avoided in breastfeeding mothers.

We conclude these general thoughts about **opioids** with one of the more debate-provoking issues. The controversy surrounding *meperidine* (*pethidine*) use in the ED is hard for acute care providers to avoid. On the one hand, concerns about *meperidine* are based on indisputable pharmacological bases (e.g. cardiac and neurological sequelae). On the other hand, it is hard to find evidence that a few doses of *meperidine* truly pose any hazard to the average ED patient. Furthermore, there is such a wealth of practical experience with safe and effective use of *meperidine* that we are uncomfortable condemning its use – especially in a text aimed in part at busy clinicians who have relieved pain with the drug on hundreds (if not thousands) of occasions. Our conclusion is that the available evidence in this book supplies no basis for an ED provider's reaching for *meperidine* as the **opioid** of choice – but that there is also little clinical basis for the opprobrium often visited upon those who administer the drug in an attempt to relieve a patient's pain.

References

1. Clark E, Plint AC, Correll R, *et al*. A randomized, controlled trial of acetaminophen, ibuprofen, and codeine for acute pain relief in children with musculoskeletal trauma. *Pediatrics*. 2007;**119**(3):460–467.

2. Henry D, Lim LL, Garcia Rodriguez LA, *et al*. Variability in risk of gastrointestinal complications with individual non-steroidal anti-inflammatory drugs: results of a collaborative meta-analysis. *BMJ*. 1996;**312**(7046):1563–1566.

3. Shrestha M, Morgan DL, Moreden JM, *et al*. Randomized double-blind comparison of the analgesic efficacy of intramuscular ketorolac and oral indomethacin in the treatment of acute gouty arthritis. *Ann Emerg Med*. 1995;**26**(6):682–686.

4. Arora S, Wagner JG, Herbert M. Myth: parenteral ketorolac provides more effective analgesia than oral ibuprofen. *CJEM*. 2007;**9**(1):30–32.

5. Navascues JA, Soleto J, Romero R, *et al.* [Impact of formation programs in initial management of injured children.] *Cir Pediatr.* 2004;**17**(1):28–32.

6. Sanchez-Borges M, Caballero-Fonseca F, Capriles-Hulett A. Tolerance of nonsteroidal anti-inflammatory drug-sensitive patients to the highly specific cyclooxygenase 2 inhibitors rofecoxib and valdecoxib. *Ann Allergy Asthma Immunol.* 2005;**94**(1):34–38.

7. Bannwarth B, Berenbaum F. Lumiracoxib in the management of osteoarthritis and acute pain. *Expert Opin Pharmacother.* 2007; **8**(10):1551–1564.

8. Bannwarth B, Berenbaum F. Clinical pharmacology of lumiracoxib, a second-generation cyclooxygenase 2 selective inhibitor. *Expert Opin Invest Drugs.* 2005;**14**(4):521–533.

9. Rainsford KD. Current status of the therapeutic uses and actions of the preferential cyclo-oxygenase-2 NSAID, nimesulide. *Inflammopharmacology.* 2006;**14**(3–4):120–137.

10. Rabb H, Colvin RB. Case records of the MGH: a 41-year-old man with abdominal pain and elevated serum creatinine. *New Eng J Med.* 2007;**357** (15):1531–1541.

11. Peura DA. Prevention of nonsteroidal anti-inflammatory drug-associated gastrointestinal symptoms and ulcer complications. *Am J Med.* 2004;**117** (Suppl 5A):63S–71S.

12. Hooper L, Brown TJ, Elliott R, *et al.* The effectiveness of five strategies for the prevention of gastrointestinal toxicity induced by non-steroidal anti-inflammatory drugs: systematic review. *BMJ.* 2004;**329**(7472):948.

13. Lane NE. Clinical practice. Osteoarthritis of the hip. *N Engl J Med.* 2007;**357** (14):1413–1421.

14. Hur C, Chan AT, Tramontano AC, *et al.* Coxibs versus combination NSAID and PPI therapy for chronic pain: an exploration of the risks, benefits, and costs. *Ann Pharmacother.* 2006;**40**(6):1052–1063.

15. Koller DM, Myers AB, Lorenz D, *et al.* Effectiveness of oxycodone, ibuprofen, or the combination in the initial management of orthopedic injury-related pain in children. *Pediatr Emerg Care.* 2007;**23**(9):627–633.

16. Chang AK, Bijur PE, Meyer RH, *et al.* Safety and efficacy of hydromorphone as an analgesic alternative to morphine in acute pain: a randomized clinical trial. *Ann Emerg Med.* 2006;**48**(2):164–172.

17. Dunbar PJ, Chapman CR, Buckley FP, *et al.* Clinical analgesic equivalence for morphine and hydromorphone with prolonged PCA. *Pain.* 1996;**68**(2–3):265–270.

18. Collins JJ, Geake J, Grier HE, *et al.* Patient-controlled analgesia for mucositis pain in children: a three-period crossover study comparing morphine and hydromorphone. *J Pediatr.* 1996;**129**(5):722–728.

19. Birnbaum A, Esses D, Bijur PE, *et al.* Randomized double-blind placebo-controlled trial of two intravenous morphine dosages (0.10 mg/kg and 0.15 mg/kg) in emergency department patients with moderate to severe acute pain. *Ann Emerg Med.* 2007;**49**(4):445–453, 453, e441-442.

20. Bailey B, Bergeron S, Gravel J, *et al.* Efficacy and impact of intravenous morphine before surgical consultation in children with right lower quadrant pain suggestive of appendicitis: a randomized controlled trial. *Ann Emerg Med.* 2007;**50**(4):371-378.

Nonstandard medication delivery

JAMES R. MINER

■ Delivery routes

- Rectal
- Nasal
- Nebulized/inhaled
- Transmucosal
- Transdermal

■ Introduction

This chapter addresses delivery of analgesics via a variety of "nonstandard" routes. Since the focus is on systemic drug delivery, useful regional approaches (e.g. locally active topical therapy, nerve blocks) are not discussed here. The vast majority of medications are administered orally or parenterally. Oral therapies are most commonly employed, since they are convenient and inexpensive for patients who can tolerate PO intake. When pain is severe, however, analgesics must be given immediately and titrated to effect.

As outlined in other chapters of this text, the IV (not IM) route is indicated in the context of need for rapid and titrateable analgesia. Injections IM may have some occasional utility when IV access is difficult, or when rapid analgesia is unnecessary. However, the IM route's ease of use is largely offset by injection pain, titration difficulty, and delayed onset of action. Unless IV access is difficult, there is usually little reason to recommend the IM route.

Situations may occasionally arise in the ED in which IV placement is either too difficult or best avoided for other reasons. This scenario is encountered most frequently in children, who often do not tolerate IV placement attempts. While non-IV routes for delivery of analgesics such as **opioids** are not superior (and sometimes do not reach equivalence) to the IV approach, "nonstandard" administration routes do have occasional ED utility.[1,2] One exception is the **NSAIDs**, for which PO administration is usually sufficient (and difficult to improve upon).

This chapter focuses on the general approach to nonstandard routes for analgesia delivery. For the most part, specific drugs and indications are left for discussion elsewhere in the text. When a particular nonstandard administration route is indicated in only a few situations, those conditions are identified.

■ Rectal

Comparative studies demonstrate that PR administration of either *morphine* (0.2 mg/kg) or *codeine* (1 mg/kg) provides equivalent analgesia to that associated with IM or PO dosing.[3-7] *Acetaminophen* and **NSAIDs** PR are also equivalent to PO dosing of the same medications. The common co-administration of sedatives with analgesics lends relevance to findings that efficacy of PR *midazolam* exceeds that of PO administration of the **benzodiazepine**.[8-11]

■ Nasal

Analgesia administration by the IN route has been most successfully described in the treatment of migraine headaches using *sumatriptan* (p. 243).[12,13] Utility of IN *butorphanol* for migraine headache is more limited, with issues of both efficacy and side effects.[14]

Morphine, fentanyl (1.7 µg/kg), and *sufentanil* (0.05 µg/kg per puff) are effective for IN administration.[15-20] Just as PR sedation is a viable adjunct to PR analgesia, IN *midazolam* (0.2 mg/kg) is an effective means to complement IN analgesia.[21, 22]

While not often used in the ED, IN salmon *calcitonin* may be useful for some conditions seen in the ED. Among the indications for which this approach has been found at least partially efficacious are vertebral compression fractures and some of the neuropathies (in particular, phantom limb pain).[23,24] Other information on these possible indications for IN therapy is found in the relevant chapters of this text.

■ Nebulized/inhaled route

The practice of delivering **opioids** via a nebulizer has been discussed in the literature for over a quarter of a century.[25] For myriad painful conditions, ranging from sickle cell crisis to cancer and even undifferentiated abdominal pain, nebulization of **opioids** such as *morphine* (10–20 mg) or *fentanyl* (1.5–3.0 µg/kg) is shown to be safe and effective.[20,26–32] Compared with IV administration, nebulization of the **opioids** achieves roughly equivalent pain relief, with similar times of onset.[20,28–31] The use of a breath-actuated delivery system has proven safe and effective and seems particularly attractive for ED patients who are old enough (about three years of age) to use the system.[32]

Nebulized *naloxone* has been described for the reversal of **opioid** toxicity.[33]

■ Oral transmucosal route

The OTM administration of *fentanyl* is perhaps the best described of the alternative dosing strategies. Since they were developed for breakthrough cancer pain, many currently available OTM *fentanyl* formulations are too potent to be safely given to **opioid**-naïve patients.[34,35] There is, however, potential utility for this administration route. For instance, one study of (opioid-naïve, noncancer) trauma patients showed OTM *fentanyl* (1600 µg) to be similarly efficacious to standard IV dosing, over a period of 5 h.[36] A recent trial in children found that OTM *fentanyl* (10–15 µg/kg) provided analgesic efficacy superior to that achieved with IV *morphine* (0.1 mg/kg).[37] The study's authors noted relatively few adverse effects (17% overall rate of nausea/vomiting or pruritis with OTM *fentanyl*), but appropriately point out that their patient sample of 87, with 47 taking OTM *fentanyl*, is too small to serve as conclusive demonstration of OTM *fentanyl*'s safety.

■ Transdermal route

The TD administration of *buprenorphine* and *fentanyl* has been been well described, but the onset of action is too prolonged for routine use of this approach in ED therapy of acute pain.[38,39] The use of iontophoresis to augment *fentanyl* delivery across the skin barrier shows promise as a means to improve TD **opioids**' acute care utility. Studies show iontophoresis-aided TD *fentanyl* delivery can achieve onset times approximating those for IV use.[40–42]

■ Summary and recommendations

First-line: IV

Reasonable: nebulized and nasal fentanyl

Pregnancy: nebulized and nasal fentanyl

Pediatric: nebulized and nasal fentanyl

Special cases:
- cancer breakthrough pain: oral transmucosal fentanyl
- migraine headache: nasal triptans
- osteoporotic vertebral compression fracture or phantom limb pain: nasal calcitonin

References

1. Asenjo JF, Brecht KM. Opioids: other routes for use in recovery room. *Curr Drug Targets*. 2005;6(7):773–779.
2. Shirk MB, Donahue KR, Shirvani J. Unlabeled uses of nebulized medications. *Am J Health Syst Pharm*. 2006;63(18):1704–1716.
3. Lundeberg S, Hatava P, Lagerkranser M, *et al*. Perception of pain following rectal administration of morphine in children: a comparison of a gel and a solution. *Paediatr Anaesth*. 2006;16(2):164–169.
4. McEwan A, Sigston PE, Andrews KA, *et al*. A comparison of rectal and intra-muscular codeine phosphate in children following neurosurgery. *Paediatr Anaesth*. 2000;10(2):189–193.
5. Owczarzak V, Haddad J, Jr. Comparison of oral versus rectal administration of acetaminophen with codeine in postoperative pediatric adenotonsillectomy patients. *Laryngoscope*. 2006;116(8):1485–1488.

6. Pannuti F, Rossi AP, Iafelice G, *et al.* Control of chronic pain in very advanced cancer patients with morphine hydrochloride administered by oral, rectal and sublingual route. Clinical report and preliminary results on morphine pharmacokinetics. *Pharmacol Res Commun.* 1982;**14**(4):369–380.

7. Pasero C, McCaffery M. Opioids by the rectal route. *Am J Nurs.* 1999;**99**(11):20.

8. Kanegaye JT, Favela JL, Acosta M, *et al.* High-dose rectal midazolam for pediatric procedures: a randomized trial of sedative efficacy and agitation. *Pediatr Emerg Care.* 2003;**19**(5):329–336.

9. Shane SA, Fuchs SM, Khine H. Efficacy of rectal midazolam for the sedation of preschool children undergoing laceration repair. *Ann Emerg Med.* 1994;**24**(6):1065–1073.

10. Jensen B, Matsson L. Oral versus rectal midazolam as a pre-anaesthetic sedative in children receiving dental treatment under general anaesthesia. *Acta Paediatr.* 2002;**91**(8):920–925.

11. Primosch RE, Bender F. Factors associated with administration route when using midazolam for pediatric conscious sedation. *ASDC J Dent Child.* 2001;**68**(4):233–238, 228.

12. Ahonen K, Hamalainen ML, Rantala H, *et al.* Nasal sumatriptan is effective in treatment of migraine attacks in children: a randomized trial. *Neurology.* 2004;**62**(6):883–887.

13. Rapoport AM, Bigal ME, Tepper SJ, *et al.* Intranasal medications for the treatment of migraine and cluster headache. *CNS Drugs.* 2004;**18**(10):671–685.

14. Goldstein J, Gawel MJ, Winner P, *et al.* Comparison of butorphanol nasal spray and fiorinal with codeine in the treatment of migraine. *Headache.* 1998;**38**(7):516–522.

15. Borland M, Jacobs I, King B, *et al.* A randomized controlled trial comparing intranasal fentanyl to intravenous morphine for managing acute pain in children in the emergency department. *Ann Emerg Med.* 2007;**49**(3): 335–340.

16. Dale O, Hjortkjaer R, Kharasch ED. Nasal administration of opioids for pain management in adults. *Acta Anaesthesiol Scand.* 2002;**46**(7):759–770.

17. Finn J, Wright J, Fong J, *et al.* A randomised crossover trial of patient controlled intranasal fentanyl and oral morphine for procedural wound care in adult patients with burns. *Burns.* 2004;**30**(3):262–268.

18. Illum L, Watts P, Fisher AN, *et al.* Intranasal delivery of morphine. *J Pharmacol Exp Ther.* 2002;**301**(1):391–400.

19. Mathieu N, Cnudde N, Engelman E, *et al.* Intranasal sufentanil is effective for postoperative analgesia in adults. *Can J Anaesth.* 2006;**53**(1):60–66.

20. Zeppetella G. Nebulized and intranasal fentanyl in the management of cancer-related breakthrough pain. *Palliat Med.* 2000;**14**(1):57–58.

21. Ljungman G, Kreuger A, Andreasson S, *et al.* Midazolam nasal spray reduces procedural anxiety in children. *Pediatrics.* 2000;**105**(1, Pt 1):73–78.

22. Primosch RE, Guelmann M. Comparison of drops versus spray administration of intranasal midazolam in two- and three-year-old children for dental sedation. *Pediatr Dent.* 2005;**27**(5):401–408.

23. Wall GC, Heyneman CA. Calcitonin in phantom limb pain. *Ann Pharmacother.* 1999;**33**(4):499–501.

24. Kanis JA, McCloskey EV. Effect of calcitonin on vertebral and other fractures. *QJ Med.* 1999;**92**(3):143–149.

25. Higgins M, Asbury A, Brodie M. Inhaled nebulised fentanyl for postoperative analgesia. *Anaesthesia.* 1991;**46**(8):973–976.

26. Ballas SK, Viscusi ER, Epstein KR. Management of acute chest wall sickle cell pain with nebulized morphine. *Am J Hematol.* 2004;**76**(2):190–191.

27. Bruera E, Sala R, Spruyt O, *et al.* Nebulized versus subcutaneous morphine for patients with cancer dyspnea: a preliminary study. *J Pain Symptom Manage.* 2005;**29**(6):613–618.

28. Bartfield JM, Flint RD, McErlean M, *et al.* Nebulized fentanyl for relief of abdominal pain. *Acad Emerg Med.* 2003;**10**(3):215–218.

29. Farr SJ, Otulana BA. Pulmonary delivery of opioids as pain therapeutics. *Adv Drug Deliv Rev.* 31 2006;**58**(9–10):1076–1088.

30. Higgins MJ, Asbury AJ, Brodie MJ. Inhaled nebulised fentanyl for postoperative analgesia. *Anaesthesia.* 1991;**46**(11):973–976.

31. Fulda GJ, Giberson F, Fagraeus L. A prospective randomized trial of nebulized morphine compared with patient-controlled analgesia morphine in the management of acute thoracic pain. *J Trauma.* 2005;**59**(2):383–388; discussion 389–390.

32. Miner J, Kletti C, Herold M, *et al.* Randomized clinical trial of nebulized fentanyl citrate versus IV fentanyl citrate in children presenting to the ED with acute pain. *Acad Emerg Med.* 2007;**14**(10):895–898.

33. Mycyk MB, Szyszko AL, Aks SE. Nebulized naloxone gently and effectively reverses methadone intoxication. *J Emerg Med.* 2003;**24**(2):185–187.

34. Aronoff GM, Brennan MJ, Pritchard DD, *et al.* Evidence-based oral transmucosal fentanyl citrate (OTFC) dosing guidelines. *Pain Med.* 2005;**6**(4):305–314.

35. Blick SK, Wagstaff AJ. Fentanyl buccal tablet: in breakthrough pain in opioid-tolerant patients with cancer. *Drugs.* 2006;**66**(18):2387–2393; discussion 2394–2395.

36. Kotwal RS, O'Connor KC, Johnson TR, *et al*. A novel pain management strategy for combat casualty care. *Ann Emerg Med*. 2004;**44**(2):121–127.

37. Mahar PJ, Rana JA, Kennedy CS, *et al*. A randomized clinical trial of oral transmucosal fentanyl citrate versus intravenous morphine sulfate for initial control of pain in children with extremity injuries. *Pediatr Emerg Care*. 2007;**23**(8):544–548.

38. Griessinger N, Sittl R, Likar R. Transdermal buprenorphine in clinical practice – a post-marketing surveillance study in 13 179 patients. *Curr Med Res Opin*. 2005;**21**(8):1147–1156.

39. Koo PJ. Postoperative pain management with a patient-controlled transdermal delivery system for fentanyl. *Am J Health Syst Pharm*. 1 2005;**62**(11):1171–1176.

40. Hartrick CT, Bourne MH, Gargiulo K, *et al*. Fentanyl iontophoretic transdermal system for acute-pain management after orthopedic surgery: a comparative study with morphine intravenous patient-controlled analgesia. *Reg Anesth Pain Med*. 2006;**31**(6):546–554.

41. Mayes S, Ferrone M. Fentanyl HCl patient-controlled iontophoretic transdermal system for the management of acute postoperative pain. *Ann Pharmacother*. 2006;**40**(12):2178–2186.

42. Sinatra R. The fentanyl HCl patient-controlled transdermal system (PCTS): an alternative to intravenous patient-controlled analgesia in the postoperative setting. *Clin Pharmacokinet*. 2005;**44**(Suppl 1):1–6.

Reflections on analgesia in emergency departments

PETER ROSEN AND STEPHEN H. THOMAS

This book is an attempt to make recommendations for safe and effective practice of pain management. As spelled out in the chapters that follow, the book has tried to base all recommendations upon evidence that is available from research and review. It is for this reason that we feel it necessary to remind our readers about some limitations of trying to produce evidence-based recommendations. These limitations do not mean that the reader should consider fruitless the attempt to generate data-driven guidelines for pain relief. Nevertheless, we do wish to offer some thoughts about integrating this text's evidence overviews into day-to-day ED practice.

First of all, there are the realities of trying to generalize recommendations from specific pieces of research evidence. Not always is this generically difficult, but extrapolation of results from pain care studies can be especially challenging.

Part of the difficulty lies in the widely varying degree to which investigators have focused upon different questions regarding acute pain management. For instance, dozens of studies address acute relief of migraine headache, but there is a paucity of data comparing ED approaches to vertebral compression fracture. Though not always the case, it is usually true that the fewer the trials assessing a particular diagnosis, the less certain the foundation for data-driven treatment guidelines. Consequently, this text – like the data upon which it is based – is uneven.

Interpretation and application of ED pain literature can be complicated by qualitative as well as quantitative issues. One does not have to search for long to identify the difficulties inherent to studying analgesia – first among them being our incomplete understanding of pain pathophysiology.

While the presence of pain makes sense from an oversimplified, evolutionary fight-or-flight point of view, it is hard to understand all the ramifications of biologic pain. At times, we inappropriately feel no pain whatsoever, and because of this enable much greater destruction of body tissues. It is as if we had total denervation, and can no longer respond to painful stimuli. Who of us has never experienced this when under the stimulation of competition, fear, or simple distraction? This is hardly a useful trait for longevity, especially when we observe it in elderly patients who may never perceive any discomfort with the acute onset of very serious disease (e.g. cholecystitis, acute myocardial infarction). Why is it that so many life-threatening diseases produce little discomfort, while trivial problems often seem to incapacitate the patient?

Pain is a cultural phenomenon as well as a physical one. Certain kinds of patient obtain more attention from their relatives or immediate companions and friends, and seem always to overreact to pain. Other patients seem to think it wrong to express discomfort and often hide the symptoms that would help in their evaluation. They often fail to request pain relief even when it is obvious they have a condition that can produce pain. Unfortunately, we in the health profession seem to expect stoicism, and respond much more positively to someone who appears to be doing his or her best to bear up under the pain than we do to the patients who complain vociferously. Moreover, there is a language barrier to the effective communication of pain. Many patients cannot describe radiation, or gradations of pain. They only know they hurt. This is also true for patients whose first language is not English. They may simply not know how to talk about their pain.

Why is it that in certain situations when we do perceive pain it is the wrong degree and the wrong location? For example, in multiple trauma victims, it is often observed that the patient complains about a trivial injury, when there are major severe injuries that the patient is totally unaware of having sustained. For example, we saw a patient, a 45-year-old man, who complained of a wrist injury (it was sprained) after a motorcycle crash. He also happened to have 12 rib fractures, a humerus fracture on the side opposite the wrist sprain, a shattered liver, and a femur fracture. Yet his only concern was the wrist, and the pain was quite mild. Through the lens of analgesia research, this patient (on the basis of his injuries) would appear to have been under-treated because he was given no **opioids**.

Imagine trying to collect evidence for the utility of any single agent when the population studied is filled with patients like the one just described. There is no shortage of other potential confounders to conducting (and interpreting) pain research. One of the most important confounders deals with the population – patients with extremity fractures – making up many pain studies. While the common practice of focusing analgesia studies on these patients is sensible, clinical experience teaches us that a significant proportion of such patients achieve pain relief if the extremity is simply left at rest (even without splinting). The smaller the study number, the more likely the presence of residual confounding that may be missed by even prospective methodology.

Therefore, in studying pain, we must allow for the fact that no two patients perceive pain in the same way; that certain kinds of injury that produce maximum pain as perceived by some patients produce none in others. We must also understand that we have no objective method of measuring pain, or its relief. We are forced to rely on what the patient tells us about the individual perception of pain.

As well, there are the methodologic difficulties in our science of pain relief. Because of issues of the type just described, it is hard to constitute a uniform control group. Nevertheless, even assuming that we have a large enough patient population to allow for these vagaries of perception in the control group, we often make errors in the study group. While we are the first to applaud planning and execution of RCTs in acute care analgesia, such trials are not infallible, and emergency physicians should be wary of common shortcomings. When an ED clinician encounters RCT results that contradict years of experience, a vigilant search for oft-encountered study flaws can be enlightening.

For example, if one attempts to compare the efficacy of *morphine* with that of *meperidine* (*pethidine*), what do you think would be the outcome if the *morphine* were administered IV in a dose of 10 mg, and the meperidine IM in a dose of 50 mg? Even if the 50 mg meperidine dose were to be given IV, the outcome of such a study is predictable. Yet there are many studies that commit precisely that kind of relative dosing error. The effective dose of meperidine is 1–1.5 mg/kg; how many patients will achieve relief from a dose of 50 mg?

Non-analgesic adjunctive care also makes a difference to a pain management study. We cannot take a population of humans and alter only one parameter, the presence or absence of pain. Any patient who is complaining of pain is having many things done to her or him for the purpose of diagnosis, and management of all diseases present, above and beyond doing something for pain relief.

Science must advance by slow incremental steps that are built upon facts and observations of prior studies. Yet in clinical medicine, we must be impatient. We wish to have an effective answer *now*, because the patient who is in pain is our immediate concern. We, therefore, are too impatient to await the future increments that might indeed give us a well-integrated program of pain management. In the meantime, we must do the best we can with what we know.

For reasons of length, and in order to maximize clinical utility, the authors of the chapters have been asked to avoid detailed discourse on individual study merits and flaws. The lack of such discussion should not be taken to imply that authors believed study methodology to be ideal. Rather, the inclusion of a particular study in a chapter should be taken as evidence that the author felt the trial's data added significantly to the relevant body of evidence. This is admittedly a subjective judgment made by chapter authors. For this reason, among others, the contributors to this text were chosen with an eye to their possessing extensive clinical and research experience in the ED.

One of the ways we can do the best we can with suboptimal evidence is to realize the risks inherent to abandoning any analgesic that has been used effectively for decades. For example, it is true that the metabolic decomposition of *meperidine* produces normeperidine, which in large enough concentration produces marked neurologic changes and probably can lead to a patient's demise. Nevertheless it is also true that the ED patient will not suffer such complications if the dosage of *meperidine* is held to reasonable levels. We make this point neither to lobby for first-line *meperidine* use nor to negate any studies that show advantages of other agents. Nevertheless, before the wholesale abandonment of *meperidine*, we must remember the clinical observations of many years of success. There appear to be many patients (e.g. some with sickle cell crisis) who prefer *meperidine* to *morphine* for pain relief. We do not have a good answer as to why this should be true, but when we are treating a phenomenon like pain, that is so subject depend-ent, how can we ignore the repeated subjective observations of the patients to whom we are trying to give pain relief?

Another tremendous problem in the satisfactory management of analgesia is the pain-pill dependency of many patients with and without chronic pain syndromes. We become jaded in our response to patients with true pain, and often do not believe the patient's complaints, especially when the history includes IV drug abuse. Yet what population is more likely to have a true medical problem, often caused by the abuse? When such a patient presents to your ED with cellulitis, is the pain complaint likely to be acted upon in the absence of significant fluctuance and sufficient localization to be perceived as an abscess? One of the presenting characteristics of epidural abscess is pain out of proportion to physical findings. Relative neglect of the pain in a IV drug-abusing patient may contribute to the often-delayed diagnosis of IV drug abuse-related problems such as epidural abscess. In fact, the pain relief usually provided such patients can only be described as oligoanalgesic.

Whether the habitual use is from IV drug abuse or chronic pain-pill use, the patient who is not opioid naïve is often given smaller doses of pain medication owing to fears of contributing to addiction. The probability, however, is that the chronic user's analgesic requirement is *greater*, not lesser. We recommend not trying to figure out the patient's underlying opioid dosage. Instead, give the standard dosage for the condition and be prepared to supplement dosing if the patient does not obtain relief. The oligoanalgesia problem is also manifest in the patient who has a known dependency and who is being discharged. To such a patient, we often mistakenly give either too many, or too few, pills. This is a situation in which we most need good coordination with a following primary care or pain management physician. Unfortunately, these are the patients who have the least access to such kinds of follow-up.

We may fear to contribute to addiction in a patient with an incurable problem, such as metastatic cancer. It is wise to remember the three missions of medicine: (1) to cure disease, (2) to relieve ongoing ravages of disease, and (3) to provide comfort. When, in cancer, we can no longer have any hope of curing the tumor, and we cannot relieve the ravages via surgery, radiation, or chemotherapy, what we have left is comfort provision. Ethically, at this point, we do not need to worry about the unwanted side effects of the analgesic. What difference does it make if it slows respirations, produces coma, or drops blood pressure? We are trying to produce comfort.

The problem is even greater when we are dealing with a chronic pain syndrome or a recurrent disease (like migraine) for which there are no cures, but for which the patient wishes pain relief. Here, it is absolutely essential that patients have a physician for ongoing care, but here it is also quite probable that the patient has no access to such care. Sometimes we are forced to make compromises in what we wish to do, because the patient is from out of town, from another community, or because the patient's physician is simply unavailable. There are no patients with greater potential for making trouble for the emergency physician, and it is simply impossible to fight with every patient over whether or not to give more opioid. Each physician has to make a judgment on which patient to accommodate, how much analgesic to give, and how to arrange follow-up. A great deal of the solution is institutionally dependent, and also financially dependent. For those patients who are clearly pain-pill seeking, we recommend the "they law." You the physician tell the patient that you would love to honor a request for pain medications, and will be happy to provide non-opioid prescriptions, but that "they" won't let you prescribe opiates. It keeps you from getting into power struggles and gives the patient a courteous way of saving face. Of course, if the physician is not sure that the patient does not, in fact, have a new condition causing pain, pain should be treated.

The somatizing patient is also a source of considerable burden to the emergency physician. It does not help the physician to do a complete workup; often these patients have had hundreds of complete workups. They frequently are incredibly savvy about the kind of history to give, which mandates yet another complete workup. Yet even if the physician falls into the trap of once again yielding to the needs to be ill, and performs yet another thorough and expensive workup, there is still no good answer for how to manage the patient's persistent symptoms. We recommend the "stupidity law." Tell the patient first of all that they have real problems. Even if their real problem is a somatizing syndrome, the patient does not want to hear that she or he has no problems, despite the extent and expense of the workup. Then tell the patient that you have probably been seen by multiple physicians, none of whom has been able to identify, never mind solve, your problems. The patient will agree. You then ask the patient: "How do you expect a stupid emergency physician, who has never seen you before, to be able to discern and solve your problems? How can I help you get through the day so you can get to see one of your superior physicians?" Though this is offered somewhat tongue-in-cheek, and we suggest some alternative less emotionally charged wording, the fact remains that the "stupidity law" can often be applied with success. When it fails, and the somatizing patient demands opiates, you can always invoke the "they law."

We, therefore, hope that you will accept the evidence presented in this book, but that you will view it through the lens of your own clinical experience. While evidence is based on populations, you must treat each patient as a unique entity. You must develop your style of transmitting concern and goodwill to every patient – even the ones you do not like. You do not have to love your patients to provide them with high-quality care, concern, and professional behavior. In fact, the main problems often occur from the patients we dislike, because they make us feel angry, inadequate, and resentful of being in a position where we have something they want but do not need. By developing personal strategies for dealing with these problem patients, you can avert your own anger and frustration, and be comfortable in finding a medical reason to satisfy the demands being placed upon you.

Finally, do not be misled by observations of other of your ED staff. The patient who was writhing in agony when you performed your evaluation may have been comfortable when the nurse was making an assessment. Such a situation is often encountered with the severe, but intermittent, pain of renal colic. You have the responsibility, and the right, to perform and rely upon your own assessment of the patient's degree of need for analgesia.

As an overarching guide, remember that because pain is subjective to the patient it is also subjective to the physician. You have the training, the experience, and the expertise to interact in a way that provides comfort. In our opinion, it never hurts to lean to the side of providing that comfort.

Chief complaints and diagnoses

Abdominal aortic aneurysm

BETH WICKLUND AND ROBERT KNOPP

■ Agents

- Opioids
- NSAIDs

■ Evidence

Abdominal aortic aneurysm (AAA) pain should be considered by the acute care provider as a harbinger of aortic leakage or rupture. Therefore, analgesic selection in AAA is influenced by the high potential for hemodynamic instability.

The high acuity and relatively low frequency of AAA pain presentations are probably responsible for the absence of clinical trials addressing preoperative analgesia in this population. The anesthesia literature addresses operative/postoperative questions (e.g. epidural versus intrathecal anesthesia), but such issues have limited relevance to the acute care provider.[1]

When treating pain in patients with suspected ruptured AAA, the most important consideration is the effect the analgesic will have on the patient's hemodynamic status. The analgesia administered should not interfere with the goal of maintaining adequate end-organ perfusion. That said, expert commentators addressing preoperative care for symptomatic patients with AAA have emphasized the importance of analgesia, since pain can cause hyperventilation, increased oxygen consumption, and augmented endocrine stress response.[2]

Opioids, in small titrated doses, are the analgesics recommended by experts in AAA pain relief.[2] Most **opioids** can cause minor reductions in heart rate (through vagomimetic action) and blood pressure (through reduction in systemic vascular resistance).[3] Hypotension is much less likely to occur with *fentanyl* since this agent does not cause the histamine release often associated with morphine.[3,4] Studies of *fentanyl* in acute care (mostly prehospital) settings have demonstrated the rarity with which hypotension occurs even in critically ill and injured patients (some of whom had ruptured AAA).[5-10] These studies and expert reviews consistently indicate that *fentanyl* can be safely titrated in doses of 25–50 µg.[11-13] Respiratory depression is dose related and extremely rare, probably because of the titrated dosing of the drug.[14] The acute care findings of *fentanyl*'s safety and efficacy are mirrored by recommendations favoring *fentanyl*'s employment for inpatient critical care use in potentially unstable patients.[7,15,16]

In patients with normal renal function, **NSAIDs** (e.g. *ketorolac*) have been used perioperatively, without sequelae, in patients undergoing abdominal and retroperitoneal procedures.[17] However, patients with symptomatic AAA are at particular risk for perioperative renal hypoperfusion. The risk of compromised renal function, in addition to the potential for increased perioperative blood loss (in a population with limited fluid-status reserves), renders **NSAIDs** a poor analgesic choice in symptomatic AAA.[17-22]

■ Summary and recommendations

First line: fentanyl (initial dose 50–100 µg IV, then titrate)

Pregnancy: fentanyl (initial dose 50–100 µg IV, then titrate)

Pediatric: fentanyl (initial dose 1–2 µg/kg IV, then titrate)

Special case:
- *no concern about hemodynamic instability*: morphine (initial dose 4–6 mg IV, then titrate) or hydromorphone (initial dose 1 mg IV, then titrate)

References

1. Marret E, Lembert N, Bonnet F. [Anaesthesia and critical care for scheduled infrarenal abdominal aortic aneurysm surgery.] *Ann Fr Anesth Reanim.* 2006;**25**:158–179.
2. Brimacombe J, Berry A. A review of anaesthesia for ruptured abdominal aortic aneurysm with special emphasis on preclamping fluid resuscitation. *Anaesth Intensive Care.* 1993;**21**:311–323.

3. Bowdle TA. Adverse effects of opioid agonists and agonist-antagonists in anaesthesia. *Drug Saf.* 1998;**19**:173–189.

4. Volles DF, McGory R. Pharmacokinetic considerations. *Crit Care Clin.* 1999;**15**:55–75.

5. Kanowitz A, Dunn TM, Kanowitz EM, *et al.* Safety and effectiveness of fentanyl administration for prehospital pain management. *Prehosp Emerg Care.* 2006;**10**:1–7.

6. Krauss B, Shah S, Thomas S. Fentanyl analgesia in the out-of-hospital setting: Variables associated with hypotension in 1091 administrations among 500 consecutive patients. *Acad Emerg Med.* 2007; **14**(5, Suppl 1): 115.

7. Thomas S, Rago O, Harrison T, *et al.* Fentanyl trauma analgesia use in air medical scene transports. *J Emerg Med.* 2005;**29**:179–185.

8. DeVellis P, Thomas S, Wedel S, *et al.* Prehospital fentanyl analgesia in air-transported pediatric trauma patients. *Pediatr Emerg Care.* 1998;**14**:321 323.

9. DeVellis P, Thomas SH, Wedel SK. Prehospital and emergency department analgesia for air-transported patients with fractures. *Prehosp Emerg Care.* 1998;**2**:293–296.

10. Thomas S, Benevelli W, Brown D, *et al.* Safety of fentanyl for analgesia in adults undergoing air medical transport from trauma scenes. *Air Med J.* 1996;**15**:57–59.

11. Hendrickson M, Naparst TR. Abdominal surgical emergencies in the elderly. *Emerg Med Clin North Am.* 2003;**21**:937–969.

12. Braude D, Richards M. Appeal for fentanyl prehospital use. *Prehosp Emerg Care.* 2004;**8**:441–442.

13. Thomas S. Fentanyl in the prehospital setting. *Am J Emerg Med.* 2007; **25**(7): 842–843.

14. Peng P, Sandler A. A review of the use of fentanyl analgesia in the management of acute pain in adults. *Anesthesiology.* 1999;**90**:576–579.

15. Jacobi J, Fraser G. Clinical practice guidelines for the sustained use of sedatives and analgesics in the critically ill adult. *Crit Care Med.* 2002;**30**:119–141.

16. Thomas SH, Rago O, Harrison T, *et al.* Fentanyl trauma analgesia use in air medical scene transports. *J Emerg Med.* 2005;**29**:179–187.

17. Lee A, Cooper MC, Craig JC, *et al.* Effects of nonsteroidal anti-inflammatory drugs on postoperative renal function in adults with normal renal function. *Cochrane Database Syst Rev.* 2004(2):CD002765.

18. McDougal WS. Reversible acute renal failure after unilateral extracorporeal shock-wave lithotripsy. *J Urol.* 2005;**174**:1024.

19. Lee A, Cooper MG, Craig JC, *et al*. Effects of nonsteroidal anti-inflammatory drugs on postoperative renal function in adults. *Cochrane Database Syst Rev.* 2000(4):CD002765.

20. Splinter WM, Rhine EJ, Roberts DW, et al. Preoperative ketorolac increases bleeding after tonsillectomy in children. *Can J Anaesth.* 1996;**43**:560–563.

21. Fragen RJ, Stulberg SD, Wixson R, *et al*. Effect of ketorolac tromethamine on bleeding and on requirements for analgesia after total knee arthroplasty. *J Bone Joint Surg Am.* 1995;**77**:998–1002.

22. Strom B, Berlin J. Parenteral ketorolac and risk of gastrointestinal and operative site bleeding: a postmarketing surveillance study. *JAMA.* 1996;**275**:376–382.

Aortic dissection

KALANI OLMSTED AND DEBORAH B. DIERCKS

■ Agents

- Opioids
- Beta-blockers
- Calcium channel blockers
- Vasodilators

■ Evidence

According to panels addressing management of aortic dissection (AD), available levels of evidence rate no higher than "expert opinion."[1] Hemodynamic (anti-impulse) therapy remains the foundation of AD care, and successful control of blood pressure and heart rate improves patient comfort. However, in most patients with AD, the inability of anti-impulse therapy to control severe pain mandates an early role for aggressive analgesia.[2]

The first step in AD care, anti-impulse therapy, serves as optimal medical management and also provides some pain relief. **Beta-blockers** (e.g. *metoprolol, propranolol, esmolol, labetalol*) decrease the force of cardiac contraction and reduce blood pressure; both of these properties make this class ideal for minimizing AD progression.[1,3,4] In patients with relative **beta blocker** intolerance, *esmolol*'s short half-life renders it the best initial choice.[1]

Ongoing pain after **beta-blocker** administration usually indicates incomplete blood pressure control. In such cases, pain relief (and optimal medical management) is facilitated by vasodilation. The traditional choice is *sodium nitroprusside*. *Fenoldopam* (a **dopamine-1 agonist** that selectively dilates arterioles and renal vasculature) may also be used. When AD is accompanied by cardiac ischemia, the **calcium channel blocker** *nicardipine* is indicated; reflex tachycardia renders *nitroglycerin* (*glyceryl trinitrate*) potentially dangerous as a treatment for chest pain when AD is suspected.[1,3-5]

Citing sedative and anxiolytic properties, expert reviewers recommend *morphine* for AD pain, but there is no evidence demonstrating its superiority over other **opioids**.[1,4] Patients in pain from AD tend to be hypertensive, but in those cases where blood pressure is borderline or low, *fentanyl*'s limited hemodynamic impact is attractive.[6,7] Anesthesiologists confirm *fentanyl*'s utility for AD, including in cases where there are complicating conditions such as subarachnoid hemorrhage or pregnancy.[8–11]

■ Summary and recommendations

First line: morphine (initial dose 4–6 mg IV, then titrate);
standard anti-impulse therapy (e.g. beta-blockers, vasodilators)

Reasonable: other opioid agonists such as hydromorphone (initial dose 1 mg IV, then titrate)

Pregnancy: fentanyl (initial dose 50–100 µgIV, then titrate); avoid nitroprusside if possible

Pediatric: morphine (initial dose 0.05–0.1 mg/kg IV, then titrate)

Special case:
■ *hypotension or concern for hemodynamic instability*: fentanyl (initial dose 50–100 µg IV, then titrate)

References

1. Erbel R, Alfonso F, Boileau C, *et al*. Diagnosis and management of aortic dissection. *Eur Heart J*. 2001;**22**:1642–1681.
2. Winsor G, Thomas S, Biddinger P, *et al*. Inadequate hemodynamic management in patients undergoing interfacility transfer for suspected aortic dissection. *Am J Emerg Med*. 2005;**23**:24–29.
3. Khoynezhad A, Plestis KA. Managing emergency hypertension in aortic dissection and aortic aneurysm surgery. *J Card Surg*. 2006;**21**(Suppl 1):S3–S7.
4. Nienaber CA, Eagle KA. Aortic dissection: new frontiers in diagnosis and management. Part II: therapeutic management and follow-up. *Circulation*. 2003;**108**:772–778.

5. Elliott WJ. Clinical features in the management of selected hypertensive emergencies. *Prog Cardiovasc Dis*. 2006;**48**:316–325.

6. Kurtz T. Safety of IV fentanyl in adults requiring analgesia during ground interfacility transports by a critical care transport team. *Prehosp Emerg Care*. 2006;**10**:140.

7. Peng P, Sandler A. A review of the use of fentanyl analgesia in the management of acute pain in adults. *Anesthesiology*. 1999;**90**:576–579.

8. Ojeda Betancor N, Garcia Cortes J, Mena Hernandez C, *et al*. [Term pregnancy and dissection of the ascending aorta.] *Rev Esp Anestesiol Reanim*. 2003;**50**:109–111.

9. Inaba S, Iwata S, Kayano T, *et al*. [Perioperative management of a patient with subarachnoid hemorrhage complicated with descending aortic dissection.] *Masui*. 2005;**54**:680–682.

10. Ben Letaifa D, Slama A, Methamem M, *et al*. [Anesthesia for cesarean section in a Marfan patient with complicated aortic dissection.] *Ann Fr Anesth Reanim*. 2002;**21**:672–675.

11. Mossop PJ, McLachlan CS, Amukotuwa SA, *et al*. Staged endovascular treatment for complicated type B aortic dissection. *Nat Clin Pract Cardiovasc Med*. 2005;**2**:316–321; quiz 322.

Arthritis

TODD M. LISTWA AND STEPHEN H. THOMAS

■ Agents

- NSAIDs
- Acetaminophen (paracetamol)
- Steroids
- Colchicine
- Local anesthetics
- Opioids
- Corticotropin

■ Evidence

In the initial part of the ED encounter, it may not be possible to distinguish between the various causes of joint pain.[1] Therefore, the acute care provider may need to begin therapy before a firm diagnosis is established. This chapter presents evidence relating to acute therapies for some of the more common arthritic conditions. For those cases where the diagnosis is uncertain, the clinician can exercise judgment and select an agent with utility in more than one disease. Some of the diagnostic workup (e.g. arthrocentesis) may contribute to pain relief.[2]

The major arthritides to be covered in this section are crystal-mediated arthropathy, osteoarthritis (OA), and rheumatoid arthritis (RA). These topics are considered in one chapter because of the commonality of their presenting symptoms, signs, and analgesic approaches. Although this text is intended to focus on pharmacological therapy, two nondrug approaches are worth special mention because of their differential effects in varying arthritides. The first nondrug approach, thermal therapy, is used differently in rheumatoid arthritis and gout; local heat is often useful for the former condition, whereas local cold may relieve pain in the crystal arthropathies. Indications for the second nondrug approach, splinting, are also diagnosis dependent. Immobilization may reduce discomfort in crystal or autoimmune arthropathies, but lack of joint use can actually worsen osteoarthritis pain.

GOUT AND CRYSTAL ARTHROPATHY

For gouty arthritis, most commentators favor **NSAIDs** as first-line therapy, but other treatment options (*colchicine*, **corticosteroids**, *corticotropin* [*adreno-corticotropic hormone*]) are also used.[3,4] Meta-analysis of the crystal arthropathy pain literature is limited by the relatively small number of high-quality studies addressing acute care analgesia.[5] There are, however, a number of therapeutic options described in the literature. Acute care providers should gain familiarity with the various approaches, since they have relatively high side effect rates that warrant careful risk-to-benefit considerations in the (often elderly) patient with crystal arthropathy.[5]

Colchicine (0.6 mg PO hourly, until pain relief or GI side effects occur) is one of the most commonly used drugs for acute gout. *Colchicine* is most effective when administered within 24–48 h of onset of pain from gout (it is much less effective for pseudogout).[4] Cochrane review concludes that one in three patients responds to *colchicine*, which reduces pain and tenderness by 30–34%.[6] The IV route of administration is not recommended for acute care providers, owing to concerning side effects (e.g. in the bone marrow and kidneys).

Even when administered PO, *colchicine*'s rate of side effects (e.g. nausea, vomiting, diarrhea) approaches 100%.[5] The side effect rate, combined with the lack of evidence supporting *colchicine*'s analgesic superiority over **NSAIDs**, underpin expert recommendations to use *colchicine* only if **NSAIDs** or **corticosteroids** are ineffective or contraindicated.[6] Given the recurrent nature of gout and the likelihood of previous use of *colchicine* in a given patient, the ED provider may find it useful to ask if the drug has been efficacious in the past. Since most alternative drug approaches for gout have their own side effect issues, a patient in whom *colchicine* has been previously well tolerated may be a good candidate for repeat use.

Two major conclusions can be drawn from the many trials of various **NSAIDs** in crystal arthropathy: (1) there is little therapeutic difference between appropriately dosed **NSAIDs**, and (2) in terms of acute care use, the **COX-2 selective**

NSAIDs *may* be safer than, while achieving similar efficacy to, nonselective **NSAIDs** such as *indomethacin*.[5,7,8]

Some illustrative **NSAID** studies demonstrate utility of this class in arthritis pain. An RCT has shown that once-daily administration of the **COX-2 selective NSAID** *lumiracoxib* (400 mg PO) provides pain relief comparable to that achieved with thrice-daily *indomethacin* (50 mg per dose).[9] Similar results were reported in a trial of *etoricoxib* (120 mg PO QD), which demonstrated the **COX-2 selective NSAID** to be as effective as *indomethacin* (50 mg PO TID).[10] In both trials, the **COX-2 selective NSAIDs** were found to have significantly fewer adverse drug events than the nonselective **NSAID**.

The cardiovascular risks associated with even brief use of **COX-2 selective NSAIDs** are not to be ignored by the acute care provider. Emergency physicians should generally try to avoid the controversy surrounding risks of **COX-2 selective NSAIDs** by choosing another therapeutic approach. However, the arthritis population may include patients for whom risk profiles of **COX-2 selective NSAIDs** are preferable to those of nonselective **NSAIDs**. While the ED physician should prescribe **COX-2 selective NSAIDs** only after careful consideration, it is incorrect to assume that the current state of the evidence refutes any short-term ED role for these agents.[11,12] The cardiovascular risks will often be the most prominent concern, but arthritis patients are also likely to be at increased risk from other well-known adverse effects (e.g. GI complications).[1] The question remains unresolved. Until more concrete data are available, the ED provider should individualize therapy, taking into consideration the planned treatment duration as well as the patient's GI and cardiovascular risk profiles. Some experts recommend prescribing a nonselective **NSAID** with a gastroprotective agent (**proton pump inhibitor**), as a cost-beneficial means to provide pain relief with acceptable risk profile. However, these reviews also concluded that there remains a role for **COX-2 selective NSAIDs** in patients with higher GI risk, and lower cardiovascular risk.[13]

Comparisons of parenteral versus PO **NSAIDs** fail to identify an advantage to the former route. An RCT found equal efficacy between pain relief from a dose of IM *ketorolac* (60 mg) or one of PO *indomethacin* (50 mg).[14]

Corticosteroids are generally rated as a second-line therapy for crystal-related arthritis, although some experts feel they are equally efficacious as either **NSAIDs** or *colchicine* (for gouty arthritis) for treating acute flares.[3,4] Those favoring the use of **corticosteroids** in acute crystal arthropathy contend that the short-term use of these agents does not incur the well-known problems occurring with longer-term use.[1] When PO **corticosteroids** are employed for crystal arthropathy, recommendation is for daily doses of 40–60 mg *prednisone*.[4] One trial suggested that the combination of an oral **corticosteroid** plus *acetaminophen* (*paracetamol*) provides equal pain relief to *indomethacin*, and is associated with fewer side effects.[1]

Corticosteroids may be given parenterally for patients who cannot tolerate PO therapy (e.g. those with post *colchicine* GI symptoms). As an example, IV *methylprednisolone* (100 mg IV) is known to ameliorate acute gout pain.[4]

If the ED provider can definitively rule out infectious arthropathy, joint injection therapy is a therapeutic alternative. Intra-articular administration of **corticosteroids** (e.g. *methylprednisolone* 10–40 mg depending on joint size) provides some pain relief in crystal arthropathy.[4]

Intramuscular *corticotropin* in two or three doses of 40–80 units given 8–12 h apart, is a useful option for pain caused by acute gout or pseudogout.[15] The two-dose regimen is necessary, since single-dose therapy is associated with higher rates of rebound pain than other approaches (e.g. intra-articular **corticosteroid** injection).[4,16] *Corticotropin* appears to relieve gout pain via a melanocortin receptor subtype, so its efficacy is unrelated to whether patients are adrenally insufficient.[17] It is reasonable to use *corticotropin* as first-line therapy in patients with acute polyarticular gout, or in those with renal impairment or other medical diseases (e.g. congestive heart failure, GI bleeding) that increase the risks from other anti-gout therapies such as **NSAIDs**.[15,18,19]

There is little evidence specifically addressing acute pain relief for other deposition-related arthropathies (e.g. from hydroxyapatite), but the general approach of **NSAIDs** or **corticosteroids** probably constitutes the best initial therapy.[20]

OSTEOARTHRITIS

For patients with OA in the acute care setting, *acetaminophen* remains a reasonable initial analgesic choice in selected patients. This is especially true for patients with high risk for **NSAID**-related side effects. Cochrane review finds acceptable efficacy for *acetaminophen* for OA, although pain relief is better with **NSAIDs**.[21] *Acetaminophen*'s main advantage is its safety and side effect profile. Even in patients with liver disease, *acetaminophen* has fewer risks than other systemic OA analgesics.[22] Finally, *acetaminophen* has additional utility as a rescue medication for patients taking **NSAIDs**.[23]

While the available evidence is limited, some commentators endorse combination therapy with *acetaminophen* plus *tramadol* as a relatively low-risk analgesic approach for OA.[24] Overall, there seems to be little role for **opioids** in OA pain management. Most expert reviews and meta-analyses find an unfavorable risk-to-benefit ratio, although some commentators do report occasional utility of the **opioids** for OA.[25–27]

When *acetaminophen* is not an option, the **NSAIDs** constitute the best choice for short-term therapy of acute OA flares.[28] As is the case with other conditions, for treatment of OA there is little difference (in either risks or efficacy) between comparably dosed **NSAIDs**. For example, *diclofenac* in a dose of 25 mg PO is at least as safe (and equally effective) as *ibuprofen* 400 mg PO.[29] Cochrane review concludes that the **NSAIDs** are a reasonable first-choice therapy for OA, given their relatively reliable relief of moderate pain and the overall side effect profile.[21] The evidence upon which the Cochrane recommendations are based includes head-to-head comparisons. One such trial finds *diclofenac* (combined with *misoprostol*) clearly superior to *acetaminophen*.[30]

Meta-analysis of four RCTs assessing a topical *diclofenac* preparation found the evidence to be of high quality and to consistently favor the use of the topical **NSAID**.[31] Other than localized skin reactions, which are mild and usually limited to dryness, topically applied *diclofenac* (1.5%) is much better tolerated than the same agent administered orally, and the level of pain relief appears to be similar with the two approaches.[31] A gel form of *diclofenac* (*diclofenac diethylamine* 1.16%, 4 g QID for three weeks) is also significantly better than placebo for pain relief, with no safety problems identified over a three week course.[23] Another preparation of topical *diclofenac* (a bio-adhesive plaster containing *diclofenac epolamine*) provides significantly better pain relief than placebo, with a pooled analysis finding 50% pain reduction achieved in a third of treated patients.[32] Although the acute care implications are uncertain, and clinicians should keep in mind the potential for systemic absorption and related side effect risk, large-scale meta-analyses consistently suggest a useful role in topical **NSAIDs** for OA therapy.[25,33,34] For the most part, these topical agents are probably best left to the longitudinal care provider, but there may be instances (e.g. when topical agents have previously been effective) when ED prescription is appropriate.

Both clinical experience and the available trial evidence reflect a growing emphasis on use of **COX-2 selective NSAIDs** for treating OA (owing to the improved GI side effect profile compared with nonspecific **NSAIDs**).[35,36] As noted above in the discussion on crystal arthropathies, the potential cardiovascular side effects of the **COX-2 selective NSAIDs** cannot be dismissed.[11] However, both meta-analysis (including OA patients and others) and individual OA trials underscore arguments that acute care clinicians should not allow cardiovascular risk concerns to blunt awareness of **NSAIDs'** GI effects.[12] A large-scale RCT, for example, found similarly low cardiovascular side effects and equivalent pain relief in OA patients taking *celecoxib* (100 mg PO BID) as taking *diclofenac* (50 mg PO BID) or *naproxen* (500 mg PO BID); the **COX-2 selective NSAID** was also found to have significantly fewer GI effects.[37] Similarly, pooled analysis of thrombotic cardiovascular events from multiple clinical trials of the **COX-2 selective NSAID** agent *etoricoxib* failed to identify a significant risk over that associated with nonselective **NSAIDs**.[38] Even after considering the recently delineated risks of the **COX-2 selective NSAIDs**, a recent expert panel review concluded that available evidence supported use of this class for treating OA.[39]

A randomized double-blind investigation reported that the **COX-2 selective NSAIDs** *valdecoxib* (10 mg PO QD) and *rofecoxib* (2.5 mg PO QD) both achieve significantly better pain relief than placebo in as little as 3 h after oral administration.[40] Trials generally indicate little analgesic difference between various **COX-2 selective NSAIDs**. Though the literature on the subject continues to evolve, it is unlikely that, as a class, the **COX-2 selective NSAIDs** consistently provide better analgesia than do the nonselective **NSAIDs**. For instance, meta-analysis and well-conducted RCTs have demonstrated that *lumaricoxib* (100 mg PO QD) relieves pain at least as well as *celecoxib,* *rofecoxib*, or *diclofenac*; all agents are consistently better than placebo.[41–43] Similarly, *valdecoxib* (10 mg PO QD) provides OA relief similar to that achieved by *naproxen* and *diclofenac*.[44]

The **COX-2 selective NSAID** *nimesulide*, with fewer GI effects than non-specific **NSAIDs** and (potentially) fewer cardiovascular risks than the coxib-type **COX-2 selective NSAIDs**, appears to be useful as an OA analgesic.[45] An RCT of another **COX-2 selective NSAID**, *aceclofenac* (100 mg PO BID), found it provided better analgesia, with fewer adverse effects (and better patient compliance), than *diclofenac* (75 mg PO BID).[46]

Injectable *hyaluronans* may have a non-ED role in the relief of OA pain, but their acute care use is limited by potentially serious (although uncommon) side effects such as pseudogout, anaphylactoid reactions, and severe inflammatory reactions.[47–49] Furthermore, the overall weight of evidence of *hyaluronans'* efficacy is insufficient to warrant their introduction into the acute care setting.[27] Similarly, while an RCT demonstrated feasibility and potential efficacy of injection therapy with **interleukin-1 antagonists**, it is premature to advocate this approach in the acute care setting.[50]

The topical agent *capsaicin*, and the related compound *ricinoleic acid*, have been investigated for treating OA.[51] The limitations of these agents lie in the potential for pain upon cream application, and in the fact that the magnitude of analgesic effect is small. One RCT of *capsaicin* (0.025%) in OA found that addition of *nitroglycerin* (*glyceryl trinitrate*; 1.33%) reduced application pain and improved analgesic effect – but analgesia from even the best-performing *capsaicin* preparation was found to be marginal.[52] In some patients, however, the failure of other agents may make *capsaicin* worth trying since there are at least some data supporting pain relief with the drug.[39]

A variety of other topical agents have been assessed for OA relief. Among the agents with potential benefit in OA are *cetylated fatty acids, glucosamine/chondroitin,* and plant-derived agents such as Arnica montana *gel*.[53–55] Given placebo-controlled studies demonstrating lack of benefit in intent-to-treat analysis, however, there is insufficient evidence basis for recommending use of these agents in the acute care setting.[27]

RHEUMATOID ARTHRITIS AND JUVENILE
RHEUMATOID ARTHRITIS

RA and juvenile RA (JRA) are treated with an array of disease-modifying agents that have secondary effects of relieving pain. The large number of these agents precludes their discussion in detail here. This chapter will address use of agents with a primary analgesic effect.

First-line analgesia for RA and JRA consists of **NSAIDs**.[56] More than 50% of patients will have significant pain relief with the first **NSAID** chosen; half of the remaining group will respond to a different **NSAID**.[56] There are few data supporting the use of one **NSAID** over another, but the agents that are available in liquid form (e.g. *naproxen, ibuprofen, indomethacin*) may be particularly useful in younger patients with JRA. *Naproxen* has an additional advantage in its twice-daily dosing; it can be administered to children in a BID regimen of 10–20 mg/kg per dose (maximum daily dose 1000 mg).[56] The lowest effective dose should be administered in order to minimize side effect risk.[56,57] Data from an RCT demonstrated the utility of *naproxen* (500 mg PO BID), which provided pain relief equivalent to that achieved with the **COX-2 selective NSAID** *valdecoxib*.[58]

The excess coronary mortality in RA patients should heighten acute care providers' awareness of the potential for **COX-2 selective NSAIDs**' cardiovascular sequelae.[59] However, as is the case for OA, there is evidence that use of **COX-2 selective NSAIDs** for RA is both effective and safe (i.e. fewer GI side effects at no cost of increased cardiovascular problems).[36] When administered at a dosage associated with relative COX-2 specificity, *meloxicam* (7.5–15 mg PO QD) achieves equal pain relief and improved GI safety, compared with *diclofenac, piroxicam*, or *naproxen*.[60] Meta-analysis concluding that *celecoxib* use incurred no significant cardiovascular risk increment (over placebo or nonselective **NSAIDs**) included trial participants with RA.[12] There is, therefore, some role for **COX-2 selective NSAIDs** in RA, particularly in patients with significant potential for GI side effects; expert rheumatology reviews suggest **COX-2 selective NSAIDs** are cost effective for patients at high risk of GI bleeding.[61] Acute care use of the **COX-2 selective NSAIDs** should be embarked upon only with appropriate consideration (and discussion) of cardiovascular risk in any patient; extra precaution is warranted in patients with RA.

For breakthrough pain for patients taking **NSAIDs**, the combination of PO *tramadol* (37.5 mg) and *acetaminophen* (325 mg) provides significant symptom relief.[62] Mild side effects (e.g. dizziness, nausea) are relatively common, but serious drug-related adverse effects are rare.[62] Meta-analysis of trials of chronic pain relief, including RA patients, endorsed the conclusion that **opioid** utility in this population is limited (owing to side effects) to short courses for breakthrough pain.[26]

Systemic or injected **glucocorticoids** are useful in RA and JRA. Although a few weeks may be required to achieve maximal pain relief, intra-articular *methylprednisolone* (40 mg) provides equal symptom relief to that achieved with *etanercept*.[63] Pooled analysis of available data for RA and JRA suggests that therapeutic efficacy of intra-articular **corticosteroids** may be enhanced with immobilization of the knee after injection, but not the wrist.[64] When more than one joint is involved, polyarticular injection of **corticosteroids** appears to achieve better pain relief than a single IM injection.[65]

The **NSAIDs** are administered for analgesia only; they do not modify the JRA or RA disease process. Other agents that do modify the disease process, but are not appropriate for ED use owing to treatment complexity or complications, include drugs such as **biologics** (e.g. *etanercept*), **cytotoxins** (e.g. *azathioprine*), and antirheumatics such as *methotrexate* and *sulfasalazine*. The **pyrimidine synthesis inhibitor** *leflunomide*, the **omega-3 polyunsaturated fatty acids**, and the antibacterial agents *levofloxacin* and *clarithromycin* have promise, but again their application is for longer-term therapy (analgesic effects can take weeks).[66–69]

■ Summary and recommendations

CRYSTAL ARTHROPATHY

First line: NSAID (e.g. indomethacin 50 mg PO TID)

Reasonable: short-course COX-2 selective NSAID therapy (e.g. celecoxib 200 mg PO BID), if favorable GI/cardiovascular risk profile

Pregnancy:

- acetaminophen (650–1000 mg PO QID)
- prednisone (1 mg/kg PO QD)
- intra-articular corticosteroid injection (if infection is ruled out) is performed at the Massachusetts General Hospital for pregnant patients with inflammatory arthritis

Pediatric: NSAID (e.g. liquid naproxen 10 mg/kg PO BID)

Special cases:

- *previous colchicine efficacy and tolerance*: colchicine 0.6 mg PO q1 h until pain relief or GI side effects (maximum 10 doses/day)
- *if NSAIDs and corticosteroids are ineffective or contraindicated*: colchicine (for gout) or corticotropin (40–80 units IM q8–12 h for two or three doses)
- *significant renal disease and gout or pseudogout*: corticotropin (two or three doses of 40–80 units IM, administered 8–12 h apart)
- *infectious arthritis ruled out with certainty*: intra-articular injection of corticosteroid (e.g. methylprednisolone 10–40 mg depending on joint size)

OSTEOARTHRITIS

First line: NSAID (e.g. diclofenac 25–50 mg PO TID)

Reasonable:

- acetaminophen (for mild pain), 650–1000 mg PO QID
- short-course COX-2 selective NSAID therapy (e.g. celecoxib 200 mg PO BID), if favorable GI/cardiovascular risk profile

Pregnancy:

- acetaminophen (650–1000 mg PO QID)
- prednisone (1 mg/kg PO QD)
- intra-articular corticosteroid injection (if infection is ruled out) is performed at the Massachusetts General Hospital for pregnant patients

Pediatric: NSAID (e.g. liquid naproxen 10 mg/kg BID)

Special cases:

- *infectious arthritis ruled out with certainty*: intra-articular injection of corticosteroid (e.g. methylprednisolone 10–40 mg depending on joint size)
- *contraindications to NSAIDs and glucocorticoids*: short-course acetaminophen (650–1000 mg PO QID) with a mild opioid (e.g. tramadol 25–50 mg PO QID)

RHEUMATOID AND JUVENILE RHEUMATOID ARTHRITIS

First line: NSAID (e.g. diclofenac 25–50 mg PO TID)

Reasonable:

- acetaminophen (650–1000 mg PO QID)
- acetaminophen (650–1000 mg PO QID) combined with tramadol (25–50 mg PO QID)

Pregnancy:

- acetaminophen (650–1000 mg PO QID)
- prednisone (1 mg/kg PO QD)
- Intra-articular corticosteroid injection (if infection is ruled out) is performed at the Massachusetts General Hospital for pregnant patients

Pediatric: NSAID (e.g. naproxen 10 mg/kg PO BID)

Special cases:

- *infectious arthritis ruled out with certainty*: intra-articular injection of corticosteroid (e.g. methylprednisolone 10–40 mg depending on joint size)
- *contraindications to NSAIDs and glucocorticoids:* short-course acetaminophen with a mild opioid (e.g. tramadol 25–50 mg PO QID)
- *high risk of GI bleeding:* short-course COX-2 selective NSAID therapy (e.g. celecoxib 200 mg PO BID)

References

1. Man C, Cheung I, Cameron P, *et al.* Comparison of oral prednisolone/ paracetamol and oral indomethacin/paracetamol combination therapy in the treatment of acute goutlike arthritis: a double-blind, randomized, controlled trial. *Ann Emerg Med.* 2007;**49**:678–681.

2. Schlesinger N. Response to application of ice may help differentiate between gouty arthritis and other inflammatory arthritides. *J Clin Rheumatol.* 2006;**12**:275–276.

3. Schlesinger N. Management of acute and chronic gouty arthritis: present state-of-the-art. *Drugs.* 2004;**64**:2399–2416.

4. Keith MP, Gilliland WR. Updates in the management of gout. *Am J Med.* 2007;**120**:221–224.

5. Sutaria S, Katbamna R, Underwood M. Effectiveness of interventions for the treatment of acute and prevention of recurrent gout: a systematic review. *Rheumatology (Oxford).* 2006;**45**:1422–1431.

6. Schlesinger N, Schumacher R, Catton M, *et al.* Colchicine for acute gout. *Cochrane Database Syst Rev.* 2006(4):CD006190.

7. Schumacher H, Boice J, Daikh D. Randomised double-blind trial of etoricoxib and indomethacin in treatment of acute gouty arthritis. *BMJ.* 2002;**324**:1488–1492.

8. Wortmann RL. Recent advances in the management of gout and hyperuricemia. *Curr Opin Rheumatol.* 2005;**17**:319–324.

9. Willburger RE, Mysler E, Derbot J, *et al.* Lumiracoxib 400 mg once daily is comparable to indomethacin 50 mg three times daily for the treatment of acute flares of gout. *Rheumatology (Oxford).* 2007; **46**(7): 1126–1132.

10. Rubin BR, Burton R, Navarra S, *et al.* Efficacy and safety profile of treatment with etoricoxib 120 mg once daily compared with indomethacin 50 mg three times daily in acute gout: a randomized controlled trial. *Arthritis Rheum.* 2004;**50**:598–606.

11. Bresalier RS, Sandler RS, Quan H, *et al.* Cardiovascular events associated with rofecoxib in a colorectal adenoma chemoprevention trial. *N Engl J Med.* 17 2005;**352**:1092–1102.

12. White WB, West CR, Borer JS, *et al.* Risk of cardiovascular events in patients receiving celecoxib: a meta-analysis of randomized clinical trials. *Am J Cardiol.* 1 2007;**99**:91–98.

13. Hur C, Chan AT, Tramontano AC, *et al.* Coxibs versus combination NSAID and PPI therapy for chronic pain: an exploration of the risks, benefits, and costs. *Ann Pharmacother.* 2006;**40**:1052–1063.

14. Shrestha M, Morgan DL, Moreden JM, *et al.* Randomized double-blind comparison of the analgesic efficacy of intramuscular ketorolac and oral indomethacin in the treatment of acute gouty arthritis. *Ann Emerg Med.* 1995;**26**:682–686.

15. Ritter J, Kerr LD, Valeriano-Marcet J, *et al.* ACTH revisited: effective treatment for acute crystal induced synovitis in patients with multiple medical problems. *J Rheumatol.* 1994;**21**:696–699.

16. Siegel LB, Alloway JA, Nashel DJ. Comparison of adrenocorticotropic hormone and triamcinolone acetonide in the treatment of acute gouty arthritis. *J Rheumatol.* 1994;**21**:1325–1327.

17. Getting SJ, Christian HC, Flower RJ, *et al.* Activation of melanocortin type 3 receptor as a molecular mechanism for adrenocorticotropic hormone efficacy in gouty arthritis. *Arthritis Rheum.* 2002;**46**:2765–2775.

18. Fang W, Zeng X, Li M, *et al.* The management of gout at an academic healthcare center in Beijing: a physician survey. *J Rheumatol.* 2006;**33**:2041–2049.

19. Taylor CT, Brooks NC, Kelley KW. Corticotropin for acute management of gout. *Ann Pharmacother.* 2001;**35**:365–368.

20. Claudepierre P, Rahmouni A, Bergamasco P, *et al.* Misleading clinical aspects of hydroxyapatite deposits: a series of 15 cases. *J Rheumatol.* 1997;**24**:531–535.

21. Towheed TE, Maxwell L, Judd MG, *et al.* Acetaminophen for osteoarthritis. *Cochrane Database Syst Rev.* 2006(1):CD004257.

22. Benson GD, Koff RS, Tolman KG. The therapeutic use of acetaminophen in patients with liver disease. *Am J Ther.* 2005;**12**:133–141.

23. Niethard FU, Gold MS, Solomon GS, *et al.* Efficacy of topical diclofenac diethylamine gel in osteoarthritis of the knee. *J Rheumatol.* 2005;**32**:2384–2392.

24. Schug SA. Combination analgesia in 2005 – a rational approach: focus on paracetamol–tramadol. *Clin Rheumatol.* 2006;**25**(Suppl 1):S16–S21.

25. Bjordal JM, Klovning A, Ljunggren AE, *et al.* Short-term efficacy of pharmacotherapeutic interventions in osteoarthritic knee pain: A meta-analysis of randomised placebo-controlled trials. *Eur J Pain.* 2007;**11**:125–138.

26. Furlan AD, Sandoval JA, Mailis-Gagnon A, *et al*. Opioids for chronic non-cancer pain: a meta-analysis of effectiveness and side effects. *CMAJ*. 2006;**174**:1589-1594.

27. Lane NE. Clinical practice. Osteoarthritis of the hip. *N Engl J Med*. 2007;**357**:1413-1421.

28. Ehrlich GE. A benefit/risk assessment of existing therapeutic alternatives for the treatment of painful inflammatory conditions. *Int J Clin Pract Suppl*. 2004;**144**:20-26.

29. Moore N. Diclofenac potassium 12.5 mg tablets for mild to moderate pain and fever: a review of its pharmacology, clinical efficacy and safety. *Clin Drug Invest*. 2007;**27**:163-195.

30. Pincus T, Wang X, Chung C, *et al*. Patient preference in a crossover clinical trial of patients with osteoarthritis of the knee or hip: face validity of self-report questionnaire ratings. *J Rheumatol*. 2005;**32**:533-539.

31. Towheed TE. Pennsaid therapy for osteoarthritis of the knee: a systematic review and metaanalysis of randomized controlled trials. *J Rheumatol*. 2006;**33**:567-573.

32. Bruhlmann P, de Vathaire F, Dreiser RL, *et al*. Short-term treatment with topical diclofenac epolamine plaster in patients with symptomatic knee osteoarthritis: pooled analysis of two randomised clinical studies. *Curr Med Res Opin*. 2006;**22**:2429-2438.

33. Biswal S, Medhi B, Pandhi P. Longterm efficacy of topical nonsteroidal anti-inflammatory drugs in knee osteoarthritis: metaanalysis of randomized placebo controlled clinical trials. *J Rheumatol*. 2006;**33**:1841-1844.

34. Andrews PA, Sampson SA. Topical non-steroidal drugs are systemically absorbed and may cause renal disease. *Nephrol Dial Transplant*. 1999;**14**:187-189.

35. Yilmaz H, Gurel S, Ozdemir O. The use and safety profile of non-steroidal antiinflammatory drugs among Turkish patients with osteoarthritis. *Turk J Gastroenterol*. 2005;**16**:138-142.

36. Eisen GM, Goldstein JL, Hanna DB, *et al*. Meta-analysis: upper gastrointestinal tolerability of valdecoxib, a cyclooxygenase-2-specific inhibitor, compared with nonspecific nonsteroidal anti-inflammatory drugs among patients with osteoarthritis and rheumatoid arthritis. *Aliment Pharmacol Ther*. 2005;**21**:591-598.

37. Singh G, Fort JG, Goldstein JL, *et al*. Celecoxib versus naproxen and diclofenac in osteoarthritis patients: SUCCESS-I Study. *Am J Med*. 2006;**119**:255-266.

38. Curtis SP, Ko AT, Bolognese JA, *et al.* Pooled analysis of thrombotic cardio-vascular events in clinical trials of the COX-2 selective Inhibitor etoricoxib. *Curr Med Res Opin.* 2006;**22**:2365–2374.

39. Zhang W, Doherty M, Leeb BF, *et al.* EULAR evidence based recommendations for the management of hand osteoarthritis: report of a Task Force of the EULAR Standing Committee for International Clinical Studies Including Therapeutics (ESCISIT). *Ann Rheum Dis.* 2007;**66**:377–388.

40. Moskowitz RW, Sunshine A, Hooper M, *et al.* An analgesic model for assessment of acute pain response in osteoarthritis of the knee. *Osteoarthritis Cartilage.* 2006;**14**:1111–1118.

41. Sheldon E, Beaulieu A, Paster Z, *et al.* Efficacy and tolerability of lumiracoxib in the treatment of osteoarthritis of the knee: a 13-week, randomized, double-blind comparison with celecoxib and placebo. *Clin Ther.* 2005;**27**:64–77.

42. Berenbaum F, Grifka J, Brown JP, *et al.* Efficacy of lumiracoxib in osteoarthritis: a review of nine studies. *J Int Med Res.* 2005;**33**:21–41.

43. Wittenberg RH, Schell E, Krehan G, *et al.* First-dose analgesic effect of the cyclo-oxygenase-2 selective inhibitor lumiracoxib in osteoarthritis of the knee: a randomized, double-blind, placebo-controlled comparison with celecoxib (NCT00267215). *Arthritis Res Ther.* 2006;**8**:R35.

44. Fenton C, Keating GM, Wagstaff AJ. Valdecoxib: a review of its use in the management of osteoarthritis, rheumatoid arthritis, dysmenorrhoea and acute pain. *Drugs.* 2004;**64**:1231–1261.

45. Rainsford KD. Current status of the therapeutic uses and actions of the preferential cyclo-oxygenase-2 NSAID, nimesulide. *Inflammopharmacology.* 2006;**14**:120–137.

46. Pareek A, Chandanwale AS, Oak J, *et al.* Efficacy and safety of aceclofenac in the treatment of osteoarthritis: a randomized double-blind comparative clinical trial versus diclofenac – an Indian experience. *Curr Med Res Opin.* 2006;**22**:977–988.

47. Hamburger MI, Lakhanpal S, Mooar PA, *et al.* Intra-articular hyaluronans: a review of product-specific safety profiles. *Semin Arthritis Rheum.* 2003;**32**:296–309.

48. Hammesfahr JF, Knopf AB, Stitik T. Safety of intra-articular hyaluronates for pain associated with osteoarthritis of the knee. *Am J Orthop.* 2003;**32**:277–283.

49. Zhang DW, Yang QS, Zhu JY, *et al.* Amelioration of osteoarthritis by intra-articular hyaluronan synthase 2 gene therapy. *Med Hypotheses.* 2007;**69**:1111–1113.

50. Chevalier X, Giraudeau B, Conrozier T, *et al.* Safety study of intraarticular injection of interleukin 1 receptor antagonist in patients with painful knee osteoarthritis: a multicenter study. *J Rheumatol.* 2005;**32**:1317–1323.

51. Vieira C, Evangelista S, Cirillo R, *et al.* Antinociceptive activity of ricinoleic acid, a capsaicin-like compound devoid of pungent properties. *Eur J Pharmacol.* 2000;**407**:109–116.

52. McCleane G. The analgesic efficacy of topical capsaicin is enhanced by glyceryl trinitrate in painful osteoarthritis: a randomized, double blind, placebo controlled study. *Eur J Pain.* 2000;**4**:355–360.

53. Kraemer WJ, Ratamess NA, Maresh CM, *et al.* Effects of treatment with a cetylated fatty acid topical cream on static postural stability and plantar pressure distribution in patients with knee osteoarthritis. *J Strength Cond Res.* 2005;**19**:115–121.

54. Cohen M, Wolfe R, Mai T, *et al.* A randomized, double blind, placebo controlled trial of a topical cream containing glucosamine sulfate, chondroitin sulfate, and camphor for osteoarthritis of the knee. *J Rheumatol.* 2003;**30**:523–528.

55. Knuesel O, Weber M, Suter A. Arnica montana gel in osteoarthritis of the knee: an open, multicenter clinical trial. *Adv Ther.* 2002;**19**:209–218.

56. Guthrie B, Rouster-Stevens KA, Reynolds SL. Review of medications used in juvenile rheumatoid arthritis. *Pediatr Emerg Care.* Jan 2007;**23**:38–46.

57. Henry D, Lim LL, Garcia Rodriguez LA, *et al.* Variability in risk of gastrointestinal complications with individual non-steroidal anti-inflammatory drugs: results of a collaborative meta-analysis. *BMJ.* 1996;**312**:1563–1566.

58. Williams GW, Kivitz AJ, Brown MT, *et al.* A comparison of valdecoxib and naproxen in the treatment of rheumatoid arthritis symptoms. *Clin Ther.* 2006;**28**:204–221.

59. Douglas KM, Pace AV, Treharne GJ, *et al.* Excess recurrent cardiac events in rheumatoid arthritis patients with acute coronary syndrome. *Ann Rheum Dis.* 2006;**65**:348–353.

60. Ahmed M, Khanna D, Furst DE. Meloxicam in rheumatoid arthritis. *Expert Opin Drug Metab Toxicol.* 2005;**1**:739–751.

61. Hochberg MC. COX-2 selective inhibitors in the treatment of arthritis: a rheumatologist perspective. *Curr Top Med Chem.* 2005;**5**:443–448.

62. Lee EY, Lee EB, Park BJ, *et al.* Tramadol 37.5 -mg/acetaminophen 325 -mg combination tablets added to regular therapy for rheumatoid arthritis pain: a 1-week, randomized, double-blind, placebo-controlled trial. *Clin Ther.* 2006;**28**:2052–2060.

63. Bliddal H, Terslev L, Qvistgaard E, *et al*. A randomized, controlled study of a single intra-articular injection of etanercept or glucocorticosteroids in patients with rheumatoid arthritis. *Scand J Rheumatol*. 2006;**35**:341–345.

64. Wallen M, Gillies D. Intra-articular steroids and splints/rest for children with juvenile idiopathic arthritis and adults with rheumatoid arthritis. *Cochrane Database Syst Rev*. 2006(1):CD002824.

65. Furtado RN, Oliveira LM, Natour J. Polyarticular corticosteroid injection versus systemic administration in treatment of rheumatoid arthritis patients: a randomized controlled study. *J Rheumatol*. 2005;**32**:1691–1698.

66. Li EK, Tam LS, Tomlinson B. Leflunomide in the treatment of rheumatoid arthritis. *Clin Ther*. 2004;**26**:447–459.

67. Ogrendik M. Effects of clarithromycin in patients with active rheumatoid arthritis. *Curr Med Res Opin*. 2007;**23**:515–522.

68. Ogrendik M. Levofloxacin treatment in patients with rheumatoid arthritis receiving methotrexate. *South Med J*. 2007;**100**:135–139.

69. Goldberg RJ, Katz J. A meta-analysis of the analgesic effects of omega-3 polyunsaturated fatty acid supplementation for inflammatory joint pain. *Pain*. 2007;**129**:210–223.

Biliary tract pain

STEPHEN H. THOMAS AND JONATHAN S. ILGEN

■ Agents

- Opioids
- NSAIDs
- Cholecystokinin receptor agents
- Spasmolytics/anticholinergics
- Calcium channel blockers

■ Evidence

OPIOIDS

Opioids are the benchmark against which other biliary tract analgesics are assessed. Historically, the distinction between **opioids** used for biliary tract pain (BTP) has been based upon differential effects on Oddi's sphincter. We believe that clinical tradition has tended to exaggerate the magnitude of, and even mischaracterize, these differential effects. The evidence reveals that, in terms of Oddi sphincter effects and induction of biliary tract spasm, there are no significant differences between *morphine* and other pure mu receptor agonists.[1] There is thus no evidence basis for the common practice of substituting *meperidine* (*pethidine*) for *morphine* when treating BTP.

While the pure mu agonists are generally equivalent for BTP, there are other **opioid** considerations that clinicians should keep in mind. *Pentazocine* is to be avoided, since it increases frequency and duration of bile duct sphincter contraction; there are no such untoward effects from *tramadol* or *buprenorphine*.[2,3,4] In fact, *buprenorphine* is arguably the **opioid** of choice for BTP, since it even relieves pain from *meperidine*-induced spasm of Oddi's sphincter.[5]

The well-known association between pure mu agonism and biliary tract spasm translates into an occasional role for *naloxone* for BTP in patients (including those post-cholecystectomy) who have received **opioids**.[6,7]

A retrospective analysis found that test characteristics of the sonographic Murphy's sign were not altered by administration of **opioids** (*morphine* or *meperidine*) before the ultrasound.[8]

NSAIDs

NSAIDs provide good analgesic effect, lack untoward effects on biliary tract pressure, and (perhaps through anti-inflammatory activity) seem to reduce the rate of progression from uncomplicated biliary colic to acute cholecystitis.[9–12] Trials of various **NSAIDs** reveal a pattern of BTP treatment effectiveness for this class.

Ketorolac (30 mg IV) provides identical biliary colic pain relief to that achieved with *meperidine* (50 mg IV), while causing less nausea and dizziness.[13] Similar results are reported in a trial of IM *ketorolac* (60 mg) versus *meperidine* (1.5 mg/kg, max dose 100 mg).[14]

Indomethacin (50 mg IV) provides BTP pain relief equivalent to that of the **opioid** combination *oxycone-papaverine* (5 + 50 mg IV).[15] *Flurbiprofen* (150 mg IM) achieves better BTP analgesia, and is associated with fewer side effects, than either *hyoscine* (20 mg IM) or *pentazocine* (30 mg IM).[16]

The piroxicam analog *tenoxicam* (20 mg IV) achieves more rapid and prolonged biliary colic relief than *hyoscine* (20 mg IV), and also reduces likelihood of progression to acute cholecystitis.[11]

Diclofenac (75 mg IM) provides significantly better BTP pain relief than *hyoscine* (20 mg IM), and (like other **NSAIDs**) is associated with a lesser likelihood of progression to cholecystitis.[10] RCT data show that *diclofenac* (75 mg IM) provides significant biliary colic pain relief, and reduces chances of progression to cholecystitis by about $2/3^{rds}$ (as compared to placebo).[12]

NSAID use has been sporadically reported to have caused surgical bleeding after cholecystectomy.[17] However, an RCT designed to assess for association between perioperative *ketorolac* use (IM followed by IV infusion) and postcholecystectomy bleeding failed to find significant **NSAID**-induced increase in operative blood loss or hemostatic dysfunction.[18]

CHOLECYSTOKININ RECEPTOR AGENTS

Drugs acting at the cholecystokinin receptor may also be useful in acute treatment of BTP. *Ceruletide* (1 ng/kg IV or 0.5 μg/kg IM) provides more analgesia than placebo and compares favorably with *pentacozine* (0.5 mg/kg IM) in efficacy and side effects.[19–21] Preliminary evidence indicates that the **cholecystokinin-1 receptor antagonist** *loxiglumide* (50 mg IV) relieves BTP faster and more effectively than *scopolamine* (*hyoscine*; 20 mg IV).[20] Data for the **cholecystokinin receptor agents** are promising, but it is premature to endorse use of these agents in the ED setting.

SPASMOLYTICS/ANTICHOLINERGICS

Spasmolytic and **anticholinergic** drugs have been investigated as treatment for biliary colic. A large placebo-controlled trial assessing three dosing levels of *pargeverine* (*propinoxate*) found pain relief (and no significant side effects) after IV administration of either 20 mg or 30 mg of the mandelic acid derivative.[22]

The **analgesic/spasmolytic** *metamizole* (2.5 g IV) fared well in a double-blinded trial comparing its efficacy with that of *tramadol* (100 mg IV) or the pure **spasmolytic** *butylscopolamine* (*hyoscine butylbromide*; 20 mg IV).[23] *Metamizole* (not available in the USA owing to bone marrow risks) is significantly more effective than both *tramadol* and *butylscopolamine* at reducing pain and preventing need for rescue medication; it also has the shortest onset time (about 10 min).

A study assessing *glycopyrrolate* (*glycopyrronium bromide*) for ED therapy of biliary colic found no benefit over placebo.[24]

CALCIUM CHANNEL BLOCKERS

Calcium channel blockers are known to relax biliary tract smooth muscle. For BTP, the most potent agent in this class appears to be *nifedipine*.[25] There is currently insufficient evidence to support use of *nifedipine* for acute treatment of BTP, and its outpatient efficacy is hindered by suboptimal pain relief and frequent headache.[26]

■ Summary and recommendations

First line: ketorolac (15–30 mg IV q6 h) buprenorphine (initial dose 0.3 mg IV, then titrate)

Reasonable: morphine (initial dose 4–6 mg IV, then titrate)

Pregnancy: buprenorphine (initial dose 0.3 mg IV, then titrate)

Pediatric:
- NSAIDs (e.g. liquid naproxen 10 mg/kg PO BID)
- buprenorphine (initial dose 2–6 µg/kg IV, then titrate)

Special cases:
- *opioid exposure prior to development of biliary colic*: naloxone (initial dose 0.4 mg IV)
- *operative intervention likely*: buprenorphine (initial dose 0.3 mg IV, then titrate); NSAIDs only after consultation with surgeon
- *failure of, or ineligibility for, NSAIDs and opioids*: propinoxate (20 mg IV)

References

1. Thompson DR. Narcotic analgesic effects on the sphincter of Oddi: a review of the data and therapeutic implications in treating pancreatitis. *Am J Gastroenterol.* 2001;**96**(4):1266–1272.
2. Staritz M, Poralla T, Manns M, *et al.* Effect of modern analgesic drugs (tramadol, pentazocine, and buprenorphine) on the bile duct sphincter in man. *Gut.* 1986;**27**(5):567–569.
3. Staritz M. Pharmacology of the sphincter of Oddi. *Endoscopy.* 1988;**20**(Suppl 1):171–174.
4. Rosow CE. The clinical usefulness of agonist–antagonist analgesics in acute pain. *Drug Alcohol Depend.* 1987;**20**(4):329–337.
5. Hubbard GP, Wolfe KR. Meperidine misuse in a patient with sphincter of Oddi dysfunction. *Ann Pharmacother.* 2003;**37**(4):534–537.
6. Druart-Blazy A, Pariente A, Berthelemy P, *et al.* The underestimated role of opiates in patients with suspected sphincter of Oddi dysfunction after cholecystectomy. *Gastroenterol Clin Biol.* 2005;**29**(12):1220–1223.

7. Butler KC, Selden B, Pollack CV, Jr. Relief by naloxone of morphine-induced spasm of the sphincter of Oddi in a post-cholecystectomy patient. *J Emerg Med.* 2001;**21**(2):129–131.

8. Nelson B, Senecal E, Hong C, *et al.* Opioid analgesia and assessment of the sonographic Murphy's sign. *J Emerg Med.* 2005;**28**(4):409–413.

9. Goldman G, Kahn PJ, Alon R, *et al.* Biliary colic treatment and acute cholecystitis prevention by prostaglandin inhibitor. *Dig Dis Sci.* 1989;**34**(6):809–811.

10. Kumar A, Deed JS, Bhasin B, *et al.* Comparison of the effect of diclofenac with hyoscine N-butylbromide in the symptomatic treatment of acute biliary colic. *ANZ J Surg.* 2004;**74**(7):573–576.

11. Al-Waili N, Saloom KY. The analgesic effect of intravenous tenoxicam in symptomatic treatment of biliary colic: a comparison with hyoscine N-butylbromide. *Eur J Med Res.* 14 1998;**3**(10):475–479.

12. Akriviadis EA, Hatzigavriel M, Kapnias D, *et al.* Treatment of biliary colic with diclofenac: a randomized, double-blind, placebo-controlled study. *Gastroenterology.* 1997;**113**(1):225–231.

13. Henderson SO, Swadron S, Newton E. Comparison of intravenous ketorolac and meperidine in the treatment of biliary colic. *J Emerg Med.* 2002;**23**(3):237–241.

14. Dula DJ, Anderson R, Wood GC. A prospective study comparing i.m. ketorolac with i.m. meperidine in the treatment of acute biliary colic. *J Emerg Med.* 2001;**20**(2):121–124.

15. Jonsson PE, Erichsen C, Holmin T, *et al.* Double-blind evaluation of intravenous indomethacin and oxycone–papaverine in the treatment of acute biliary pain. *Acta Chir Scand.* 1985;**151**(6):561–564.

16. Camp Herrero J, Artigas Raventos V, M111a Santos J, *et al.* [The efficacy of injectable flurbiprofen in the symptomatic treatment of biliary colic.] *Med Clin (Barc).* 1992;**98**(6):212–214.

17. Vuilleumier H, Halkic N. Ruptured subcapsular hematoma after laparoscopic cholecystectomy attributed to ketorolac-induced coagulopathy. *Surg Endosc.* 2003;**17**(4):659.

18. Varrassi G, Panella L, Piroli A, *et al.* The effects of perioperative ketorolac infusion on postoperative pain and endocrine-metabolic response. *Anesth Analg.* 1994;**78**(3):514–519.

19. Lishner M, Lang R, Jutrin I, *et al.* Analgesic effect of ceruletide compared with pentazocine in biliary and renal colic: a prospective, controlled, double-blind study. *Drug Intell Clin Pharm.* 1985;**19**(6):433–436.

20. Malesci A, Pezzilli R, D'Amato M, *et al*. CCK-1 receptor blockade for treatment of biliary colic: a pilot study. *Aliment Pharmacol Ther.* 2003;**18**(3):333–337.

21. Pizzuto G, Surgo D, Nasorri L, *et al*. [Echographic and ERCP–manometric study of gallbladder and Oddi's sphincter behavior in biliary colic in patients with cholelithiasis. Effects of cerulein.] *Minerva Chir.* 1996;**51**(12):1145–1149.

22. de los Santos AR, Marti ML, Di Girolamo G, *et al*. Propinox in biliary colic: a multicenter, randomized, prospective and parallel double-blind study of three doses of propinox versus placebo in acute biliary colic pain. *Int J Tissue React.* 1999;**21**(1):13–18.

23. Schmieder G, Stankov G, Zerle G, *et al*. Observer-blind study with metamizole versus tramadol and butylscopolamine in acute biliary colic pain. *Arzneimittelforschung.* 1993;**43**(11):1216–1221.

24. Antevil JL, Buckley RG, Johnson AS, *et al*. Treatment of suspected symptomatic cholelithiasis with glycopyrrolate: a prospective, randomized clinical trial. *Ann Emerg Med.* 2005;**45**(2):172–176.

25. Dehpour AR, Samini M, Rastegar H, *et al*. Comparison of various calcium channel blockers on guinea-pig isolated common bile duct. *Gen Pharmacol.* 1994;**25**(8):1655–1660.

26. Peng P, Sandler A. A review of the use of fentanyl analgesia in the management of acute pain in adults. *Anesthesiology.* 1999;**90**(2):576–579.

Bites and stings – marine

STEPHEN H. THOMAS AND CIARAN J. BROWNE

■ Agents

- ■ Antivenom
- ■ Opioids
- ■ Magnesium
- ■ Local anesthetics
- ■ Acetic acid (vinegar)
- ■ Papain (proteolytic meat tenderizer)
- ■ Slurry of bicarbonate (baking soda)

■ Evidence

Marine envenomation can result from discharging nematocysts (e.g. jellyfish, fire coral), puncturing spines (e.g. sea urchins, stingrays), or actual bites (e.g. blue octopus, sea snakes). The preponderance of the evidence, and thus most of this chapter's focus, addresses jellyfish (*Cnidaria* or *Coelenterates*) envenomation.

In keeping with this text's aim, this discussion emphasizes pharmacotherapy, but one physical modality deserves mention. For most marine envenomations, hot water immersion (40–45 °C via immersion or shower, for up to 90 min) can inactivate venom and achieve better pain relief than alternative approaches such as *acetic acid*, *papain*, or **opioids**.[1] [5] One recent US series of over 100 stingray envenomations found that hot water immersion alone was sufficient for pain therapy in nearly 90% of patients.[6]

Whether considering physical interventions (e.g. hot water immersion), topical therapies (e.g. *acetic acid* dousing), or IV drug therapy (e.g. with **antivenom**), treatments for different marine envenomations – even those from different members of the same genus – can vary significantly. Be aware of local species, and be wary of overextrapolating clinical trials data. Although it may be impossible to identify the organism responsible for a given envenomation, the differences in therapeutic approach justify attempts at such identification.

For jellyfish stings, prophylaxis may be an option. Application of a sunscreen containing a sting inhibitor decreases frequency and severity of stings from a sea nettle common along the US Pacific coast (*Chrysaora fuscescens*), and also from one of the more dangerous box jellyfish, the sea wasp *Chiropsalmus quadrumanus* (found in the US southern coasts and in the Pacific).[7]

Before removing remnant marine tissue, consider topical approaches such as hot water immersion and other therapies outlined below. Pretreatment maximizes chances of venom inactivation and may prevent further venom delivery. Of course, application of topical therapies intended to inactivate nematocysts will have no effect on pain from venom that has already been delivered. Consequently, nematocyst inhibition therapies should be accompanied by attempts at venom inactivation, and clinicians should be prepared to administer adjuvant analgesia. Immobilization, compression bandages, and other medical approaches outside the realm of this text (e.g. hemodialysis) may also decrease pain.[1]

Antivenoms (or **antivenins**) may be an option for some species of sea snakes, jellyfish (e.g. box jellyfish *Chironex fleckeri*), and stonefish. When they are available, **antivenoms** are known to have rapid and profound effects upon pain.[8] Prehospital administration of jellyfish **antivenom** is demonstrated to be a safe and effective means of treating pain.[9] While there is no RCT evidence for **antivenom**'s analgesic effects, the case series and expert opinion evidence is consistently positive. In fact, Australian clinicians have acknowledged for decades that "early administration of the specific antivenom appears to be the best treatment for the savage pain of the sting."[10] The importance of **antivenom** therapy for *C. fleckeri* is augmented by the fact that rapidity of systemic envenomation limits efficacy of hot water immersion.[11]

Injections of **local anesthetics** are occasionally mentioned as a means to alleviate marine envenomation pain.[1,12,13] However, there is little or no high-quality evidence addressing the subject. For envenomations in which sympathetic overactivity is a problem (e.g. Irukandji syndrome), the use of *epinephrine*-containing local anesthetics seems unwise.

For jellyfish stings worldwide, the most useful topical agent appears to be *acetic acid* topically applied in the 4–5% concentration found in vinegar.[14–18] *Acetic acid* controls pain by deactivating nematocysts, thus limiting continued envenomation from attached stinging cells.[1,2] *Acetic acid* seems to be effective with most jellyfish, although there is conflicting evidence for some types. For example, while *acetic acid* is recommended for *Physalia* species indigenous to US coasts (e.g. Portuguese man-of-war [*Physalia physalis*] or bluebottle), *acetic acid* dousing is reported to cause nematocyst *discharge* in some Australian *Physalia*.[19,20] Some Australians recommend withholding *acetic acid* in patients lacking severe pain and having no visualizable retained tentacles, since such cases are less likely to involve sea wasps (cubozoan species such as *C. fleckeri*) for which *vinegar* dousing is very helpful.

Although less effective than *acetic acid*, a slurry of *bicarbonate* (water and baking soda) also relieves pain from the sting of the Portuguese man-of-war.[20,21] The *bicarbonate* slurry has been reported more useful than *acetic acid* in pain due to stings from one of the sea nettles found commonly on the US Atlantic coast (*Chrysaora quinquecirrha*).[21]

The proteolytic enzyme *papain* has historically been reported to relieve jellyfish sting pain. However, for the sting of the Hawaiian box jellyfish *Carybdea alata*, *acetic acid* is more useful.[5] In fact, a randomized double-blind assessment of *C. alata* stings found no utility for topical spray with *fresh water*, *papain*, or *aluminum sulfate*.[22] A multitude of other proposed remedies (e.g. micturating on the sting site) are reported; none have evidence support – though the urine of an individual with fever (at least 40 °C) may be efficacious.

Though the evidence is inconclusive, authorities recommend IV *magnesium* (up to 0.05 g/kg to a maximum dose of 2.5 g) as a treatment of the pain and cardiovascular aspects of Irukandji syndrome (severe diffuse pain, diaphoresis, GI symptoms, and cardiovascular stimulation).[14] Although reported failures of *magnesium* temper enthusiasm, the cation's safety and the lack of clearly effective alternatives translate into some role for its use for Irukandji pain.[14,23] The possible indication for *magnesium* treatment extends far beyond Australian shores, since Irukandji-like syndrome occurs in jellyfish other than the classic Australian cubozoan (box) culprit, the tiny *Carukia barnesi*; the syndrome has been reported around the world (e.g. in Florida).[24]

Therapies for the Irukandji syndrome tend to focus on systemic complications such as hypertension. Severe muscle cramping, which can present in delayed fashion, is treated with **benzodiazepines**.[25,26] There is no role for either **antihistamines** or **corticosteroids**.[26–28]

No RCT data address use of **opioids** for marine envenomation, but case series consistently demonstrate this class' utility in treating refractory pain from a variety of marine-inflicted bites and stings. Analysis of a large series of *C. fleckeri* stings found that parenteral **opioids** were required in nearly a third of patients.[29] Nearly all clinicians with experience in treating Irukandji syndrome consider IV **opioids** part of the standard treatment.[14,30] Stonefish envenomation, notable for its severe pain, is often controllable with **opioids** (and hot water immersion).[31,32] Hot water immersion and **opioids** are also recommended for pedicellarial stings from sea urchins.[33] There is no guiding trial evidence, but if allergic or anaphylactic symptoms are present it may be prudent to use *fentanyl* (which does not release histamine) rather than *morphine*.

There are no data on use of **NSAIDs** for marine envenomation, but there are theoretical reasons to avoid this class. Most notably, the antiplatelet effects of the **NSAIDs** may be problematic in situations where punctures have occurred.

■ Summary and recommendations

First line: hot water immersion or shower (40–45 °C as tolerated, for 90 min); jellyfish: acetic acid dousing with 4–5% solution (household vinegar)

Reasonable: morphine (initial dose 4-6 mg IV, then titrate)

Pregnancy: topical hot water and acetic acid dousing with 4–5% solution (household vinegar)

Pediatric: topical hot water and acetic acid dousing with 4–5% solution (household vinegar)

Special cases:

- *antivenom available*: consider for intractable pain or severe toxicity
- *Irukandji-like syndrome*: magnesium (0.05 g/kg IV, maximum 2.5 g over 20–30 min, with repeat dosing and infusion rates guided by side effects and magnesium levels); benzodiazepines (e.g. diazepam 5–10 mg IV q3–4 h) for cramping
- *failure of acetic acid, especially for stings of the sea nettle*: slurry of bicarbonate (baking soda) in water

References

1 Watters MR, Stommel EW. Marine neurotoxins: envenomations and contact toxins. *Curr Treat Options Neurol*. 2004;**6**(2):115–123.

2. Perkins RA, Morgan SS. Poisoning, envenomation, and trauma from marine creatures. *Am Fam Physician*. 15 2004;**69**(4):885–890.

3. Atkinson PR, Boyle A, Hartin D, *et al*. Is hot water immersion an effective treatment for marine envenomation? *Emerg Med J*. 2006;**23**(7):503–508.

4. Yoshimoto CM, Yanagihara AA. Cnidarian (coelenterate) envenomations in Hawai'i improve following heat application. *Trans R Soc Trop Med Hyg*. 2002;**96**(3):300–303.

5. Nomura JT, Sato RL, Ahern RM, *et al*. A randomized paired comparison trial of cutaneous treatments for acute jellyfish (*Carybdea alata*) stings *Am J Emerg Med*. 2002,**20**(7):624–626.

6. Clark RF, Girard RH, Rao D, *et al*. Stingray envenomation: a retrospective review of clinical presentation and treatment in 119 cases. *J Emerg Med*. 2007;**33**(1):33–37.

7. Kimball AB, Arambula KZ, Stauffer AR, *et al*. Efficacy of a jellyfish sting inhibitor in preventing jellyfish stings in normal volunteers. *Wilderness Environ Med*. 2004;**15**(2):102–108.

8. Currie BJ. Marine antivenoms. *J Toxicol Clin Toxicol*. 2003;**41**(3):301–308.

9. Fenner PJ, Williamson JA, Blenkin JA. Successful use of Chironex antivenom by members of the Queensland Ambulance Transport Brigade. *Med J Aust*. 1989;**151**(11–12):708–710.

10. Williamson JA, Le Ray LE, Wohlfahrt M, *et al*. Acute management of serious envenomation by box-jellyfish (*Chironex fleckeri*). *Med J Aust*. 1984;**141**(12–13):851–853.

11. Carrette TJ, Cullen P, Little M, *et al*. Temperature effects on box jellyfish venom: a possible treatment for envenomed patients? *Med J Aust*. 2002;**177** (11–12):654–655.

12. Mann JW, 3rd, Werntz JR. Catfish stings to the hand. *J Hand Surg (Am)*. 1991;**16**(2):318–321.

13. Sein Anand J, Chodorowski Z, Waldman W. Hand wound caused by an active sting with a toxin spine of a catfish (*Heteropneustes fossilis*): a case report. *Przegl Lek*. 2005;**62**(6):526–527.

14. Barnett FI, Durrheim DN, Speare R, *et al*. Management of Irukandji syndrome in northern Australia. *Rural Remote Health*. 2005;**5**(3):369.

15. Hartwick R, Callanan V, Williamson J. Disarming the box-jellyfish: nematocyst inhibition in *Chironex fleckeri*. *Med J Aust*. 1980;**1**(1):15–20.

16. Beadnell CE, Rider TA, Williamson JA, *et al*. Management of a major box jellyfish (*Chironex fleckeri*) sting. Lessons from the first minutes and hours. *Med J Aust*. 1992;**156**(9):655–658.

17. Haddad V, Jr., da Silveira FL, Cardoso JL, *et al*. A report of 49 cases of cnidarian envenoming from southeastern Brazilian coastal waters. *Toxicon*. 2002;**40** (10):1445–1450.

18. Lee NS, Wu ML, Tsai WJ, *et al*. A case of jellyfish sting. *Vet Hum Toxicol*. 2001;**43**(4):203–205.

19. Fenner P, Williamson J, Burnett J, *et al*. First aid treatment of jellyfish stings in Australia. Response to a newly differentiated species. *Med J Aust*. 1993;**158** (7):498–501.

20. Kaufman MB. Portuguese man-of-war envenomation. *Pediatr Emerg Care*. 1992;**8**(1):27–28.

21. Burnett J, Rubinstein H, Carlton G. First aid for jellyfish envenomation. *South Med J*. 1983;**76**(7):870–872.

22. Thomas CS, Scott SA, Galanis DJ, *et al*. Box jellyfish (*Carybdea alata*) in Waikiki. The analgesic effect of sting-aid, Adolph's meat tenderizer and fresh water on their stings: a double-blinded, randomized, placebo-controlled clinical trial. *Hawaii Med J*. 2001;**60**(8):205–207, 210.

23. Little M. Failure of magnesium in treatment of Irukandji syndrome. *Anaesth Intensive Care*. 2005;**33**(4):541–542.

24. Grady JD, Burnett JW. Irukandji-like syndrome in South Florida divers. *Ann Emerg Med*. 2003;**42**(6):763–766.

25. Tibballs J. Australian venomous jellyfish, envenomation syndromes, toxins and therapy. *Toxicon*. 2006;**48**(7):830–859.

26. Fenner PJ, Williamson J, Callanan VI, *et al.* Further understanding of, and a new treatment for, "Irukandji" (*Carukia barnesi*) stings. *Med J Aust.* 1986;**145**(11–12):569, 572–574.

27. Little M, Pereira P, Mulcahy R, *et al.* Severe cardiac failure associated with presumed jellyfish sting. Irukandji syndrome? *Anaesth Intensive Care.* 2003;**31**(6):642–647.

28. Huynh TT, Seymour J, Pereira P, *et al.* Severity of Irukandji syndrome and nematocyst identification from skin scrapings. *Med J Aust.* 2003;**178**(1):38–41.

29. Currie BJ, Jacups SP. Prospective study of *Chironex fleckeri* and other box jellyfish stings in the "Top End" of Australia's Northern Territory. *Med J Aust.* 2005;**183**(11–12):631 636.

30. Winkel KD, Hawdon GM, Ashby K, *et al.* Eye injury after jellyfish sting in temperate Australia. *Wilderness Environ Med.* 2002;**13**(3):203 205.

31. Brenneke F, Hatz C. Stonefish envenomation: a lucky outcome. *Travel Med Infect Dis.* 2006;**4**(5):281–285.

32. Lee JY, Teoh LC, Leo SP. Stonefish envenomations of the hand – a local marine hazard: a series of 8 cases and review of the literature. *Ann Acad Med Singapore.* 2004;**33**(4):515–520.

33. Wu ML, Chou SL, Huang TY, *et al.* Sea-urchin envenomation. *Vet Hum Toxicol.* 2003;**45**(6):307–309.

Bites and stings – terrestrial

FRANK LOVECCHIO AND STEPHEN H. THOMAS

■ Agents

- Antivenom
- Opioids
- Antihistamines
- Calcium
- Benzodiazepines
- NSAIDs
- Local anesthetics
- Corticosteroids

■ Evidence

A multitude of land-based animals can produce an envenomation. Snakes are of particular clinical importance, and severe pain is a consequence of envenomation from members of the orders *Hymenoptera, Araneae* (spiders), and *Scorpiones*.[1-3] Given the wide variety of causes of envenomation, it is important to know the local probable sources.

Treating the pain of land-based envenomations is an acute care priority, since the discomfort may be both severe and long lasting. Even in cases where there is no risk of major morbidity or mortality (e.g. *Chilopoda* centipede envenomation), terrestrial envenomations can cause unbearable pain. The control of symptoms is not limited to the first-aid or wilderness clinic setting, since pain can be delayed in onset (e.g. from the brown recluse spider), and symptoms can be long lasting. A review of snakebite cases by one poison control center found that the average patient has over a week of significant pain.[4]

Topical therapies, often useful for marine envenomations, have little role in pain control for terrestrial bites and stings. There is no high-quality evidence supporting either hot or cold therapy for the majority of land-based envenomations. (Potential exceptions include ice for *Hymenoptera* and heat for *Chilopoda* envenomation.[5,6]) Clinical trials show that *nitroglycerin (glyceryl trinitrate)*, recommended by some sources for brown recluse spider bites, controls neither symptoms nor necrosis caused by loxoscelism.[7,8] Evidence from RCTs assessing other topical therapies for a variety of envenomations (e.g. *Hymenoptera*, *Solenopsis invicta* fire ants) has found no benefit in application of *aspirin, aluminum sulfate, papain,* or *bicarbonate*.[5,9–11]

The failure of topical approaches and the severity of pain from terrestrial envenomations translate into need for IV analgesics. (Most patients with potentially serious envenomation require IV access anyway.) The need for the IV approach is reinforced by the fact that many envenomation syndromes, such as latrodectism, include delay of gastric emptying.[12]

In some cases, administration of **antivenom** (or **antivenin**) can dramatically relieve pain and other symptoms of envenomation, even after failure of other approaches (e.g. **opioids, muscle relaxants**).[13] Owing to a misconception that an envenomation that is nonfatal does not require **antivenom**, this therapy is sometimes inappropriately withheld; such withholding of **antivenom** is particularly problematic in envenomation syndromes that are predictably prolonged and severe.[14,15] The presence of distressing symptoms should be a sufficient trigger to consider **antivenom** therapy.[16] Even when administered many hours (up to a day or more) after envenomation, **antivenom** may produce profound relief of pain and systemic symptoms and prevent progression (especially for latrodectism) to days of severe pain.[13,17–20]

Patient characteristics, as well as the particular type of bite or sting, influence the decision as to whether **antivenom** is indicated. While the use of **antivenom** is controversial, it may be the only effective method of pain relief.[21–23] If **antivenom** is to be used, IV (rather than IM) administration achieves maximal pain relief.[24] Subcutaneous *epinephrine (adrenaline)* pretreatment can enhance patient comfort by reducing incidence and severity of **antivenom** reactions.[25] Case reports and expert opinion argue for the safety (and efficacy) of **antivenom** in pregnant patients and in children.[26–29]

The utility of **opioids** for terrestrial envenomations is supported by many case series covering a wide variety of arachnids, caterpillars, and reptiles – including those (e.g. *Micrurus*) with primarily neurotoxic venoms.[30–35]

While neurotoxic envenomation should prompt close respiratory monitoring, **opioids** should be administered if clinically indicated for pain relief.[36] The mixed-mechanism **opioid** *tramadol* is effective in painful ant envenomation.[37] One large-series review of *Latrodectus* (widow) envenomation demonstrated utility of IV *morphine* as a single or adjuvant agent to pain relief; *morphine* was found in this study to be much more effective than *calcium*.[38] Data from animal models, while preliminary, suggest utility for **opioids** in scorpion envenomation.[39]

There is probably little difference in the pain relief afforded by different **opioids** for terrestrial bites and stings. There are potential benefits to use of *fentanyl*. Its potency and ease of titration are noteworthy, and lack of histamine release makes *fentanyl* an excellent choice when histaminic pathways are a major part of the envenomation syndrome (e.g. *Hymenoptera* stings). *Fentanyl* is also recommended as the **opioid** of choice when **antivenom** is administered.[17,21,38,40] *Fentanyl* appears at least as safe as other **opioids** in pregnancy, and may in fact be less likely than *morphine* to cause fetal–placental hemodynamic problems in patients with envenomation.[41]

The histamine pathway's contributions to terrestrial envenomation symptoms create a role for **antihistamines** (e.g. *diphenhydramine*) in treating land-based bites and stings. Animal data support the theory that **antihistamines** can ameliorate symptoms of envenomation.[39] The utility of **antihistamines** in *Hymenoptera* stings is well described, and case series evidence points to consistent (although moderate) benefits from **antihistamine** use for scorpion, caterpillar, and centipede envenomation.[42–46]

For decades, authorities have recommended *calcium* for envenomations associated with painful muscle cramps.[47,48] Particularly in the treatment of latrodectism, case series evidence indicates continued worldwide use (and reported salutary effect) of *calcium*.[20,31,49] It is not easy to dismiss years of experience with *calcium*, since there are so many anecdotal reports of immediate (if often short-lived) analgesia after its administration. Although the best large-series review found no significant analgesia from *calcium* use, the cation's relative safety renders a therapeutic trial reasonable.[38]

Evidence from multiple case series suggests that, instead of *calcium*, **muscle relaxants** (particularly the **benzodiazepines**) should be used for treatment for severe cramps associated with terrestrial envenomation.[31,38] Though there are no RCTs comparing *calcium* and **muscle relaxants**, case report data in latrodectism indicate superiority of *diazepam* over *calcium* preparations.[50] There is no good evidence supporting use of non-benzodiazepine muscle relaxants (e.g. *methocarbamol*); these agents are not recommended.

NSAIDs have been reported useful in small case series of bites from spiders such as brown recluses and tarantulas.[51,52] Preliminary evidence from animal models and case reports suggests a role for **NSAIDs** for scorpion envenomation.[39,53] The use of **NSAIDs** in snakebites is discouraged, since many snake venoms inhibit the arachidonic acid cascade (**NSAID** administration can theoretically worsen bleeding and renal complications).[54] Safety considerations aside, trials of **NSAIDs** suggest they provide less-effective snakebite pain relief than **antivenom**.[55]

Case series evidence supports consideration of injecting **local anesthetics** (e.g. *lidocaine*, *mepivacaine*) for bites of some spiders, scorpions, and centipedes.[44,56–59] Limited case report evidence supports use of Bier's block regional anesthesia for *Latrodectus* species, but caution is recommended owing to the risk of worsening toxicity.[60,61]

A large randomized double-blind trial demonstrated no utility for **corticosteroids** in scorpion envenomation.[62] Case series suggest that **corticosteroids** are occasionally useful for some centipede bites, especially in cases in which Wells' syndrome (eosinophilic cellulitis) develops.[44,58]

■ Summary and recommendations

First line: fentanyl (initial dose 50–100 µg IV, then titrate)

Reasonable:

- antihistamines (e.g. diphenhydramine 25–50 mg IV q4–6 h)
- morphine (initial dose 4–6 mg IV, then titrate) *if* antivenom will not be administered for severe symptoms
- local anesthetic (e.g. bupivacaine 0.25%) injection unless snakebite

Pregnancy:

- fentanyl (initial dose 50–100 µg, then titrate)
- local anesthetic (e.g. bupivacaine 0.25%) injection unless snakebite

Pediatric:

- fentanyl (initial dose 1–2 μg/kg IV, then titrate)
- consider local anesthetic injection (e.g. bupivacaine 0.25%) unless snakebite

Special cases:

- *administering serum-based antivenom*: epinephrine pretreatment (0.25 mg SC)
- *abdominal or other painful muscle cramps*: diazepam (5–10 mg IV q3–4 h)
- *non-snakebite envenomation*: NSAIDs (e.g. ibuprofen 400–600 mg PO q6–8 h)
- *oral therapy appropriate*: oxycodone or hydrocodone (5–10 mg of either drug PO q4–6 h)

References

1. Hodgson WC. Pharmacological action of Australian animal venoms. *Clin Exp Pharmacol Physiol*. 1997;**24**(1):10–17.
2. White J, Warrell D, Eddleston M, *et al*. Clinical toxinology: where are we now? *J Toxicol Clin Toxicol*. 2003;**41**(3):263–276.
3. Isbister GK, Volschenk ES, Balit CR, *et al*. Australian scorpion stings: a prospective study of definite stings. *Toxicon*. 2003;**41**(7):877–883.
4. Spiller HA, Bosse GM. Prospective study of morbidity associated with snakebite envenomation. *J Toxicol Clin Toxicol*. 2003;**41**(2):125–130.
5. Balit CR, Isbister GK, Buckley NA. Randomized controlled trial of topical aspirin in the treatment of bee and wasp stings. *J Toxicol Clin Toxicol*. 2003;**41**(6):801–808.
6. Balit CR, Harvey MS, Waldock JM, *et al*. Prospective study of centipede bites in Australia. *J Toxicol Clin Toxicol*. 2004;**42**(1):41–48.
7. Forks TP. Brown recluse spider bites. *J Am Board Fam Pract*. 2000;**13**(6):415–423.
8. Lowry BP, Bradfield JF, Carroll RG, *et al*. A controlled trial of topical nitroglycerin in a New Zealand white rabbit model of brown recluse spider envenomation. *Ann Emerg Med*. 2001;**37**(2):161–165.
9. Bruce S, Tschen EH, Smith EB. Topical aluminum sulfate for fire ant stings. *Int J Dermatol*. Apr 1984;**23**(3):211.

10. Ross EV, Jr., Badame AJ, Dale SE. Meat tenderizer in the acute treatment of imported fire ant stings. *J Am Acad Dermatol*. 1987;**16**(6):1189–1192.

11. Hile DC, Coon TP, Skinner CG, *et al*. Treatment of imported fire ant stings with mitigator sting and bite treatment: a randomized control study. *Wilderness Environ Med*. 2006;**17**(1):21–25.

12. Kleiner-Baumgarten A. [Black widow spider bite in the Negev.] *Harefuah*. 1991;**120**(5):257–260.

13. Hoover NG, Fortenberry JD. Use of antivenin to treat priapism after a black widow spider bite. *Pediatrics*. 2004;**114**(1):e128–e129.

14. Isbister GK, Gray MR. A prospective study of 750 definite spider bites, with expert spider identification. *Q J Med*. 2002;**95**(11):723–731.

15. Dzelalija B, Medic A. Latrodectus bites in northern Dalmatia, Croatia: clinical, laboratory, epidemiological, and therapeutical aspects. *Croat Med J*. 2003;**44** (2):135–138.

16. Graudins A, Gunja N, Broady KW, *et al*. Clinical and in vitro evidence for the efficacy of Australian red-back spider (*Latrodectus hasselti*) antivenom in the treatment of envenomation by a cupboard spider (*Steatoda grossa*). *Toxicon*. 2002;**40**(6):767–775.

17. Suntorntham S, Roberts JR, Nilsen GJ. Dramatic clinical response to the delayed administration of black widow spider antivenin. *Ann Emerg Med*. 1994;**24**(6):1198–1199.

18. Lira-da-Silva RM, Matos GB, Sampaio RO, *et al*. [Retrospective study on *Latrodectus* stings in Bahia, Brazil.] *Rev Soc Bras Med Trop*. 1995;**28**(3):205–210.

19. Muller GJ. Black and brown widow spider bites in South Africa. A series of 45 cases. *S Afr Med J*. 1993;**83**(6):399–405.

20. Bucur IJ, Obasi OE. Spider bite envenomation in Al Baha Region, Saudi Arabia. *Ann Saudi Med*. 1999;**19**(1):15–19.

21. Isbister GK, Graudins A, White J, *et al*. Antivenom treatment in arachnidism. *J Toxicol Clin Toxicol*. 2003;**41**(3):291–300.

22. Dart RC, Goldfrank LR, Chyka PA, *et al*. Combined evidence-based literature analysis and consensus guidelines for stocking of emergency antidotes in the United States. *Ann Emerg Med*. 2000;**36**(2):126–132.

23. el Hafny B, Ghalim N. [Clinical evolution and circulating venom levels in scorpion envenomations in Morocco.] *Bull Soc Pathol Exot*. 2002;**95**(3):200–204.

24. Ellis RM, Sprivulis PC, Jelinek GA, *et al*. A double-blind, randomized trial of intravenous versus intramuscular antivenom for red-back spider envenoming. *Emerg Med Australas*. 2005;**17**(2):152–156.

25. Premawardhena AP, de Silva CE, Fonseka MM, *et al.* Low dose subcutaneous adrenaline to prevent acute adverse reactions to antivenom serum in people bitten by snakes: randomised, placebo controlled trial. *BMJ.* 1999;**318** (7190):1041–1043.

26. Sherman RP, Groll JM, Gonzalez DI, *et al.* Black widow spider (*Latrodectus mactans*) envenomation in a term pregnancy. *Curr Surg.* 2000;**57**(4):346–348.

27. Mead HJ, Jelinek GA. Red-back spider bites to Perth children, 1979–1988. *J Paediatr Child Health.* 1993;**29**(4):305–308.

28. Bailey B. Are there teratogenic risks associated with antidotes used in the acute management of poisoned pregnant women? *Birth Defects Res A Clin Mol Teratol.* 2003;**67**(2):133–140.

29. Trinh HH, Hack JB. Use of CroFab antivenin in the management of a very young pediatric copperhead envenomation. *J Emerg Med.* 2005;**29**(2):159–162.

30. Isbister GK, Gray MR. Effects of envenoming by comb-footed spiders of the genera *Steatoda* and *Achaearanea* (family Theridiidae: Araneae) in Australia. *J Toxicol Clin Toxicol.* 2003;**41**(6):809–819.

31. Diez Garcia F, Laynez Bretones F, Galvez Contreras MC, *et al.* [Black widow spider (*Latrodectus tredecimguttatus*) bite. Presentation of 12 cases.] *Med Clin (Barcelona).* 1996;**106**(9):344–346.

32. Morgan DL, Borys DJ, Stanford R, *et al.* Texas coral snake (*Micrurus tener*) bites. *South Med J.* 2007;**100**(2):152–156.

33. Thorson A, Lavonas EJ, Rouse AM, *et al.* Copperhead envenomations in the Carolinas. *J Toxicol Clin Toxicol.* 2003;**41**(1):29–35.

34. Cantrell FL. Envenomation by the Mexican beaded lizard: a case report. *J Toxicol Clin Toxicol.* 2003;**41**(3):241–244.

35. Isbister GK, Whelan PI. Envenomation by the billygoat plum stinging caterpillar (*Thosea penthima*). *Med J Aust.* 2000;**173**(11–12):654–655.

36. Gold BS, Barish RA, Dart RC. North American snake envenomation: diagnosis, treatment, and management. *Emerg Med Clin North Am.* 2004;**22**(2):423–443, ix.

37. Haddad Junior V, Cardoso JL, Moraes RH. Description of an injury in a human caused by a false tocandira (*Dinoponera gigantea*, Perty, 1833) with a revision on folkloric, pharmacological and clinical aspects of the giant ants of the genera *Paraponera* and *Dinoponera* (sub-family Ponerinae). *Rev Inst Med Trop Sao Paulo.* 2005;**47**(4):235–238.

38. Clark RF, Wethern-Kestner S, Vance MV, *et al.* Clinical presentation and treatment of black widow spider envenomation: a review of 163 cases. *Ann Emerg Med.* 1992;**21**(7):782–787.

39. Nascimento EB, Jr., Costa KA, Bertollo CM, *et al.* Pharmacological investigation of the nociceptive response and edema induced by venom of the scorpion *Tityus serrulatus*. *Toxicon.* 2005;**45**(5):585–593.

40. Moss HS, Binder LS. A retrospective review of black widow spider envenomation. *Ann Emerg Med.* 1987;**16**(2):188–192.

41. Collins LR, Hall RW, Dajani NK, *et al.* Prolonged morphine exposure in utero causes fetal and placental vasoconstriction: a case report. *J Matern Fetal Neonatal Med.* 2005;**17**(6):417–421.

42. Binder LS. Acute arthropod envenomation. Incidence, clinical features and management. *Med Toxicol Adverse Drug Exp.* 1989;**4**(3):163–173.

43. McFee RB, Caraccio TR, Mofenson HC, *et al.* Envenomation by the Vietnamese centipede in a Long Island pet store. *J Toxicol Clin Toxicol.* 2002;**40**(5):573–574.

44. Knysak I, Martins R, Bertim CR. Epidemiological aspects of centipede (Scolopendromorphae: Chilopoda) bites registered in greater S. Paulo, SP, Brazil. *Rev Saude Publica.* 1998;**32**(6):514–518.

45. Balit CR, Geary MJ, Russell RC, *et al.* Prospective study of definite caterpillar exposures. *Toxicon.* 2003;**42**(6):657–662.

46. Kuspis DA, Rawlins JE, Krenzelok EP. Human exposures to stinging caterpillar: *Lophocampa caryae* exposures. *Am J Emerg Med.* 2001;**19**(5):396–398.

47 Wilson DC, King LE, Jr. Spiders and spider bites. *Dermatol Clin.* 1990;**8**(2):277–286.

48. Neustater BR, Stollman NH, Manten HD. Sting of the puss caterpillar: an unusual cause of acute abdominal pain. *South Med J.* 1996;**89**(8):826–827.

49. de Haro L, David JM, Jouglard J. [Latrodectism in southern France. A series of cases from the poisoning center of Marseille.] *Presse Med.* 1994;**23**(24):1121–1123.

50. Casha P, Griscelli JM, Fanton Y, *et al.* [Latrodectism in a child.] *Arch Pediatr.* 1998;**5**(5):510–512.

51. Takaoka M, Nakajima S, Sakae H, *et al.* [Tarantulas bite: two case reports of finger bite from *Haplopelma lividum*.] *Chudoku Kenkyu.* 2001;**14**(3):247–250.

52. Sams HH, Hearth SB, Long LL, *et al.* Nineteen documented cases of *Loxosceles reclusa* envenomation. *J Am Acad Dermatol.* 2001;**44**(4):603–608.

53. Alvares ES, De Maria M, Amancio FF, *et al.* [First record of scorpionism caused by *Tityus adrianoi* Lourenco (Scorpiones: Buthidae).] *Rev Soc Bras Med Trop.* 2006;**39**(4):383–384.

54. Teixeira CF, Landucci EC, Antunes E, *et al.* Inflammatory effects of snake venom myotoxic phospholipases A_2. *Toxicon.* 2003;**42**(8):947–962.

55. Jacome D, Melo MM, Santos MM, *et al.* Kinetics of venom and antivenom serum and clinical parameters and treatment efficacy in *Bothrops alternatus* envenomed dogs. *Vet Hum Toxicol.* 2002;**44**(6):334–338.

56. Al-Asmari AK, Al-Saif AA. Scorpion sting syndrome in a general hospital in Saudi Arabia. *Saudi Med J.* 2004;**25**(1):64–70.

57. Bucaretchi F, Deus Reinaldo CR, Hyslop S, *et al.* A clinico-epidemiological study of bites by spiders of the genus *Phoneutria*. *Rev Inst Med Trop Sao Paulo.* 2000;**42**(1):17–21.

58. Mohri S, Sugiyama A, Saito K, *et al.* Centipede bites in Japan. *Cutis.* 1991;**47**(3):189–190.

59. Zancada Diaz de Entre-Sotos F, Fernandez Ballesteros A, Roldan Montaud A, *et al.* [Local anesthesia in scorpion stings.] *Rev Clin Esp.* 1991;**189**(5):247–248.

60. Winkel KD. Caution regarding Bier's block technique for redback spider bite. *Med J Aust.* 1999;**171**(4):220–221.

61. Fatovich DM, Dunjey SJ, Constantine CJ, *et al.* Successful treatment of red-back spider bite using a Bier's block technique. *Med J Aust.* 1999;**170**(7):342–343.

62. Abroug F, Nouira S, Haguiga H, *et al.* High-dose hydrocortisone hemisuccinate in scorpion envenomation. *Ann Emerg Med.* 1997;**30**(1):23–27.

Breast pain

JANET SIMMONS YOUNG

■ Agents

- NSAIDs
- Opioids
- Gonadotropin release inhibitors
- Selective estrogen receptor modulators

■ Evidence

Pain of the breast is commonly classified as cyclic or noncyclic, depending on its temporal association with menstruation. Visits to ED typically involve acute, noncyclic breast pain, with the most common etiologies being blunt trauma or infection. In all cases, treatment of pain is important. Additionally, follow-up is vital to provide opportunity for advanced pain therapy (e.g. *tamoxifen*, see below) and to assure appropriate evaluation for neoplastic mastalgia.

Other than discussions of pain associated with cancer or postoperative discomfort, there are few clinical analyses of medication effectiveness in relieving mastalgia. The agents most often mentioned are **NSAIDs**, including the **COX-2 selective NSAIDs**, and **opioids**.

NONCYCLIC MASTALGIA

Ketorolac (10 mg PO every 4–6 h) is useful for acute mastalgia and extra-mammary pain, especially in instances of breast pain complicated by blunt thoracic trauma.[1,2] Although *ketorolac*'s parenteral availability is a potential advantage, it is reasonable to extend the available evidence on *ketorolac*'s efficacy to other **NSAIDs**.[2]

The **COX-2 selective NSAIDs** are also effective in anti-nociception for breast pain. There is little available evidence directly addressing acute care use of

COX-2 selective NSAIDs for acute mastalgia. Relevant information is found in the breast augmentation literature. A controlled trial demonstrated that a single 400 mg PO preoperative dose of *celecoxib* effectively reduced postoperative breast pain (i.e. resulted in less **opioid** requirement).[3] Since the cardiovascular adverse effects of the **COX-2 selective NSAIDs** (see the Arthritis chapter, p. 94) may be less applicable to short-term use in patients with breast pain, *celecoxib* remains a potentially useful approach to mastalgia.

Assessment in an RCT found relief of mastalgia with topical application of the **NSAID** *diclofenac diethylammonium* (2% gel, 11.6 mg/g, 50 mg *diclofenac* component TID).[4]

All **NSAIDs** are contraindicated in pregnancy. For mild pain in pregnant patients, *acetaminophen* (*paracetamol*) is a good choice, although it will often need to be combined with an **opioid** for more severe pain.[5,6]

As is the case with **NSAIDs**, there is little clinical trial evidence addressing use of **opioids** for breast pain. Potentially useful data include demonstrations of efficacy, for breast cancer pain, of *hydrocodone* or *oxycodone*; the available evidence does support a role for oral **opioid** use for treating breast pain (e.g. from inflammatory carcinoma) too severe for **NSAID** monotherapy.[7] Breast pain from infections ranging from cellulitis to abscess can also be severe; **opioids** may be used to complement appropriate medical and surgical therapy.[8]

Lactation pain, caused by a combination of breast overfilling, nipple cracking, and ulceration (with occasional fungal or bacterial overgrowth owing to the presence of breast milk "culture media") is treated with breast pumping and occasional antimicrobials.[9] Nipple vasospasm, an unusual but probably underappreciated cause of lactation-related pain, is successfully (and safely, for mother and infant) treated with once-daily *nifedipine* if warm compresses fail to alleviate symptoms.[10]

CYCLIC (PREMENSTRUAL) MASTALGIA

The unclear etiology of cyclic breast pain (i.e. usually presenting during luteal phase and resolving with onset of menses) translates into lack of consensus on treatment of this form of mastalgia. The current focus of therapy is based on use of systemic or topical **NSAIDs**.

A clinical trial found reduction or resolution of cyclic mastalgia with 15 days of therapy with the **COX-2 selective NSAID nimesulide** (100 mg PO BID).[11] *Nimesulide*'s effectiveness is cited by those supporting its use for cyclic mastalgia, but the drug's hepatic side effect risk precludes a recommendation for its use from the ED.[12]

RCT assessment found relief of cyclic (as well as noncyclic) mastalgia with topical application of *diclofenac diethylammonium* (2% gel, 11.6 mg/g, 50 mg *diclofenac* component TID).[4]

Danazol (200 mg PO daily), a **gonadotropin secretion inhibitor** that reduces ovarian estrogen production, is effective in reducing severe, cyclic mastalgia.[13] *Danazol* is FDA-approved for treatment of mastalgia, although it should be used for less than 6 months' duration. Androgenic side effects (e.g. hot flashes, acne, weight gain, GI disturbances) may be reduced by limiting *danazol* administration to the patient's luteal phase (i.e. days 15–25 for a 28 day menstrual cycle).[13]

Selective estrogen receptor modulators such as *tamoxifen* (administered PO) and *afimoxifene* (4-hydroxytamoxifen, applied topically as a gel) may have a role in chronic therapy of mastalgia.[14] At this time, the risks of these agents (e.g. venous thrombosis, gynecologic cancer) are either incompletely characterized (with *afimoxefene*) or outweigh the benefits of therapy as used in the ED setting. Thus, the acute care provider is advised to avoid prescribing the **selective estrogen receptor modulators** for mastalgia.

■ Summary and recommendations

NONCYCLIC MASTALGIA

First line:

- NSAID (e.g. ketorolac 30 mg IV every 6 h)
- topical diclofenac (2% gel, 11.6 mg/g, 50 mg diclofenac component TID)

Reasonable:

- other NSAIDs (e.g. ibuprofen 400–600 mg PO q6–8 h)
- opioids (e.g. hydromorphone 1 mg IV, then titrate)

Pregnancy: acetaminophen (650–1000 mg PO q4–6 h), with as-needed opioid (e.g. hydrocodone 5–10 mg PO q4–6 h)

Pediatric:

- NSAID (e.g. ketorolac 0.25 mg/kg PO q6 h)
- acetaminophen 15 mg/kg PO q4–6 h

Special circumstances:

- *susceptibility to GI NSAID side effects and wish to avoid opioids:* celecoxib (400 mg PO followed by 200 mg PO QD–BID)
- *nipple blanching/vasospasm-mediated mastalgia*: once-daily PO sustained release nifedipine 30 mg

CYCLIC MASTALGIA

First line:

- NSAID (e.g. ibuprofen 400–600 mg PO q6–8 h)
- topical diclofenac (2% gel, 11.6 mg/g, 50 mg diclofenac component TID)

Reasonable:

- danazol (200 mg PO daily)
- opioids (e.g. hydromorphone 5–10 mg PO q4–6 h)

Pregnancy: not applicable

Pediatric: not applicable

References

1. Mahabir RC, Peterson BD, Williamson JS, *et al.* Locally administered ketorolac and bupivacaine for control of postoperative pain in breast augmentation patients. *Plast Reconstr Surg.* 2004;**114**(7):1910–1916.
2. Pavlin DJ, Chen C, Penaloza DA, *et al.* Pain as a factor complicating recovery and discharge after ambulatory surgery. *Anesth Analg.* 2002;**95**(3):627–634, table of contents.

3. Parsa AA, Soon CW, Parsa FD. The use of celecoxib for reduction of pain after subpectoral breast augmentation. *Aesthetic Plast Surg.* 2005;**29**(6):441–444; discussion 445.

4. Colak T, Ipek T, Kanik A, *et al.* Efficacy of topical nonsteroidal antiinflammatory drugs in mastalgia treatment. *J Am Coll Surg.* 2003;**196**(4):525–530.

5. Davis MP, Walsh D, Lagman R, *et al.* Controversies in pharmacotherapy of pain management. *Lancet Oncol.* 2005;**6**(9):696–704.

6. Macdonald R. Steering Committee on Clincal Practice Guidelines for the Care and Treatment of Breast Cancer: the management of chronic pain in patients with breast cancer. *CMAJ.* 1998;**158**:S71–S81.

7. Kampe S, Warm M, Kaufmann J, *et al.* Clinical efficacy of controlled-release oxycodone 20 mg administered on a 12-h dosing schedule on the management of postoperative pain after breast surgery for cancer. *Curr Med Res Opin.* 2004;**20**(2):199–202.

8. Hamed H, Fentiman IS. Benign breast disease. *Int J Clin Pract.* 2001;**55** (7):461–464.

9. Amir LH, Pakula S. Nipple pain, mastalgia and candidiasis in the lactating breast. *Aust N Z J Obstet Gynaecol.* 1991;**31**(4):378–380.

10. Page SM, McKenna DS. Vasospasm of the nipple presenting as painful lactation. *Obstet Gynecol.* 2006;**108**(3, Pt 2):806–808.

11. Gabrielli G, Binazzi P, Scaricabarozzi I, *et al.* Nimesulide in the treatment of mastalgia. *Drugs.* 1992;**46**(Suppl 1):137–139.

12. Rainsford KD. Nimesulide: a multifactorial approach to inflammation and pain: scientific and clinical consensus. *Curr Med Res Opin.* 2006;**22** (6):1161–1170.

13. O'Brien PM, Abukhalil IE. Randomized controlled trial of the management of premenstrual syndrome and premenstrual mastalgia using luteal phase-only danazol. *Am J Obstet Gynecol.* 1999;**180**(1, Pt 1):18–23.

14. Mansel R, Goyal A, Nestour EL, *et al.* A phase II trial of afimoxifene (4-hydroxytamoxifen gel) for cyclical mastalgia in premenopausal women. *Breast Cancer Res Treat.* 2007;**106**(3):389–397.

Burns

JEREMY ACKERMAN AND ADAM J. SINGER

■ Agents

- Opioids
- NSAIDSs
- Topical and IV lidocaine
- Gabapentin
- Benzodiazepines

■ Evidence

Management of burn pain remains difficult and poorly investigated. For all but the most inconsequential of burns, factors such as burn type, burn area, burn depth, and patient demographics are of little help in predicting the pain control requirements. Control of pain from burns in the ED setting is complicated by a high incidence of preexisting intoxication, the need to assess for additional injuries, and concern about the adequacy of ventilation and oxygenation.

Though it may be challenging, pain management in the ED is important for patient comfort acutely, and it may have important implications for the duration of management of the burn injury.[1-3] For those managed on an outpatient basis, providers should keep in mind that many burns cause significant pain in the days after the initial injury, as a result of dressing changes and nerve regeneration.

This chapter focuses primarily on thermal burns, but some brief points about related injuries are warranted. Electrical burns are similar to thermal burns, but special attention should be paid to pain out of proportion to the visualized degree of injury; such unremitting pain may indicate vascular compromise. For chemical burns, decontamination and agent-specific therapy (e.g. *calcium* for hydrofluoric acid exposure) are of paramount importance. For most (but not all) chemical burns, irrigation will reduce pain as well as assist in decontamination. In cold-induced injury (e.g. chilblain, frostbite), the severe pain of rewarming will usually require **NSAID** and **opioid** supplementation of regional analgesia, *nifedipine*, or **prostaglandins**. There is very limited high-quality evidence comparing various therapeutic approaches for cold-induced injury. An animal study suggests that the mechanical allodynia and thermal hyperalgesia associated with frostbite may be ameliorated with **opioids** such as *fentanyl*.[4]

While the burn itself can cause intense pain, thermal injury causes significant local and systemic responses that may both potentiate the pain from additional stimuli and alter the physiologic response to medication. In order to obtain pain relief, patients with burns frequently require higher doses of pain medication than would be needed for other patients with similar pain levels. In addition, anxiety associated with the burn injury and manipulation of the burn during ED evaluation may further increase the patient's pain response.

Although this discussion focuses on pharmacologic approaches to analgesia, burn pain is a case in which adjunctive therapies such as covering and cooling the burn can be critical to optimal pain management.[5-7] Local cooling applied immediately following a burn may contribute significantly to pain relief, in part by reducing further injury to (and pain from) nearby tissue.[8] Optimal cooling is performed by continuous irrigation with tap water, but cooling with saline soaked gauze is far simpler.[9] Either technique is acceptable, as long as care is taken to avoid overzealous cooling that can lead to systemic hypothermia or worsen injury to viable tissue.[10]

A survey of North American burn centers found that IV *morphine* is the most frequently used analgesic for wound care.[11] The survey reported that the most common background pain medications are IV *morphine* and PO *acetaminophen* (*paracetamol*) (with or without *codeine*). Although supporting high-level evidence is lacking, case reports from the USA and other areas with more limited healthcare resources indicate the utility of *ketamine* (e.g. 1.5 mg/kg IV) analgesia for burn care.[12-14]

While minor burn pain may be managed with *acetaminophen* (1 g [or 15 mg/kg in children] every 4–6 h) or **NSAIDs** (e.g. *ibuprofen* 400–800 mg [or 10 mg/kg in children] every 6–8 h), **opioids** are the mainstay of therapy for moderate-to-severe burn-associated pain. The IV route for **opioid** analgesics is preferred over PO administration because of the rapidity and consistency of absorption and onset. This makes titration to an effective dose easier, but care must be taken to provide dosing with appropriate frequency to maintain the analgesic effect (a particular issue if *fentanyl* is used). The fact that control of burn pain often requires relatively higher doses of **opioid** analgesia may be in part related to changes in volume of distribution, protein binding, and clearance.[15]

For some **opioids**, other sites of rapid absorption may also be utilized. For example, IN *fentanyl* has been favorably compared to PO and IV **opioids** for control of procedural pain in burn patients. A small double-blind RCT suggested that IN *fentanyl* (1.4 μg/kg) was as effective as PO *morphine* (1 mg/kg) in reducing the pain of dressing changes in 24 children with burns.[16] Similar results were reported in a study of 26 adult burn patients treated with IN *fentanyl* (1.48 μg/kg) or PO *morphine* (0.35 mg/kg).[17] Preliminary assessment of the use of topical *morphine* for burn analgesia had disappointing results.[18]

A small pilot study of 10 patients suggested that the analgesic qualities of oral *controlled-release morphine* were comparable to those of continuous IV *morphine sulfate* infusions.[19]

In addition to the general risk of respiratory depression with **opioids**, their use in patients with burns may have some association with the immune suppression frequently seen in severely burned patients. However, evidence on this subject is conflicting.[20,21]

Intravenous infusion of *lidocaine* (1 mg/kg bolus followed by 2–4 mg/min infusion) and other **local anesthetics** has also been investigated with some promising results.[22–26] Although timely provision of regional nerve blocks may not be feasible in many ED settings, this approach can provide exceptional relief of burn pain.

Topical application of **local anesthetics** or **opioids** may have salutary effects on local physiology, but this approach has not otherwise been successful, and it is not recommended for pain management.[27]

Anxiolytics, particularly **benzodiazepines**, have been shown to be useful adjuncts to pain therapy in burns. Care must be exercised in administering

opioids and **benzodiazepines** together as they may act synergistically in reducing respiratory drive and causing hypotension as well. *Lorazepam* (1 mg IV or PO) and *midazolam* (IV or IN) are both widely reported for use in burn patients.[28-31]

Several other agents have been investigated for use in controlling burn pain. These agents have primarily been studied for the management of pain in the burn center and for the long-term management of chronic pain sometimes associated with burns. Such agents include *gabapentin*, **stimulants**, **beta-blockers**, **antidepressants**, and **NSAIDs**. While several of these agents have been shown to have an **opioid**-sparing effect, and some agents have additional indications for use in burn patients, there is insufficient evidence to support their routine use in the ED.[32-39]

■ Summary and recommendations

First line: morphine (initial dose 4-6 mg IV, then titrate)

Reasonable: oral opioids (e.g. hydrocodone 5-10 mg PO q4-6 h)

Pregnancy: morphine (initial dose 4-6 mg IV, then titrate)

Pediatric: morphine (initial dose 0.05-0.1 mg/kg IV, then titrate)

Special cases:
- *concern for hemodynamic instability:* fentanyl (initial dose 1-2 µg/kg IV, then titrate)
- *lack of IV access:* transmucosal or IN fentanyl (1-2 µg/kg q1-2 h)
- *burn with amenable anatomic distribution:* regional nerve block with local anesthetic
- *chemical burns:* agent-appropriate irrigation (often with water or saline); specific therapy
- *cold-induced injury:* regional anesthesia (particularly during rewarming); morphine (initial dose 4-6 mg IV, then titrate) and NSAIDs (e.g. ibuprofen 400-600 mg PO q6 h) in addition to "tissue therapy" (calcium channel blockers or prostaglandins)

References

1. Singer AJM, Thode HCJP. National analgesia prescribing patterns in emergency department patients with burns. *J Burn Care Rehabil.* 2002;**23**(6):361–365.

2. Stoddard FJ, Sheridan RL, Saxe GN, *et al.* Treatment of pain in acutely burned children. *J Burn Care Rehabil.* 2002;**23**(2):135–156.

3. Summer GJ, Puntillo KA, Miaskowski C, *et al.* Burn injury pain: the continuing challenge. *J Pain.* 2007;**8**(7):533–548.

4. Ta LE, Dionne RA, Fricton JR, *et al.* SYM-2081, a kainate receptor antagonist, reduces allodynia and hyperalgesia in a freeze injury model of neuropathic pain. *Brain Res.* 2000;**858**(1):106–120.

5. O'Neill AC, Purcell E, Jones D, *et al.* Inadequacies in the first aid management of burns presenting to plastic surgery services. *Ir Med J.* 2005;**98**(1):15–16.

6. Nguyen NL, Gun RT, Sparnon AL, *et al.* The importance of immediate cooling: a case series of childhood burns in Vietnam. *Burns.* 2002;**28**(2):173–176.

7. Gallagher G, Rae CP, Kinsella J. Treatment of pain in severe burns. *Am J Clin Dermatol.* 2000;**1**(6):329–335.

8. Yuan J, Wu C, Harvey JG, *et al.* Assessment of cooling on an acute scald burn injury in a porcine model. *J Burn Care Res.* 2007;**28**(3):514–520.

9. Jandera V, Hudson DA, de Wet PM, *et al.* Cooling the burn wound: evaluation of different modalites. *Burns.* 2000;**26**(3):265–270.

10. Sawada Y, Urushidate S, Yotsuyanagi T, *et al.* Is prolonged and excessive cooling of a scalded wound effective? *Burns.* 1997;**23**(1):55–58.

11. Martin-Herz SP, Patterson DR, Honari S, *et al.* Pediatric pain control practices of North American burn centers. *J Burn Care Rehabil.* 2003;**24**(1):26–36.

12. Batta SK. Low-dose ketamine analgesia for use in under-developed countries. *Anesth Analg.* 2007;**104**(1):232.

13. Owens VF, Palmieri TL, Comroe CM, *et al.* Ketamine: a safe and effective agent for painful procedures in the pediatric burn patient. *J Burn Care Res.* 2006;**27**(2):211–216; discussion 217.

14. Edrich T, Friedrich AD, Eltzschig HK, *et al.* Ketamine for long-term sedation and analgesia of a burn patient. *Anesth Analg.* 2004;**99**(3):893–895; table of contents.

15. Han T, Harmatz JS, Greenblatt DJ, *et al.* Fentanyl clearance and volume of distribution are increased in patients with major burns. *J Clin Pharmacol.* 2007;**47**(6):674–680.

16. Blanda M, Rench T, Gerson LW, *et al.* Intranasal lidocaine for the treatment of migraine headache: a randomized, controlled trial. *Acad Emerg Med.* 2001;**8**(4):337–342.

17. Finn J, Wright J, Fong J, *et al.* A randomised crossover trial of patient controlled intranasal fentanyl and oral morphine for procedural wound care in adult patients with burns. *Burns.* 2004;**30**(3):262–268.

18. Welling A. A randomised controlled trial to test the analgesic efficacy of topical morphine on minor superficial and partial thickness burns in accident and emergency departments. *Emerg Med J.* 2007;**24**(6):408–412.

19. Alexander L, Wolman R, Blache C, *et al.* Use of morphine sulfate (MS Contin) in patients with burns: a pilot study. *J Burn Care Rehabil.* 1992;**13**(5):581–583.

20. Schwacha MG, McGwin G, Jr., Hutchinson CB, *et al.* The contribution of opiate analgesics to the development of infectious complications in burn patients. *Am J Surg.* 2006;**192**(1):82–86.

21. Alexander M, Daniel T, Chaudry IH, *et al.* Opiate analgesics contribute to the development of post-injury immunosuppression. *J Surg Res.* 2005;**129**(1):161–168.

22. Cassuto J, Tarnow P. Potent inhibition of burn pain without use of opiates. *Burns.* 2003;**29**(2):163–166.

23. Dahl JB, Brennum J, Arendt-Nielsen L, *et al.* The effect of pre- versus post-injury infiltration with lidocaine on thermal and mechanical hyperalgesia after heat injury to the skin. *Pain.* 1993;**53**(1):43–51.

24. Holthusen H, Irsfeld S, Lipfert P. Effect of pre- or post-traumatically applied i.v. lidocaine on primary and secondary hyperalgesia after experimental heat trauma in humans. *Pain.* 2000;**88**(3):295–302.

25. Jonsson A, Cassuto J, Hanson B. Inhibition of burn pain by intravenous lignocaine infusion. *Lancet.* 1991;**338**(8760):151–152.

26. Mattsson U, Cassuto J, Tarnow P, *et al.* Intravenous lidocaine infusion in the treatment of experimental human skin burns: digital colour image analysis of erythema development. *Burns.* 2000;**26**(8):710–715.

27. Jonsson A, Brofeldt BT, Nellgard P, *et al.* Local anesthetics improve dermal perfusion after burn injury. *J Burn Care Rehabil.* 1998;**19**(1, Pt 1):50–56.

28. Carrougher GJ, Ptacek JT, Honari S, *et al.* Self-reports of anxiety in burn-injured hospitalized adults during routine wound care. *J Burn Care Res.* 2006;**27**(5):676–681.

29. Ratcliff SL, Brown A, Rosenberg L, *et al.* The effectiveness of a pain and anxiety protocol to treat the acute pediatric burn patient. *Burns.* 2006;**32**(5):554–562.

30. Patterson DR, Ptacek JT, Carrougher GJ, *et al.* Lorazepam as an adjunct to opioid analgesics in the treatment of burn pain. *Pain.* 1997;**72**(3):367–374.

31. Rice TL, Kyff JV. Intranasal administration of midazolam to a severely burned child. *Burns.* 1990;**16**(4):307–308.

32. Werner MU, Perkins FM, Holte K, *et al.* Effects of gabapentin in acute inflammatory pain in humans. *Reg Anesth Pain Med.* 2001;**26**(4):322–328.

33. Cuignet O, Pirson J, Soudon O, *et al.* Effects of gabapentin on morphine consumption and pain in severely burned patients. *Burns.* 2007;**33**(1):81–86.

34. Pereira CT, Jeschke MG, Herndon DN. Beta-blockade in burns. *Novartis Found Symp.* 2007;**280**:238–248; discussion 248–251.

35. Aarsland A, Chinkes D, Wolfe RR, *et al.* Beta-blockade lowers peripheral lipolysis in burn patients receiving growth hormone. Rate of hepatic very low density lipoprotein triglyceride secretion remains unchanged. *Ann Surg.* 1996;**223**(6):777–787; discussion 787–779.

36. Enkhbaatar P, Murakami K, Shimoda K, *et al.* Ketorolac attenuates cardiopulmonary derangements in sheep with combined burn and smoke inhalation injury. *Clin Sci (Lond).* 2003;**105**(5):621–628.

37. Tan Q, Lin Z, Ma W, *et al.* Failure of Ibuprofen to prevent progressive dermal ischemia after burning in guinea pigs. *Burns.* 2002;**28**(5):443–448.

38. Barrow RE, Ramirez RJ, Zhang XJ. Ibuprofen modulates tissue perfusion in partial-thickness burns. *Burns.* 2000;**26**(4):341–346.

39. Petersen KL, Brennum J, Dahl JB. Experimental evaluation of the analgesic effect of ibuprofen on primary and secondary hyperalgesia. *Pain.* 1997;**70**(2–3):167–174.

Bursitis and periarticular inflammation

NATHANAEL WOOD AND JOHN H. BURTON

■ Agents

- ■ NSAIDs
- ■ Corticosteroids
- ■ Local anesthetics
- ■ Hyaluronate

■ Evidence

There are few rigorously conducted clinical trials assessing specific therapy for nonseptic bursitis. In fact, many "bursitis" studies actually include patients with various related periarticular inflammatory disorders (e.g. bursitis, capsulitis, tendinitis). First-line treatments of nonseptic bursitis include **NSAIDs**, aspiration, and injection therapy with **corticosteroids** and **local anesthetics**. Disease processes in the periarticular regions (e.g. epicondylitis) are usually treated with **NSAIDs**, in similar fashion to the recommendations outlined for bursitis. Some periarticular conditions warranting special mention are included in the following discussion.

With regard to systemic drug therapy, **NSAIDs** are the analgesic mainstay, with much of the available evidence addressing use of *diclofenac*. An illustrative study examined patients with acute shoulder tendinitis or bursitis and showed that nearly all patients (90%) had pain reduction after two weeks of *diclofenac* (50 mg PO BID or TID, with *misoprostol* added for GI protection).[1] An RCT enrolling patients who failed with other **NSAIDs** found that once-daily PO *oxaprozin* (1200 mg) provided pain relief equivalent to that achieved by PO *diclofenac* TID (50 mg per dose); patients receiving *oxaprozin* showed improved overall function scores on a variety of measures.[2] Results for periarticular inflammation other than bursitis are similar to the findings for bursitis. For example, Cochrane review of lateral epicondylitis trials found no evidence of difference between **NSAIDs**, or for use of topical rather than PO **NSAIDs**.[3]

The treatment of patellofemoral pain syndrome has been overviewed in a 2004 Cochrane review.[4] Notable from the report are findings that while there is no difference in pain relief achieved with *diflunisal* or *naproxen*, *aspirin* is no better than placebo for pain relief in this indication.[4]

For patients with shoulder bursitis, oral **corticosteroids** (*prednisolone*, 30 mg PO QD) provide early improvement over placebo, but treatment benefit is lost after the first few weeks of therapy.[5]

There are no RCTs that demonstrate a therapeutic difference between nonselective **NSAIDs** and **COX-2 selective NSAIDs**.[6–9] Patients treated for a week with either *celecoxib* (400 mg PO followed by 200 mg PO BID) or *naproxen* (500 mg PO BID) experienced similar pain relief benefit over placebo.[6] After a more prolonged treatment period (14 days), patients receiving *celecoxib*, but not those taking *naproxen*, maintained pain score reductions exceeding those seen in patients taking placebo.[6] Two studies assessing short-term treatment of bursitis and tendinitis showed therapeutic equivalence for the **COX-2 selective NSAID** *nimesulide* (100 mg PO BID), *diclofenac* (75 mg PO BID), and *naproxen* (500 mg PO BID).[8,9] Issues regarding **COX-2 selective NSAIDs** and cardiovascular toxicity, which may be relevant even to the ED provider prescribing a short course of therapy, are discussed in detail in the Arthritis chapter (p. 94).

Evidence addressing use of topical agents for bursitis is sparse. *Diclofenac epolamine* (*2-hydroxyethyl-pyrrolidine*, *DHEP*), an enhanced-permeation lecithin-enriched *diclofenac* salt gel, shows potential for clinical utility. An RCT assessing a 10 day (TID) course of 1.3% gel for shoulder or elbow inflammatory pain found a persistent and significant pain score improvement, although rescue medication need was not reduced compared with placebo.[10]

Once septic bursitis has been excluded, intrabursal **corticosteroid** injections are recommended for acute management. Injection therapy is particularly useful for bursitis of the elbow, knee, and shoulder; subacromial injection results are improved with ultrasound guidance.[11] Hip and ankle injections may be useful, but the former are technically difficult and the latter risk steroid-associated Achilles tendon rupture. Other areas of inflammation, such as the wrist or anserine bursae, may be amenable to **corticosteroid**

Injection but performance of such injections in the acute care setting is uncommon, in part owing to technical difficulties.[12,13] No more than two injections (per bursa) should be administered during a single episode of bursitis.

Many **corticosteroids** have demonstrated effectiveness for injection of subacromial inflammation. *Triamcinolone* (20 mg) provides persistent pain relief that is additive to that achieved by outpatient physical therapy.[14] Cochrane review of literature addressing pain relief in patients with lateral epicondylitis ("tennis elbow") concluded that **corticosteroid** injection provides better short-term analgesia than oral **NSAIDs.**[3]

The most relevant RCT investigating intrabursal injections for olecranon bursitis demonstrated improved clinical response from combination therapy with intrabursal *methylprednisolone* (20 mg) and oral *naproxen* (500 mg PO bid for 10 days), compared with monotherapy with PO *naproxen* or placebo.[15]

For trochanteric bursitis, studies investigating intrabursal injection of **corticosteroids** have found efficacy similar to that reported for other bursal injection sites.[16-18] For example, one investigation found benefit in two thirds to three quarters of patients after injection of *betamethasone* (6, 12, or 24 mg) mixed with 4 mL of 1% *lidocaine*; the higher response rates are seen with the higher doses of **corticosteroid**.[16]

Radiographic guidance (i.e. fluoroscopy) significantly improves the success rates of injection therapy for trochanteric injection.[19] Fluoroscopy may also be necessary to guide **corticosteroid** injection for bursitis in unusual locations (e.g. interspinous).[20]

Adjuvant therapy with *sodium hyaluronidate* (20 mg injected into the bursa) may be useful in the long-term management of bursitis, but in the acute care setting is unnecessary.[21]

A wide variety of medical conditions, each with disease-specific therapy, can predispose patients to bursitis and related inflammatory conditions. One long-recognized and commonly encountered medication-related etiology of subacromial inflammation is the use of protease inhibitors (e.g. indinavir, lamivudine).[22] Given the obvious risks in altering these medication regimens, the ED provider should reduce dosages only after consultation with patients' physicians.

■ Summary and recommendations

First line: NSAID (e.g. naproxen 500 mg PO BID)

Reasonable: aspiration and intrabursal injection (e.g. with methylprednisolone 20 mg plus 1–4 mL 1% lidocaine)

Pregnancy:

- NSAIDs should generally be avoided; therefore, injection therapy would be appropriate in cases of failure of acetaminophen (1000 mg PO q4–6 h);
- corticosteroid can be used with clinician discretion injection; injection of corticosteroids for bursitis treatment in pregnant patients is standard practice at the Massachusetts General Hospital; the low-range dose of steroids is recommended (e.g. betamethasone 6 mg *plus* 4 mL 1% lidocaine)

Pediatric: NSAIDs (e.g. ibuprofen 5–10 mg/kg PO q6–8 h)

Special cases:

- *calcaneal bursitis*: avoid intrabursal infiltration
- *possible septic bursitis*: corticosteroid injection contraindicated
- *subacromial inflammation in patients taking protease inhibitors* (e.g. *indinavir, lamivudine*): consult longitudinal care physician regarding medication alteration
- *favorable GI/cardiovascular risk profile*: COX-2 selective NSAID (e.g. celecoxib 200 mg PO BID)

References

1. Zuinan C. Diclofenac/misoprostol vs diclofenac/placebo in treating acute episodes of tendinitis/bursitis of the shoulder. *Drug*. 1993;**45**:12–23.
2. Heller B, Tarricone R. Oxaprozin versus diclofenac in NSAID-refractory periarthritis pain of the shoulder. *Curr Med Res Opin*. 2004;**20**:1279–1290.
3. Green S, Buchbinder R, Barnsley L, *et al*. Non-steroidal anti-inflammatory drugs (NSAIDs) for treating lateral elbow pain in adults. *Cochrane Database Syst Rev*. 2002(4):CD003686.
4. Heintjes E, Berger MY, Bierma-Zeinstra SM, *et al*. Pharmacotherapy for patellofemoral pain syndrome. *Cochrane Database Syst Rev*. 2004(3):CD003470.

5. Buchbinder R, Hoving JL, Green S, *et al.* Short course prednisolone for adhesive capsulitis (frozen shoulder or stiff painful shoulder): a randomised, double blind, placebo controlled trial. *Ann Rheum Dis.* 2004;**63**:1460–1469.

6. Petri M, Hufman SL, Waser G, *et al.* Celecoxib effectively treats patients with acute shoulder tendinitis/bursitis. *J Rheumatol.* 2004;**31**:1614–1620.

7. Bertin P, Behier JM, Noel E, *et al.* Celecoxib is as efficacious as naproxen in the management of acute shoulder pain. *J Int Med Res.* 2003;**31**:102–112.

8. Wober W, Rahlfs VW, Buchl N, *et al.* Comparative efficacy and safety of the non-steroidal anti-inflammatory drugs nimesulide and diclofenac in patients with acute subdeltoid bursitis and bicipital tendinitis. *Int J Clin Pract.* 1998;**52**:169–175.

9. Lecomte J, Buyse H, Taymans J, *et al.* Treatment of tendinitis and bursitis: a comparison of nimesulide and naproxen sodium in a double blind parallel trial. *Eur J Rheumatol Inflamm.* 1994;**14**:29–32.

10. Spacca G, Cacchio A, Forgacs A, *et al.* Analgesic efficacy of a lecithin-vehiculated diclofenac epolamine gel in shoulder periarthritis and lateral epicondylitis: a placebo-controlled, multicenter, randomized, double-blind clinical trial. *Drugs Exp Clin Res.* 2005;**31**:147–154.

11. Chen MJ, Lew HL, Hsu TC, *et al.* Ultrasound-guided shoulder injections in the treatment of subacromial bursitis. *Am J Phys Med Rehabil.* 2006;**85**:31–35.

12. Hahn P, Schmitt R. [Bursitis of the ulnar recess.] *Handchir Mikrochir Plast Chir.* 2000;**32**:375–378.

13. Kang I, Han SW. Anserine bursitis in patients with osteoarthritis of the knee. *South Med J.* 2000;**93**:207–209

14. Ryans I, Montgomery A, Galway R, *et al.* A randomized controlled trial of intra-articular triamcinolone and/or physiotherapy in shoulder capsulitis. *Rheumatology (Oxford).* 2005;**44**:529–535.

15. Smith DL, McAfee JH, Lucas LM, *et al.* Treatment of nonseptic olecranon bursitis. A controlled, blinded prospective trial. *Arch Intern Med.* 1989;**149**:2527–2530.

16. Shbeeb MI, O'Duffy JD, Michet CJ, Jr., *et al.* Evaluation of glucocorticosteroid injection for the treatment of trochanteric bursitis. *J Rheumatol.* 1996;**23**:2104–2106.

17. Ege Rasmussen KJ, Fano N. Trochanteric bursitis. Treatment by corticosteroid injection. *Scand J Rheumatol.* 1985;**14**:417–420.

18. Schapira D, Nahir M, Scharf Y. Trochanteric bursitis: a common clinical problem. *Arch Phys Med Rehabil.* 1986;**67**:815–817.

19. Cohen SP, Narvaez JC, Lebovits AH, *et al.* Corticosteroid injections for trochanteric bursitis: is fluoroscopy necessary? A pilot study. *Br J Anaesth.* 2005;**94**:100–106.

20. DePalma MJ, Slipman CW, Siegelman E, *et al.* Interspinous bursitis in an athlete. *J Bone Joint Surg Br.* 2004;**86**:1062–1064.

21. Rovetta G, Monteforte P. Intraarticular injection of sodium hyaluronate plus steroid versus steroid in adhesive capsulitis of the shoulder. *Int J Tissue React.* 1998;**20**:125–130.

22. Leone J, Beguinot I, Dehlinger V, *et al.* Adhesive capsulitis of the shoulder induced by protease inhibitor therapy. Three new cases. *Rev Rhum Engl Ed.* 1998;**65**:800–801.

Cancer and tumor pain

MICHAEL WALTA AND STEPHEN H. THOMAS

■ Agents

- NSAIDs
- Opioids
- Anticonvulsants
- Antidepressants
- Local anesthetics
- Neuroleptics
- *N*-Methyl-ᴅ-aspartate (NMDA) antagonists
- Bisphosphonates
- Calcitonin
- Corticosteroids
- Octreotide
- Anticholinergic drugs

■ Evidence

Cancer and tumor pain (CTP) is traditionally described as resulting from somatic, visceral, or neuropathic origins.[1] Somatic pain is believed to result from stimulation of peripheral nociceptors by direct tumor invasion or compression (e.g. as occurs in bone metastases). Visceral pain is thought to result from ischemia, inflammation, or direct mechanical stimulation produced by an invading tumor; visceral nociceptor stimulation is associated with a classic radiating pain with accompanying nausea and diaphoresis.[2] Neuropathic pain is produced by a tumor's direct compression and stimulation of nerve fibers, producing pain that is often described as burning or lancinating.[3] The ED physician should keep in mind that non-analgesic approaches may be needed for some causes of oncologic pain (e.g. hypercalcemia).

Clinical practice with respect to CTP management historically followed this taxonomy of pain origin. **NSAIDs** have been deemed the preferred class for bony (or somatic) pain. **Opioids** have been considered beneficial for visceral, but not bony or neuropathic CTP.[1] In recent years, pain severity has supplanted CTP type as the primary determinant of analgesic therapy. Pain is treated as recommended by the World Health Organization (WHO) "analgesic ladder." The evolution of pain treatment guided by pain level is an important step in the right direction for a number of reasons. At least two are noteworthy. First, some cancers may simultaneously cause different types of pain (e.g. breast cancer with bony and solid organ metastases). Second, the clinician's focus on relieving pain should not be overly distracted by concerns about its categorization – which may not be easy.

The WHO ladder emphasizes the stepwise titration of scheduled doses of **NSAIDs**, to which are added first mild **opioids** (e.g. *hydrocodone*) and then more potent agents (e.g. *morphine, fentanyl*). The WHO model also encourages the use of adjuvant medications, as discussed below. While the WHO approach is reasonable for CTP, it should be noted that no trials have compared the efficacy of **NSAIDs** with **opioids** as the initial CTP analgesic therapy.[4]

For a variety of reasons, CTP therapy should be coordinated with longitudinal care providers. Most importantly, there is obvious benefit in having patients' physicians aware of changes in pain management plans. Additionally, discussion of therapeutic alternatives may benefit the ED provider less experienced with CTP pharmacotherapy. Some approaches discussed here (e.g. **bisphosphonates**, transmucosal *fentanyl*) lie outside the daily use patterns of most acute care providers. Even for those drugs ED physicians are accustomed to using, some of this chapter's recommended regimens (e.g. high-dose or sustained-release **opioids**) may be unfamiliar.

NSAIDs AND OPIOIDS

NSAIDs' efficacy in controlling mild CTP is demonstrated in at least eight RCTs, overviewed by the National Cancer Institute (NCI) and by the Cochrane Collaboration.[4,5] On a 10-point scale, the average CTP pain score reductions achieved with **NSAIDs** were 2–3 points better than placebo.[4]

Neither NCI nor Cochrane reviews find evidence to favor one **NSAID** over another for CTP. Conclusions as to **NSAIDs**' broad equivalence are based on 14 head-to-head trials of the following PO medications: *ketorolac* (60–90 mg/day), *naproxen* (550 mg/day), *ketoprofen* (400 mg/day), *aspirin* (600–1000 mg/day), *indomethacin* (100 mg/day), *diflunisal* (500–1000 mg/ day), and *ibuprofen* (1600–2400 mg/day). No trial shows that parental administration of **NSAIDs** is superior to PO administration.[5]

The **COX-2 selective NSAIDs piroxicam** (20 mg/day) and *nimesulide* (200 mg/day) are no more effective than nonselective **NSAIDs** for CTP; there is little or no role for these agents in ED management.[5] The safety issues with respect to **COX-2 selective NSAIDs** are outlined in more detail in the Arthritis chapter (p. 94).

There are mixed results from combination therapy with **NSAIDs** plus **opioids** in treating CTP, but the aggregate data suggest little synergism between these two classes. Data from at least 25 trials compare **NSAID** monotherapy with a dual-drug approach combining **NSAIDs** and **opioids** (either weak or strong agents). Addition of the **opioid** to **NSAIDs** is found to accrue only a modest analgesic improvement over monotherapy with either class.[4,6–8] These results cast some doubt, at least in CTP, on the value of the WHO-endorsed strategy of adding **NSAIDs** to **opioids** for added effect. The short duration of nearly all of the existing studies improves their relevance to the ED setting, but it also leaves uncertainty about whether **NSAIDs** are effective for long-term CTP management.[5,9]

Opioids have been extensively studied. On the standard 10-point pain scale, this class achieves moderate (4–6 units) to substantial (> 6 units) pain score reductions over those achieved by placebo.[4,10,11] Since the trials have involved titrating the **opioid** to effect, the studies lack uniformity with respect to dosage strength, schedule, or routes of administration.

The following **opioids** are effective, with no analgesic advantage demonstrated by any particular agent: PO *morphine* (30–90 mg every 3–6 h), IV *morphine* (10–30 mg every 3–4 h), PO controlled-release *morphine* (180–240 mg/day), PO *hydromorphone* (7.5 mg every 3–4 h), IV *hydromorphone* (1.5 mg every 3–4 h), PO levophenol (2 mg every 4–6 h), IV levophenol (4 mg every 4–6 h), IV *meperidine* (*pethidine*; 100 mg every 3 h), PO *methadone*

(20 mg every 4–6 h), IV *methadone* (10 mg every 4–6 h), PO *codeine* (180–200 mg every 3–4 h), IV *codeine* (75 mg every 3–4 h), PO *oxycodone* (30 mg every 3–4 h).[12] The dosages may seem high to the ED provider, but concerns about toxicity and addiction tend to be exaggerated, especially in patients who are not **opioid** naïve. Physicians in ED should be prepared to prescribe **opioids** in dosages that work.

Nearly all studies (28 of 29 RCTs in one review) fail to identify a safety or efficacy advantage of one route of **opioid** administration over others.[4] One of the few major differences is the IV route's advantage of shorter time to analgesia onset.[13]

Some trials address utility of agents that are not traditionally considered **opioids** but which have some **opioid** agonism. Available data do not support use of these agents at this time. As an example, *proglumide* (50 mg/day), a **cholecystokinin (CCK) antagonist** with some mu activity, provides no more pain relief than placebo when assessed as add-on therapy to a baseline **opioid** CTP regimen.[14]

No data specifically address the efficacy of long-term **opioid** use.[15] At least eight clinical trials of PO **opioid** analgesics have compared controlled-release with immediate-release *morphine*. Neither formulation demonstrates analgesic superiority as defined by pain relief onset or duration. The consistent finding of decreased dosing frequency accomplished by controlled-release formulations is the principle advantage of these dosage forms.[16]

There is one **opioid**, *methadone*, that is less preferred than other mu agonists. Even though *methadone* provides useful pain relief and has an overall side effect profile (when used appropriately) similar to that of other mu agonists, we do not recommend its use in acute care. The problem, as highlighted in a 2004 Cochrane review, is that most studies demonstrating *methadone*'s safety and efficacy assessed only brief therapeutic courses.[11] Longer-term use is associated with risk of drug buildup and unwanted side effects. The pharmacokinetics of *methadone* render use of the drug problematic, with initiation and titration of the drug best left to those with experience in its monitoring.[11] There is no evidence to support contentions that *methadone* has any effectiveness (compared with other **opioids**) in CTP, including neuropathy.[11]

Breakthrough pain is defined as intense episodic pain thought to result from a decrease in circulating levels of longer-acting (controlled-release) **opioids**. The current management of breakthrough pain tends to be prescription of a shorter-acting rescue **opioid** to supplement the longer-acting regimen. A 2006 Cochrane review identified a promising approach, involving OTM *fentanyl* for breakthrough pain. Head-to-head trial data show that, compared with immediate-release PO *morphine* (15–60 mg/dose), OTM *fentanyl* (200–1600 µg/dose) is superior in both pain relief and time to onset of action (about 5–10 min).[17,18]

ADJUVANT MEDICATIONS

Drugs other than analgesics are often of utility in the oncology setting. While agents such as sedatives may be helpful in patient management, the adjuvant medications discussed here are those believed to augment efficacy of coadministered **opioids** or **NSAIDs**. Adjuncts are tailored depending on the mechanism-based classification of CTP, as outlined in this chapter's introduction. Medications that have been specifically advocated for neuropathic CTP include **anticonvulsants**, **local anesthetics**, and **N-methyl-D-aspartate (NMDA) receptor antagonists**. Bony pain is treated with *calcitonin* and **bisphosphonates**. Studies focusing on bowel obstruction symptoms have tested utility of **corticosteroids**, *octreotide*, and **anticholinergics**. Cancer-related muscle pain is often treated with *cyclobenzaprine*, *baclofen*, and **benzodiazepines**, but there are no data supporting specific utility of these agents in CTP.[19] In general, use of adjuvants to treat CTP follows the patterns outlined in other chapters of this text (e.g. Neuropathy). This chapter presents some topics with specificity to CTP.

Although **antidepressants** are frequently prescribed for CTP, scant evidence exists to support their use.[19] In one clinical trial, *trazadone* (100 mg/day) and *amitriptyline* (50–150 mg/day) were found of borderline assistance for relieving neuropathic CTP in patients taking **opioids**.[20] Another trial including patients with neuropathic CTP found *trazadone* (100 mg/day) and *amitriptyline* (50–150 mg/day) to be similarly beneficial.[4] The ED provider should be wary prescribing **antidepressants** to patients with CTP. The existing evidence fails to demonstrate this class' safety with respect to side effects such as orthostasis or cardiotoxicity in CTP patients, who often have significant comorbidities.[19]

Anticonvulsants are frequently used as an adjunct for the treatment of neuropathic CTP. In one trial of 121 patients with neuropathic CTP, *gabapentin* (600–1800 mg/day) reduced pain scores to a degree (0.8 units on a 10-point scale) that was statistically, but not clinically, significant.[21] Overviewing evidence from this and other trials in which *gabapentin* was found of some utility in neuropathic CTP, a 2005 Cochrane review concluded that *gabapentin* is efficacious for oncologic neuropathy (but not for non-neuropathic CTP).[22]

At least two studies have assessed **local anesthetics** as adjuvant agents for neuropathic CTP. *Lidocaine* (5 mg/kg infused IV over 30 min) has not been found effective for cancer-related neuropathic pain in two clinical trials (one was an RCT).[23,24]

One trial of mixed-etiology CTP compared *phenytoin* (50 mg/dose), sublingual *buprenorphine* (0.2 mg/dose), and combination therapy with both agents. The results indicated that addition of *phenytoin* to the **opioid** achieved no significant analgesic benefit.[25]

There are inadequate data to support the use of **neuroleptics** in the treatment of CTP of various causes. The available evidence is from small studies. For acute care management of CTP, concerns with side effects currently outweigh any likely benefit of agents such as *olanzapine* (studied in doses of 2.5–7.5 mg/day).[26,27]

Among the **NMDA receptor antagonists**, *ketamine* has been studied most extensively (often for neuropathic pain). Results are mixed. In an open-label trial of PO *ketamine* (100–500 mg/day) given to patients with refractory CTP over three to five days, three quarters were found to have pain score improvement but nearly half had significant unpleasant side effects (e.g. hallucinations, confusion).[28] Another study of PO *ketamine* (0.5 mg/kg per dose) given three times daily had similar results: significant pain reduction with a high rate of unacceptable side effects.[29] One assessment of IV *ketamine* (0.25–0.50 mg/kg per dose) as an adjuvant to *morphine* found borderline pain relief efficacy, but a high (60%) rate of emergence symptoms.[30] Another trial of *ketamine* (1 mg/kg daily) administered via a TD *nitroglycerin (glyceryl trinitrate)* polymer patch (5 mg/day) found that this novel approach significantly reduced the requirements for oral morphine.[31] Overall, the use of *ketamine* for acute care management of CTP would seem limited by side effects, but there may be a role for the **NMDA receptor antagonist** in refractory cases.

Aggregate evidence from three trials comparing the CNS stimulant *methylphenidate* (2.5–5 mg/day) with placebo showed no benefit of *methylphenidate* for CTP.[4]

For bone pain, **bisphosphonates**, in particular *pamidronate* (90–120 mg/dose) and *zoledronic acid* (4 mg/dose), are shown in multiple trials to be effective in reducing bony CTP from metastatic disease.[19] Cochrane review in 2002 concluded that there is an analgesic role for **bisphosphonates** in relieving bony cancer pain, but that the role of this class lies outside the realm of acute pain relief.[32] Rather, the **bisphosphonates** are found to be of potential use when other analgesic regimens (including radiotherapy) fail.[32]

Calcitonin (100 units/day SC) provides marginal, if any, relief in patients with metastatic bone pain.[33] Although one dated trial found *calcitonin* (200 units/day SC) reduced bony pain, a 2006 Cochrane review concluded that *calcitonin* neither relieves bony pain nor reduces need for **opioids**.[34,35]

Gastrointestinal CTP is commonly encountered and inoperable bowel obstruction is a significant source of patient discomfort. Some agents have been found helpful. While **corticosteroids** are, at best, marginally effective as an **opioid**-sparing adjunct for CTP in general, this class may have a role in tumor-related bowel obstruction.[46] A 2000 Cochrane review showed a tendency towards pain relief in malignant bowel obstruction with administration of IV *dexamethasone* (6–16 mg/dose).[37] Other cancer-related uses of **corticosteroids** (e.g. in steroid-responsive tumors) fall outside this review's scope.

The **antisecretory** agents aim to relieve bowel obstruction CTP, and also to eliminate the need for uncomfortable nasogastric tubes. The most useful such agent is *octreotide* IV (600–800 µg/day), which significantly relieves pain from inoperable malignant bowel obstruction.[23,38] Some efficacy is also likely with the **antisecretory** drug *butylscopolamine (hyoscine butylbromide*; 60 mg/day).[23]

■ Summary and recommendations

First line:

- NSAID (e.g. ibuprofen 400–600 mg PO q6 h)
- oxycodone (5–10 mg PO q6 h; higher dose may be needed if patient is opioid tolerant)

Reasonable: short-course combination therapy with opioids (e.g. oxycodone 5–10 mg PO q4–6 h) and NSAIDs (e.g. ibuprofen 400–600 mg PO q6 h)

Pregnancy: opioid (e.g. oxycodone 5–10 mg PO q4–6 h)

Pediatric:

- NSAIDs (e.g. ibuprofen 10 mg/kg q6–8 h)
- Opioids (e.g. oxycodone 0.1–0.3 mg/kg PO q6 h)

Special cases:

- *for severe rapid-onset (breakthrough) pain*: IV opioids (e.g. morphine initial dose 4–6 mg IV, then titrate) or oral transmucosal fentanyl (200 µg)
- *cancer-related neuropathy*: gabapentin (300 mg PO day one, then 300 mg PO BID day two, then 300 mg PO TID)
- *refractory bone pain*: pamidronate (90–120 mg IV) or other bisphosphonate
- *bowel obstruction in cancer*: steroids (dexamethasone 10 mg IV), octreotide (25 µg/h IV)

References

1. Meldrum ML. A capsule history of pain management. *JAMA*. 2003;**290**(18):2470–2475.
2. Alter CL. Palliative and supportive care of patients with pancreatic cancer. *Semin Oncol*. 1996;**23**(2):229–240.
3. Weinstein SM. Phantom pain. *Oncology (Williston Park)*. 1994;**8**(3):65–70; discussion 70, 73–74.
4. Carr DB, Goudas LC, Balk EM, *et al*. Evidence report on the treatment of pain in cancer patients. *J Natl Cancer Inst Monogr*. 2004(32):23–31.

5. McNicol E, Strassels SA, Goudas L, *et al.* NSAIDS or paracetamol, alone or combined with opioids, for cancer pain. *Cochrane Database Syst Rev.* 2005(1): CD005180.

6. Frankendal B. [Clinical testing of a new analgesic combination on cancer patients in chronic pain.] *Lakartidningen.* 1973;**70**(10):949–951.

7. Stambaugh JE, Jr., Drew J. The combination of ibuprofen and oxycodone/ acetaminophen in the management of chronic cancer pain. *Clin Pharmacol Ther.* 1988;**44**(6):665–669.

8. Stockler M, Vardy J, Pillai A, *et al.* Acetaminophen (paracetamol) improves pain and well-being in people with advanced cancer already receiving a strong opioid regimen: a randomized, double-blind, placebo-controlled cross-over trial. *J Clin Oncol.* 2004;**22**(16):3389–3394.

9. Jenkins CA, Bruera E. Nonsteroidal anti-inflammatory drugs as adjuvant analgesics in cancer patients. *Palliat Med.* 1999;**13**(3):183–196.

10. Wiffen PJ, Edwards JE, Barden J, *et al.* Oral morphine for cancer pain. *Cochrane Database Syst Rev.* 2003(4):CD003868.

11. Nicholson AB. Methadone for cancer pain. *Cochrane Database Syst Rev.* 2004 (2):CD003971.

12. Quigley C. Hydromorphone for acute and chronic pain. *Cochrane Database Syst Rev.* 2002(1):CD003447.

13. Jacox A, Carr DB, Payne R. New clinical-practice guidelines for the management of pain in patients with cancer. *N Engl J Med.* 1994;**330**(9):651–655.

14. Bernstein ZP, Yucht S, Battista E, *et al.* Proglumide as a morphine adjunct in cancer pain management. *J Pain Symptom Manage.* 1998;**15**(5):314–320.

15. Hojsted J, Sjogren P. Addiction to opioids in chronic pain patients: a literature review. *Eur J Pain.* 2007;**11**(5):490–518.

16. Goudas L, Carr DB, Bloch R, *et al.* Management of cancer pain. *Evid Rep Technol Assess (Summ).* 2001(35):1–5.

17. Zeppetella G, Ribeiro MD. Opioids for the management of breakthrough (episodic) pain in cancer patients. *Cochrane Database Syst Rev.* 2006(1):CD004311.

18. Fine PG, Streisand JB. A review of oral transmucosal fentanyl citrate: potent, rapid and noninvasive opioid analgesia. *J Palliat Med.* 1998;**1**(1):55–63.

19. Lussier D, Huskey AG, Portenoy RK. Adjuvant analgesics in cancer pain management. *Oncologist.* 2004;**9**(5):571–591.

20. Ventafridda V, Bonezzi C, Caraceni A, *et al.* Antidepressants for cancer pain and other painful syndromes with deafferentation component: comparison of amitriptyline and trazodone. *Ital J Neurol Sci.* 1987;**8**(6):579–587.

21. Caraceni A, Zecca E, Bonezzi C, *et al.* Gabapentin for neuropathic cancer pain: a randomized controlled trial from the Gabapentin Cancer Pain Study Group. *J Clin Oncol.* 2004;**22**(14):2909–2917.

22. Wiffen PJ, McQuay HJ, Edwards JE, *et al.* Gabapentin for acute and chronic pain. *Cochrane Database Syst Rev.* 2005(3):CD005452.

23. Bruera E, Ripamonti C, Brenneis C, *et al.* A randomized double-blind crossover trial of intravenous lidocaine in the treatment of neuropathic cancer pain. *J Pain Symptom Manage.* 1992;**7**(3):138–140.

24. Ellemann K, Sjogren P, Banning AM, *et al.* Trial of intravenous lidocaine on painful neuropathy in cancer patients. *Clin J Pain.* 1989;**5**(4):291–294.

25. Yajnik S, Singh GP, Singh G, *et al.* Phenytoin as a coanalgesic in cancer pain. *J Pain Symptom Manage.* 1992;**7**(4):209–213.

26. Khojainova N, Santiago-Palma J, Kornick C, *et al.* Olanzapine in the management of cancer pain. *J Pain Symptom Manage.* 2002;**23**(4): 346–350.

27. Patt RB, Proper G, Reddy S. The neuroleptics as adjuvant analgesics. *J Pain Symptom Manage.* 1994;**9**(7):446–453.

28. Jackson K, Ashby M, Martin P, *et al.* "Burst" ketamine for refractory cancer pain: an open-label audit of 39 patients. *J Pain Symptom Manage.* 2001;**22** (4):834–842.

29. Kannan TR, Saxena A, Bhatnagar S, *et al.* Oral ketamine as an adjuvant to oral morphine for neuropathic pain in cancer patients. *J Pain Symptom Manage.* 2002;**23**(1):60–65.

30. Mercadante S, Arcuri E, Tirelli W, *et al.* Analgesic effect of intravenous ketamine in cancer patients on morphine therapy: a randomized, controlled, double-blind, crossover, double-dose study. *J Pain Symptom Manage.* 2000;**20**(4):246–252.

31. Lauretti GR, Lima IC, Reis MP, *et al.* Oral ketamine and transdermal nitroglycerin as analgesic adjuvants to oral morphine therapy for cancer pain management. *Anesthesiology.* 1999;**90**(6):1528–1533.

32. Wong R, Wiffen PJ. Bisphosphonates for the relief of pain secondary to bone metastases. *Cochrane Database Syst Rev.* 2002(2):CD002068.

33. Roth A, Kolaric K. Analgetic activity of calcitonin in patients with painful osteolytic metastases of breast cancer. Results of a controlled randomized study. *Oncology.* 1986;**43**(5):283–287.

34. Martinez-Zapata MJ, Roque M, Alonso-Coello P, *et al.* Calcitonin for metastatic bone pain. *Cochrane Database Syst Rev.* 2006(3):CD003223.

35. Hindley AC, Hill EB, Leyland MJ, *et al*. A double-blind controlled trial of salmon calcitonin in pain due to malignancy. *Cancer Chemother Pharmacol*. 1982;**9**(2):71–74.

36. Bruera E, Roca E, Cedaro L, *et al*. Action of oral methylprednisolone in terminal cancer patients: a prospective randomized double-blind study. *Cancer Treat Rep*. 1985;**69**(7–8):751–754.

37. Feuer DJ, Broadley KE. Corticosteroids for the resolution of malignant bowel obstruction in advanced gynaecological and gastrointestinal cancer. *Cochrane Database Syst Rev*. 2000(2):CD001219.

38. Mystakidou K, Tsilika E, Kalaidopoulou O, *et al*. Comparison of octreotide administration vs conservative treatment in the management of inoperable bowel obstruction in patients with far advanced cancer: a randomized, double-blind, controlled clinical trial. *Anticancer Res*. 2002;**22**(2B):1187–1192.

Cardiac chest pain

KALANI OLMSTED AND DEBORAH B. DIERCKS

■ Agents

- Oxygen
- Beta-blockers
- Nitrates
- Opioids
- Benzodiazepines

■ Evidence

Though *oxygen* has long been used for patients with acute coronary syndrome (ACS), its use for ACS has become somewhat controversial. Intuitively, it seems that increasing blood oxygenation would decrease both ischemia and pain. However, studies are contradictory, and some suggest supplemental *oxygen* may exacerbate ischemia by decreasing coronary perfusion.[1] Coronary perfusion decrease could be a result of *oxygen*'s hemodynamic effects of decreased stroke volume and cardiac output (accompanied by increased vascular resistance).[1]

The American College of Cardiology/American Heart Association (ACC/AHA) guidelines recommend supplemental *oxygen* for peripheral S_pO_2 less than 90%.[2,3] This may be a reasonable strategy but acute care clinicians are (appropriately) uncomfortable with values in the low 90s S_pO_2 in patients with ACS. The extensive use of short-term *oxygen* therapy in ACS, with rarely reported adverse effects and frequent cases of anecdotal benefit, supports *oxygen* administration as a benign intervention for cardiac patients with pain and subnormal peripheral pulse oximetry (S_pO_2).[4] *Oxygen* administration may, in fact, be associated with a significant "placebo" effect in reducing anginal pain.[1]

Intuitively, the short-term use of *oxygen* in the highest-risk ACS group – those with refractory pain and the need for thrombolysis or cardiac catheterization – is an indicated intervention. Accordingly, the ACC/AHA guidelines conclude that the weight of evidence favors *oxygen* use in ST-elevation myocardial infarction (STEMI), although they acknowledge the lack of unanimity on the subject and note that available evidence is limited to consensus opinion, case studies, and standard-of-care practice. For patients with ACS and with S_pO_2 less than 90%, a stronger ACC/AHA recommendation reflects a higher level of evidentiary support and general agreement on *oxygen* use.[2] The 2005 AHA guidelines for ACS endorse the position of *oxygen* administration for the acute phase of chest pain care.[5]

The pain of ACS is effectively decreased by **beta-blockers**.[6] Though their exact analgesia mechanism is not known, there are several possible routes by which **beta-blockers** could reduce pain. Pain and myocardial ischemia cause sympathetic stimulation, which increases catecholamine levels.[6,7] Furthermore, ischemic myocardium is characterized by increased beta-adrenoceptor density and an increased excitatory response to catecholamines.[6] By reducing contractility, heart rate, blood pressure, and oxygen demand, and by lengthening perfusion time for ischemic myocardial tissue, **beta-blockers** reduce pain and decrease the area of ischemia.[6,7] Given the mortality benefit of **beta-blockers** in ACS, the added benefit of analgesia adds to the already strong case for beta-blockade in any ACS patient lacking contraindications (e.g. bronchospasm).[3,4,6,8] In ACS, **beta-blockers** should be administered IV with PO dosing commenced after parenteral loading. *Metoprolol*, *propranolol*, and *atenolol* are the agents that have been most commonly reported in the ACS literature.[3,4,8]

Nitrates dilate the epicardial coronary arteries, their collaterals, and peripheral vessels, thus improving coronary perfusion and potentiating a favorable ratio of subendocardial-to-epicardial flow.[7,9] The decrease in myocardial oxygen demand, combined with the improved coronary blood flow, eases the pain associated with myocardial ischemia.[5] In patients with suspected ischemic chest pain, sublingual *nitroglycerin* (*glyceryl trinitrate*) should be given every 5 min for three doses; if pain persists *nitroglycerin* should be administered by infusion.[3,8] Oral or transdermal *nitroglycerin* is reserved for patients without ongoing chest pain.[3]

Opioids have long been a part of the ACS treatment armamentarium. Because of its properties as a pulmonary venodilator and anxiolytic, *morphine* has traditionally been the analgesic of choice for ACS pain.[8,10] Recent trial evidence, however, suggests that *morphine* administration to patients with non-STEMI ACS may worsen outcomes.[11] The pertinent data, from the CRUSADE trial, have prompted much theorizing. For instance, decreases in cortisol have been proposed as a mechanism by which *morphine* worsens outcomes.[12] What seems more plausible, however, is the evidence indicating that *morphine* is simply a marker for higher acuity: those patients with larger areas of ischemia require higher doses of *morphine*.[13] Furthermore, CRUSADE's analysis may fail to adjust properly for confounding variables that could explain higher mortality independent of **opioid** analgesia.[10] While the question continues to be investigated, acute care providers are advised to continue using *morphine* as per ACC/AHA guidelines, which confirm (post-CRUSADE) that "*morphine sulfate* is the analgesic of choice for continuing pain unresponsive to **nitrates**."[5]

The ACC/AHA recommends *meperidine* (*pethidine*) for patients allergic to *morphine*, but other opioids (e.g. *hydromorphone*) are equally effective.[2,14] *Fentanyl*'s hemodynamic stability forms the foundation for its popularity in acute care analgesia, and this rapid-acting, easily titratable agent is potentially useful in ACS where hypotension is a concern.[15–18] Studies of acute care *fentanyl* use have often included patients with cardiac chest pain, and one trial has specifically focused on patients with ACS. The use of *alfentanil*, pharmacologically similar to *fentanyl*, has been demonstrated effective for ACS pain in a physician-staffed prehospital setting. *Alfentanil* (0.5 mg IV with repeat dose in 2 min) provides faster relief of ischemic chest pain than does *morphine* (5.0 mg IV with repeat dose in 2 min).[19]

There is one subgroup of the ACS pain population that warrants special mention: patients with cocaine-associated cardiac chest pain. In this population, the risk of vasospasm from **beta-blockers** is such that these agents (even those with mixed alpha- and beta-antagonist properties) should be avoided.[20] In addition to standard therapies as noted above, **benzodiazepines** should be used in this patient population. Intravenous **benzodiazepines** (e.g. *lorazepam*) indirectly counteract cocaine's cardiotoxicity, and thus relieve pain, via a mechanism of decreasing central excitation.[20]

■ Summary and recommendations

First line:

- nitrates: SL nitroglycerin (0.4 mg SL every 5 min); for continuing pain after three doses of SL nitroglycerin: IV nitroglycerin infusion (begin infusion at 5 µg/min and titrate to pain and blood pressure, maximum dose usually 100 µg/min but up to 200 µg/min sometimes used)
- beta-blockers: metoprolol (5 mg IV every 5 min to 15 mg total; follow with PO load of 50 mg 15 min after last IV dose); other beta-blockers may also be used
- oxygen: administer oxygen to maintain S_pO_2 at least 95%
- opioids: morphine (initial dose 4–6 mg IV, then titrate); other opioids may also be used

Pregnancy: importance of maternal analgesia (and associated salutary effects on outcome) outweighs fetal concerns; ACS pain therapy in pregnancy is thus unchanged from that in other situations

Pediatric: children with ACS will probably be suffering from congenital anomalies or metabolic syndromes; therefore, pain management is best coordinated with subspecialists; fentanyl (initial dose 1–2 µg/kg IV, then titrate) may be preferred owing to its minimal hemodynamic effects

Special cases:

- *cocaine-associated chest pain*: avoid beta-blockers (including mixed alpha- and beta-blockers) and instead use benzodiazepines (e.g. lorazepam 1 mg IV with repeat doses as needed)
- *hemodynamic concerns*: Use fentanyl (initial dose 1–2 µg/kg IV, then titrate)

References

1. Nicholson C. A systematic review of the effectiveness of oxygen in reducing acute myocardial ischaemia. *J Clin Nurs*. 2004;**13**(8):996–1007.
2. Braunwald E, Antman EM, Beasley JW, *et al*. ACC/AHA guidelines for the management of patients with unstable angina and non-ST-segment elevation myocardial infarction: executive summary and recommendations. A report of the American College of Cardiology/American Heart Association Task Force on

Practice Guidelines (Committee on the Management of Patients with Unstable Angina). *Circulation.* 2000;**102**(10):1193–1209.

3. Pollack CV, Jr., Gibler WB. 2000 ACC/AHA guidelines for the management of patients with unstable angina and non-ST-segment elevation myocardial infarction: a practical summary for emergency physicians. *Ann Emerg Med.* 2001;**38**(3):229–240.

4. Quinn T. Commentary on Nicholson C (2004) A systematic review of the effectiveness of oxygen in reducing acute myocardial ischaemia. Journal of Clinical Nursing 13, 996–1007. *J Clin Nurs.* 2006;**15**(1):121–122.

5. American Heart Association. 2005 guidelines for cardiopulmonary resuscitation and emergency cardiovascular care. *Circulation.* 2005;**112**(24):89–111.

6. Everts B, Karlson B, Abdon NJ, *et al.* A comparison of metoprolol and morphine in the treatment of chest pain in patients with suspected acute myocardial infarction: the MEMO study. *J Intern Med.* 1999;**245**(2):133–141.

7. Haro LH, Decker WW, Boie ET, *et al.* Initial approach to the patient who has chest pain. *Cardiol Clin.* 2006;**24**(1):1–17, v.

8. Pollack CV, Jr., Diercks DB, Roe MT, *et al.* 2004 American College of Cardiology/American Heart Association guidelines for the management of patients with ST-elevation myocardial infarction: implications for emergency department practice. *Ann Emerg Med.* 2005;**45**(4):363–376.

9. Frishman WH. Pharmacology of the nitrates in angina pectoris. *Am J Cardiol.* 1985;**56**(17):8I-13I.

10. Verheugt FW. Morpheus, god of sleep or god of death? *Am Heart J.* 2005;**149**(6):945–946.

11. Meine TJ, Roe MT, Chen AY, *et al.* Association of intravenous morphine use and outcomes in acute coronary syndromes: results from the CRUSADE quality improvement initiative. *Am Heart J.* 2005;**149**(6):1043–1049.

12. Daniell HW. Opioid-induced cortisol deficiency may explain much of the increased mortality after the use of morphine during treatment of acute myocardial infarction. *Am Heart J.* 2005;**150**(6):e1.

13. Herlitz J, Richter A, Hjalmarson A, *et al.* Variability of chest pain in suspected acute myocardial infarction according to subjective assessment and requirement of narcotic analgesics. *Int J Cardiol.* 1986;**13**(1):9–26.

14. Chang AK, Bijur PE, Meyer RH, *et al.* Safety and efficacy of hydromorphone as an analgesic alternative to morphine in acute pain: a randomized clinical trial. *Ann Emerg Med.* 2006;**48**(2):164–172.

15. Thomas S. Fentanyl in the prehospital setting. *Am J Emerg Med.* 2007;**25**(7) 842–843.

16. Borland M, Jacobs I, King B, *et al.* A randomized controlled trial comparing intranasal fentanyl to intravenous morphine for managing acute pain in children in the emergency department. *Ann Emerg Med.* 2007;**49**(3):335–340.

17. Chudnofsky C, Wright S, Dronen S. The safety of fentanyl use in the emergency department. *Ann Emerg Med.* 1989;**18**:635–639.

18. Kanowitz A, Dunn TM, Kanowitz EM, *et al.* Safety and effectiveness of fentanyl administration for prehospital pain management. *Prehosp Emerg Care.* 2006;**10**(1):1–7.

19. Silfvast T, Saarnivaara L. Comparison of alfentanil and morphine in the pre hospital treatment of patients with acute ischemic-type pain. *Euro J Emerg Med.* 2001;**8**:275–278.

20. Hollander JE, Henry TD. Evaluation and management of the patient who has cocaine-associated chest pain. *Cardiol Clin.* 2006;**24**(1):103–114.

Chest wall trauma

MICHEL GALINSKI

■ Agents

- Opioids
- NSAIDs
- Local anesthetic agents (variety of administration routes)

■ Evidence

Thoracic trauma constitutes 10–15% of all injuries, with rib fractures (RF) being especially common, and particularly painful.[1,2] Pain from RF (and its exacerbation by deep breathing or coughing) is a major concern, since difficulties with pain relief contribute to splinting, ventilatory impairment, atelectasis, sputum retention, and pneumonia-associated morbidity and mortality.[2] At particular risk are the elderly, in whom RF is associated with a 31% rate of nosocomial pneumonia.[3,4]

Given the usual nonoperative management of RF, pain control constitutes one of the major foci of overall management of this condition.[5,6] The severity and duration of RF pain render effective analgesia a challenge in the ED. The recommendations of this chapter generally follow those of surgical/trauma consensus panel recommendations for RF pain management.[7]

Historically, the initial ED approach to RF is administration of **opioids**. First given by IV bolus, and then (in some settings) by PCA, the **opioids** are a reasonable means to institute analgesia.[7] However, there is debate over the risk-to-benefit ratio for **opioid** administration. The main problem is the well-known potential for **opioid**-mediated respiratory depression, but **opioids** can also cause sedation and cough suppression. Studies have begun to address the risks and benefits of **opioids** in RF, but definitive data are lacking.

Fentanyl administered as a continuous IV infusion improves pain scores and vital capacity but also results in respiratory depression and hypoxemia.[8] *Alfentanil*, another potent short-acting IV **opioid**, is successful when used as bolus therapy (100 μg every 2–3 min up to maximum dose of 800 μg) to allow chest physiotherapy in the setting of multiple chest wall fractures.[9] The hemodynamic profile of *fentanyl* makes this agent attractive in the setting of multitrauma, as in these patients *morphine*-mediated histamine release could cause or exacerbate hypotension.[10] Administration of *morphine* as PCA is slightly less effective, but causes no more side effects, than an epidural infusion regimen of *bupivacaine* and *fentanyl*.[11]

Given the lack of PCA capability in most EDs, recent data demonstrating utility for nebulized *morphine* are attractive. For the endpoint of managing RF pain (to keep pain scores below 4 on a 10-point scale), the inhaled *morphine* is found to be comparable to PCA administration of the same drug.[12] Although the existing evidence does not address use of the nebulized **opioid** in the ED setting, it appears possible there may be an occasional role for inhaled *morphine* in acute care. Until more data are available, however, the IV route for **opioid** administration will remain the mainstay of systemic RF analgesia.

If pain is controlled adequately, and if patients do not otherwise require hospitalization, a transition to PO **opioids** may be appropriate. Although there is no high-level evidence guiding selection of a PO **opioid**, *oxycodone* (with or without *acetaminophen* [*paracetamol*]) is among the agents most commonly prescribed from the ED setting. The choice of *oxycodone* may be theoretically advantageous in that this agent has relatively less antitussive effects (and thus less chance of contributing to pneumonia development) than some other **opioids** (e.g. *codeine*).

The intrathecal injection of *morphine* has been studied for patients with multiple RFs. Compared with the epidural administration route for **local anesthetics** (see below), intrathecal injection of *morphine* is less well studied, but it appears to be associated with more complications and less efficacy.[13,14] This administration route has no role in acute care.

For the majority of patients with RF, who will be managed on an outpatient basis, the controversy surrounding **NSAIDs** and delayed bone fracture healing (discussed in the chapter on extremity fractures, p. 323) is relevant.[15] Even independent of bone healing issues, the extended course of therapy necessary for managing RF pain increases relative risks of

NSAIDs. As is the case for other (non-rib) fractures, the acute care provider must weigh the risks and benefits of agents such as *ibuprofen* on a case-by-case basis. There are few high-level data investigating the various oral analgesic approaches to RF.[16]

When conditions are suitable for their use, the **local anesthetics** are perhaps the most efficacious mechanism for managing RF pain. Intercostal blocks entail injection of agents such as *bupivacaine* into the posterior aspect of the intercostal space (not at the RF site). Because of overlapping innervation, it is necessary to block the intercostal nerves above and below the fracture site.[7] Therefore, multiple RFs necessitate multiple intercostal injections, and the more intercostal injections required, the greater the procedural difficulty and risk of adverse events (e.g. pneumothorax, drug toxicity).[16,17] Adding *epinephrine* (*adrenaline*; 1:200 000) to *bupivacaine* (0.5%) used for intercostal block results in lower peak blood *bupivacaine* levels and may reduce the potential for toxicity.[18] In practice, provision of intercostal nerve blocks is rational for patients with three or fewer RFs, but dosage issues dictate epidural injection for four or more (most of these patients need admission anyway).

The intercostal block approach is attractive for application in the ED, where monitoring for adverse effects is not usually problematic. Effects of the block tend to begin to wane after about 6 h (although analgesia may be more long lasting if *epinephrine* is co-injected). In some cases, the initial pain relief provided by an intercostal block will get pain under control and allow transition to other analgesic techniques (e.g. outpatient medications). One solution to the waning drug effect is to leave an intercostal catheter in place at one level, to enable infusion for continuous nerve block; such an infusion carries its own catheter misplacement and adverse effect risks and lies outside the scope of most ED physicians' practice.[7]

Related to the intercostal nerve block approach is that of interpleural (i.e. between the parietal and visceral pleural spaces) administration of **local anesthetics**. This technique produces multiple unilateral intercostal nerve blockade by gravity-dependent retrograde diffusion of the local anesthetic.[7] The interpleural infusion approach is probably less efficacious than epidural drug administration, and it seems to be generally equal in pain relief to systemically administered **opioids**.[19,20] The success of interpleural analgesia can be affected by a number of factors, including catheter position, patient position, presence of hemothorax, location of RFs, characteristics of the **local anesthetic** used, and the co-administration of *epinephrine*.[20] Because of diaphragmatic uptake of *bupivacaine* after interpleural administration, respiratory excursion may be affected.[21] Interpleural catheter placement can be technically difficult and can result in symptomatic pneumothorax, intrapulmonary catheter placement, or misplacement into the chest wall or in an extrapleural plane. **Local anesthetic** agents are rapidly absorbed from the intrapleural space, resulting in high plasma concentration, with potential for systemic toxicity. Interpleural instillation of local anesthetic can also cause phrenic nerve paralysis and Horner's syndrome.[16]

Local anesthetics (sometimes co-administered with **opioids**) have also been used by the epidural administration route. This approach is associated with decreased pulmonary morbidity and mortality in patients older than 60 years of age with RF.[7] Used in patients with chest wall trauma, epidural analgesia produces pain relief that is dramatic and superior to that produced by systemic **opioids** or other **local anesthetic** approaches.[5,8,11,22–24] Even though the epidural route is not used by the ED provider, the evidence comparing its (favorable) performance to that of systemically administered **opioids** cannot be ignored. Particularly for patients with multiple RFs, epidural regimens' advantages of improved analgesia and decreased complication rates warrant early consideration of this approach (usually after the ED setting) in patients who have been adequately resuscitated for fluid.[22]

Local anesthetic administration via thoracic paravertebral block entails injecting an agent such as *bupivacaine* alongside the thoracic vertebrae. This produces multidermatomal ipsilateral somatic and sympathetic nerve blockade in contiguous thoracic dermatomes. There are few publications describing the use of this method in patients with blunt thoracic trauma, and there is a lack of comparative data.[16] Paravertebral administration of **local anesthetics** likely has efficacy, and low complication rates, for multiple RFs, but the technique is outside most ED providers' practice scope.[25–27]

■ Summary and recommendations

First line: morphine (initial dose 4–6 mg IV, then titrate)

Reasonable:

- opioid agonists such as hydromorphone (initial dose 1 mg IV, then titrate)
- 1–3 rib fractures: intercostal nerve block (bupivacaine with epinephrine)

Pregnancy:

- morphine (initial dose 4–6 mg IV, then titrate)
- intercostal nerve block (bupivacaine with epinephrine)

Pediatric:

- morphine (initial dose 0.05–0.1 mg/kg IV, then titrate)
- intercostal nerve block (bupivacaine with epinephrine)

Special cases:

- *multiple trauma or risk of hypotension*: fentanyl (initial dose 50–100 μg IV, then titrate)
- *multiple rib fractures (especially if four or more)*: epidural (first choice) or regional anesthesia (e.g. with bupivacaine) after adequate fluid resuscitation

References

1. Sirmali M, Turut H, Topcu S, *et al.* A comprehensive analysis of traumatic rib fractures: morbidity, mortality and management. *Eur J Cardiothorac Surg.* 2003;**24**(1):133–138.
2. Ziegler DW, Agarwal NN. The morbidity and mortality of rib fractures. *J Trauma.* 1994;**37**(6):975–979.
3. Shorr RM, Rodriguez A, Indeck MC, *et al.* Blunt chest trauma in the elderly. *J Trauma.* 1989;**29**(2):234–237.
4. Bulger EM, Arneson MA, Mock CN, *et al.* Rib fractures in the elderly. *J Trauma.* 2000;**48**(6):1040–1046; discussion 1046–1047.
5. Moon MR, Luchette FA, Gibson SW, *et al.* Prospective, randomized comparison of epidural versus parenteral opioid analgesia in thoracic trauma. *Ann Surg.* 1999;**229**(5):684–691; discussion 691–692.

6. Mayberry JC, Trunkey DD. The fractured rib in chest wall trauma. *Chest Surg Clin North Am.* 1997;**7**(2):239–261.

7. Simon BJ, Cushman J, Barraco R, *et al.* Pain management guidelines for blunt thoracic trauma. *J Trauma.* 2005;**59**(5):1256–1267.

8. Mackersie RC, Karagianes TG, Hoyt DB, *et al.* Prospective evaluation of epidural and intravenous administration of fentanyl for pain control and restoration of ventilatory function following multiple rib fractures. *J Trauma.* 1991;**31**(4):443–449; discussion 449–451.

9. Ravalia A, Suresh D. I.V. alfentanil analgesia for physiotherapy following rib fractures. *Br J Anaesth.* 1990;**64**(6):746–748.

10. Thomas S. Fentanyl in the prehospital setting. *Am J Emerg Med.* 2007; **25** (7):842–843.

11. Wu CL, Jani ND, Perkins FM, *et al.* Thoracic epidural analgesia versus intravenous patient-controlled analgesia for the treatment of rib fracture pain after motor vehicle crash. *J Trauma.* 1999;**47**(3):564–567.

12. Fulda G, Giberson F, Fagraeus L. A prospective randomized trial of nebulized morphine compared with patient-controlled analgesia morphine in the management of acute thoracic pain. *J Trauma.* 2005;**59**(2):382–389.

13. Kennedy BM. Intrathecal morphine and multiple fractured ribs. *Br J Anaesth.* 1985;**57**(12):1266–1267.

14. Dickson GR, Sutcliffe AJ. Intrathecal morphine and multiple fractured ribs. *Br J Anaesth.* 1986;**58**(11):1342–1343.

15. Giannoudis P, Furlong A, Macdonald D, *et al.* Nonunion of the femoral diaphysis. the influence of reaming and non-steroidal anti-inflammatory drugs. *J Bone Joint Surg.* 2000;**82B**(5):655–658.

16. Karmakar MK, Ho AM. Acute pain management of patients with multiple fractured ribs. *J Trauma.* 2003;**54**(3):615–625.

17. Shanti CM, Carlin AM, Tyburski JG. Incidence of pneumothorax from intercostal nerve block for analgesia in rib fractures. *J Trauma.* 2001;**51**(3):536–539.

18. Johnson MD, Mickler T, Arthur GR, *et al.* Bupivacaine with and without epinephrine for intercostal nerve block. *J Cardiothorac Anesth.* 1990;**4**(2):200–203.

19. Luchette FA, Radafshar SM, Kaiser R, *et al.* Prospective evaluation of epidural versus intrapleural catheters for analgesia in chest wall trauma. *J Trauma.* 1994;**36**(6):865–869; discussion 869–870.

20. Short K, Scheeres D, Mlakar J, *et al.* Evaluation of intrapleural analgesia in the management of blunt traumatic chest wall pain: a clinical trial. *Am Surg.* 1996;**62**(6):488–493.

21. Seltzer JL, Larijani GE, Goldberg ME, *et al.* Intrapleural bupivacaine: a kinetic and dynamic evaluation. *Anesthesiology.* 1987;**67**(5):798–800.

22. Mackersie RC, Shackford SR, Hoyt DB, *et al.* Continuous epidural fentanyl analgesia: ventilatory function improvement with routine use in treatment of blunt chest injury. *J Trauma.* 1987;**27**(11):1207–1212.

23. Bulger EM, Edwards T, Klotz P, *et al.* Epidural analgesia improves outcome after multiple rib fractures. *Surgery.* 2004;**136**(2):426–430.

24. Dittmann M, Keller R, Wolff G. A rationale for epidural analgesia in the treatment of multiple rib fractures. *Intensive Care Med.* 1978;**4**(4):193–197.

25. Haenel JB, Moore FA, Moore EE, *et al.* Extrapleural bupivacaine for amelioration of multiple rib fracture pain. *J Trauma.* 1995;**38**(1):22–27.

26. Richardson J, Lonnqvist PA. Thoracic paravertebral block. *Br J Anaesth.* 1998;**81**(2):230–238.

27. Lonnqvist PA, MacKenzie J, Soni AK, *et al.* Paravertebral blockade. Failure rate and complications. *Anaesthesia.* 1995;**50**(9):813–815.

Chronic low-back pain

DAVID CLINE

■ Agents

- Opioids
- NSAIDs
- Muscle relaxants
- Cyclic antidepressants

■ Evidence

Therapy for low-back pain (LBP) that is chronic (CLBP) differs in many respects from the approach to acute back pain. In the nonpharmacologic arena, for instance, there is much better evidence supporting exercise for CLBP than there is for its use in acute back disorders.[1] This chapter focuses on the pharmacological approaches to CLBP (defined as back pain lasting for at least three months). For optimal application of the evidence addressing drug therapy of CLBP, acute care providers should adhere to the general approach for patients with chronic pain as outlined in other chapters. One of the most important tenets is that any therapy prescribed for CLBP should be part of a longitudinal care plan that includes appropriate follow-up and monitoring for both efficacy and safety.

In CLBP, one of the major issues for the ED caregiver is use of **opioids**. The proportion of patients with CLBP who are prescribed **opioids** ranges widely – from 3% to 66% depending on the setting.[2] As outlined in other chapters in this text, there is a potential role for **opioids** in acute flares of spine pain (e.g. spinal spondylitic syndromes), but the use of **opioids** for other neck and back conditions (e.g. radicular syndromes) is not supported by available evidence.

Meta-analysis overviewing 38 studies initially, with nine high-quality investigations included in the final calculations, found only a very limited role for **opioids** in CLBP.[2] If **opioids** do have a role in this condition, it is limited to short-term use for acute exacerbations.[2] No significant long-term benefit is identified when **opioid** use is compared with placebo or non-opioid therapy.[4–7] It is noteworthy that the majority of the individual studies from the meta-analysis identified some benefit from various **opioid** preparations. Among these are were *acetaminophen* (*paracetamol*) plus *oxycodone*, *acetaminophen* plus *codeine*, sustained-release *oxycodone* or *oxymorphone*, and transdermal *fentanyl*.[2]

The utility of **opioids** in CLBP is limited not only by their marginal analgesic efficacy but also by the risk of addictive behavior. As the introductory chapters state, concerns about drug-seeking behavior are inappropriately exaggerated as applied to the general ED population. Furthermore, all patients should get the benefit of the doubt. With that caveat, it should be noted that clinical experience and available data corroborate an impression that the patient population with CLBP constitutes a high-risk group for "aberrant medication behavior" (i.e. manifestations of inappropriate drug seeking). Meta-analysis assessing nine studies in which aberrant medication behaviors were reported found such behaviors occurred in 5–24% of patients receiving **opioids**.[2]

The meta-analysis' final recommendation was that, although **opioids** are commonly prescribed for CLBP, the limited efficacy of **opioids** also comes with an appreciable cost of addiction.[2] **Opioids** cannot be recommended as first-line agents for patients with CLBP.

While **NSAIDs** have a well-established place in the management of some forms of acute LBP, extended-duration prescription of these agents for CLBP lacks solid evidence basis. The limited chronic-use efficacy of **NSAIDs** for CLBP is, in part, the result of the agents' side effect profile. Besides well-publicized ulcer, renal, and cardiovascular risk, long-term **NSAID** use risks abdominal pain, diarrhea, edema, dry mouth, rash, dizziness, headache, and tiredness.[3] In the past, some experts have recommended **NSAIDs** for CLBP; these recommendations were modified by the reviewers' subsequent clarification that the supporting evidence came from studies of six (or fewer) weeks of **NSAID** use.[4,5]

With the caveat that available data are derived from studies of somewhat limited duration, there are data supporting use of various **NSAIDs** for treating

LBP for durations up to four to six weeks. *Diclofenac, piroxicam, indomethacin, ibuprofen, ketoprofen,* and *naproxen* are all reasonable choices for treatment of LBP of up to six weeks' duration.[4,6] Although studies of truly chronic (i.e. three months or more duration) LBP are lacking, it is reasonable to use **NSAIDs** provided that potential side effects risks are incorporated into therapeutic decision-making.

As discussed in other chapters, there is little supporting evidence for use of **COX-2 selective NSAIDs** in acute treatment of neck and back pain syndromes. For longer-term therapy, there are at least two RCTs that find a reduction in pain symptoms associated with three months' use of once-daily *etoricoxib.*[7,8] Although analgesic utility is maintained over a period of months, maximal efficacy is seen approximately four weeks after institution of therapy.

Some authors recommend avoiding the potential cardiovascular risk with **COX-2 selective NSAIDs** by instead prescribing dual therapy with a nonselective **NSAID** and a **proton pump inhibitor**.[9] This decision is not an easy one and should be informed by case-specific variables such as cost and GI and cardiovascular risk profiles (see Arthritis chapter for related discussion, p. 94).

The role of **muscle relaxants** in acute LBP is addressed in other chapters. For CLBP, there is no evidence supporting use of agents of this class; none can be recommended. Even for agents that are acutely effective – and most of these are only marginally better than placebo – there is no supporting evidence for more than one or two weeks of use of either **benzodiazepines** (e.g. *diazepam, tetrazepam*) or other relaxants (e.g. *cyclobenzaprine, flupirtine*).[10,11]

A 2003 meta-analysis found five RCTs demonstrating some CLBP relief with **cyclic antidepressants**.[12] Demonstration of benefit was most pronounced in two methodologically rigorous studies assessing *nortriptyline* (25–100 mg PO daily) and *maprotiline* (50–150 mg PO daily); either drug can be administered once daily at bedtime or in divided doses.[12] The benefits of these **cyclic antidepressants** are independent of their antidepressant effects, since studies demonstrating the agents' efficacy excluded patients with clinical depression.

The **heterocyclic antidepressant** *trazodone* and the **SSRI** *paroxetine* are ineffective in CLBP, providing no added benefit over placebo.[13–15]

■ Summary and recommendations

First line: nortriptyline (initial dose 25 mg PO HS, titrated up to 100 mg/day PO HS or divided BID–TID) *or* maprotiline (initial dose 50 mg PO HS, titrated up to 150 mg/day PO HS or divided BID–TID)

Reasonable: NSAIDs (e.g. diclofenac 50 mg PO BID or TID)

Pediatrics: NSAIDs (e.g. ibuprofen 5–10 mg/kg PO q6–8 h)

Pregnancy: acetaminophen 1000 mg PO QID
short-term opioids (e.g. hydrocodone 5–10 mg PO q4–6 h)

Special case:

■ *Patient with acute flare*: acute flares may be treated in line with specific LBP diagnoses as outlined in other chapters; opioids may be indicated in some instances

References

1. Hayden JA, van Tulder MW, Malmivaara AV, *et al*. Meta-analysis: exercise therapy for nonspecific low back pain. *Ann Intern Med*. 2005;**142**(9):765–775.
2. Martell BA, O'Connor PG, Kerns RD, *et al*. Systematic review: opioid treatment for chronic back pain: prevalence, efficacy, and association with addiction. *Ann Intern Med*. 2007;**146**(2):116–127.
3. Koes BW, Scholten RJ, Mens JM, *et al*. Efficacy of non-steroidal anti-inflammatory drugs for low back pain: a systematic review of randomised clinical trials. *Ann Rheum Dis*. 1997;**56**(4):214–223.
4. van Tulder MW, Koes BW, Bouter LM. Conservative treatment of acute and chronic nonspecific low back pain. A systematic review of randomized controlled trials of the most common interventions. *Spine*. 1997;**22**(18):2128–2156.
5. van Tulder MW, Scholten RJ, Koes BW, *et al*. Nonsteroidal anti-inflammatory drugs for low back pain: a systematic review within the framework of the Cochrane Collaboration Back Review Group. *Spine*. 2000;**25**(19):2501–2513.
6. Zerbini C, Ozturk ZE, Grifka J, *et al*. Efficacy of etoricoxib 60 mg/day and diclofenac 150 mg/day in reduction of pain and disability in patients with

chronic low back pain: results of a 4-week, multinational, randomized, double-blind study. *Curr Med Res Opin.* 2005;**21**(12):2037–2049.

7. Birbara CA, Puopolo AD, Munoz DR, *et al.* Treatment of chronic low back pain with etoricoxib, a new cyclo-oxygenase-2 selective inhibitor: improvement in pain and disability – a randomized, placebo-controlled, 3-month trial. *J Pain.* 2003;**4**(6):307–315.

8. Pallay RM, Seger W, Adler JL, *et al.* Etoricoxib reduced pain and disability and improved quality of life in patients with chronic low back pain: a 3 month, randomized, controlled trial. *Scand J Rheumatol.* 2004;**33**(4):257–266.

9. Hur C, Chan AT, Tramontano AC, *et al.* Coxibs versus combination NSAID and PPI therapy for chronic pain: an exploration of the risks, benefits, and costs. *Ann Pharmacother.* 2006;**40**(6):1052–1063.

10. van Tulder MW, Touray T, Furlan AD, *et al.* Muscle relaxants for nonspecific low back pain: a systematic review within the framework of the Cochrane Collaboration. *Spine.* 2003;**28**(17):1978–1992.

11. Worz R, Bolten W, Heller B, *et al.* [Flupirtine in comparison with chlormeza-none in chronic musculoskeletal back pain. Results of a multicenter random-ized double-blind study.] *Fortschr Med.* 1996;**114**(35–36):500–504.

12. Staiger TO, Gaster B, Sullivan MD, *et al.* Systematic review of antidepressants in the treatment of chronic low back pain. *Spine.* 2003;**28**(22):2540–2545.

13. Goodkin K, Gullion CM, Agras WS. A randomized, double-blind, placebo-controlled trial of trazodone hydrochloride in chronic low back pain syn-drome. *J Clin Psychopharmacol.* 1990;**10**(4):269–278.

14. Dickens C, Jayson M, Sutton C, *et al.* The relationship between pain and depression in a trial using paroxetine in sufferers of chronic low back pain. *Psychosomatics.* 2000;**41**(6):490–499.

15. Atkinson JH, Slater MA, Wahlgren DR, *et al.* Effects of noradrenergic and serotonergic antidepressants on chronic low back pain intensity. *Pain.* 1999;**83**(2):137–145.

Cluster headache

SOHAN PAREKH AND ANDY JAGODA

■ Agents

- Triptans
- Oxygen
- Octreotide
- Dihydroergotamine
- Olanzapine

■ Evidence

Serotonin 5-HT1$_{B/D}$ agonists, collectively known as the **triptans,** are a first-line abortive treatment for cluster headache (CH). The most-studied agent for CH pain is *sumatriptan* (which can be administered subcutaneously in a dose of 6 mg). *Sumatriptan* is known to provide significantly better pain relief than placebo.[1,2] Importantly (since CHs present in groups), tachyphylaxis does not occur with multiple uses of *sumatriptan* for recurrent CHs over a short time span.[3]

Oral *zolmitriptan* (10 mg PO) also relieves CH pain better than placebo, albeit with slower time to relief than that achieved with SC *sumatriptan*.[4] Two intranasal **triptan** formulations, *sumatriptan* (20 mg IN) and *zolmitriptan* (10 mg IN), also provide effective relief of CH pain.[5,6]

While few comparison data assess CH relief by the various **triptans,** SC *sumatriptan* is shown in placebo-controlled trials to perform as well as other **triptans,** as assessed by response rate and time to pain relief. While there is insufficient evidence of safety to recommend **triptans** for routine use in children, reviews suggest this class is safe for occasional use.[7,8]

Long experience supports use of inhaled *oxygen* therapy for treatment of debilitating cluster attacks. The anecdotal evidence is complemented by a non-placebo controlled trial showing that inhaled *oxygen* (6 L/min by non-rebreather mask) is effective in CH.[9] A subsequent double-blind trial comparing *oxygen* with inhaled room air provided further evidence of *oxygen*'s superiority over placebo in CH therapy.[10] Given these data and the safety profile of inhaled *oxygen*, it should be used as an adjunctive treatment in virtually all cases of CH.

While *hyperbaric oxygen* has been investigated for CH treatment, the current evidence provides insufficient basis for recommending its use for this indication.[11]

The **somatostatin analog** *octreotide* has been shown to inhibit vasopeptides released during CH episodes. An RCT showed that *octreotide* (100 mcg SC) was superior to placebo in aborting CH pain.[12] Although there is no direct comparison between *octreotide* and the **triptans**, testing of these agents against placebo suggests that the **triptans** are superior in both number of responders and the time to onset of action. However, given the contraindications of **triptan** use in patients with vascular disease, there is at least an occasional role for *octreotide* in CH.

Numerous **ergot alkaloids** have been used for treatment of CH. The only agent that has been recently studied is the inhaled form of the ergot derivative *dihydroergotamine*. An RCT found 1 mg IN superior to placebo for relief of CH.[13]

Results from an uncontrolled, open-label study suggest a potential role for the atypical antipsychotic *olanzapine* in CH. The data are preliminary, so recommendation for *olanzapine* in acute therapy of CH must await further evidence.[14]

NSAIDs are potentially useful in some rare headache types (e.g. chronic paroxysmal hemicrania) that are similar to CH, but the current balance of evidence argues against utility of *indomethacin* or other **NSAIDs** in true CH.[15,16] Though the literature (and even the nosology) of acute hemicrania continues to evolve, there is at this time little basis for use of **NSAIDs** in acute presentations of CH.

Although there is anecdotal experience with use of **benzodiazepines**, no supporting evidence exists for their use in CH.

The use of **opioids** for CH is anecdotally reported for CH and variants.[17,18] Although there is no evidence supporting a recommendation for routine use of this class in CH, there may be occasional utility of **opioids** for severe or refractory CH.

■ Summary and recommendations

First line: oxygen (6 L by non-rebreather mask) *plus* sumatriptan (6 mg SC)

Reasonable: zolmitriptan (10 mg PO or 10 mg IN) or sumatriptan (20 mg IN)

Pregnancy: oxygen (6 L by non-rebreather mask); the pregnancy category B rating for octreotide renders this agent preferable to the category C agents olanzapine and the triptans; dihydroergotamine is pregnancy category X.

Pediatric: oxygen (6 L by non-rebreather mask); there is insufficient clinical evidence demonstrating safety of octreotide, triptans, or olanzapine to recommend their routine use in children, although reviews suggest triptans are safe for use in pediatric migraineurs

Special case:
■ *patients with vascular disease (including cardiovascular disease) and oxygen-refractory headache*: octreotide 100 mcg SC

References

1. The Sumatriptan Cluster Headache Study Group. Treatment of acute cluster headache with sumatriptan. *N Engl J Med.* 1991;**325**:322–326.
2. Ekbom K. Sumatriptan Cluster Headache Long-term Study Group. Cluster headache attacks treated for up to three months with subcutaneous sumatriptan (6 mg). *Cephalalgia.* 1995;**15**:230–236.
3. Gobel H, Lindner V, Heinze A, *et al.* Acute therapy for cluster headache with sumatriptan: findings of a one-year long-term study. *Neurology.* 1998;**51**: 908–911.
4. Bahra A. Oral zolmitriptan is effective in the acute treatment of cluster headache. *Neurology.* 2000;**54**:1832–1839.
5. van Vliet J. Intranasal sumatriptan in cluster headache: randomized placebo-controlled double-blind study. *Neurology.* 2003;**60**:630–633.
6. Cittadini E. Effectiveness of intranasal zolmitriptan in acute cluster headache: a randomized, placebo-controlled, double-blind crossover study. *Arch Neurol.* 2006;**63**:1537–1542.

7. Yonker ME. Pharmacologic treatment of migraine. *Curr Pain Headache Rep.* 2006;**10**:377–381.

8. Lewis DW, Yonker M, Winner P, *et al.* The treatment of pediatric migraine. *Pediatr Ann.* 2005;**34**:448–460.

9. Kudrow L. Response of cluster headache attacks to oxygen inhalation. *Headache.* 1981;**21**:1–4.

10. Fogan L. Treatment of cluster headache. A double-blind comparison of oxygen versus air inhalation. *Arch Neurol.* 1985;**42**:362–363.

11. Nilsson A, Ansjon R, Lind F, *et al.* Hyperbaric oxygen treatment of active cluster headache: a double-blind placebo-controlled crossover study. *Cephalalgia.* 2002;**22**:730–739.

12. Matharu M, Levy M, Meeran K, *et al.* Subcutaneous octreotide in cluster headache. randomized placebo-controlled double-blind crossover study. *Ann Neurol.* 2004;**56**:488–494.

13. Andersson P, Jespersen L. Dihydroergotamine nasal spray in the treatment of attacks of cluster headache. A double-blind trial versus placebo. *Cephalalgia.* 1986;**6**:51–54.

14. Rozen T. Olanzapine as an abortive agent for cluster headache. *Headache.* 2001;**41**:813–816.

15. Antonaci F, Costa A, Ghirmai S, *et al.* Parenteral indomethacin (the INDOTEST) in cluster headache. *Cephalalgia.* 2003;**23**:193–196.

16. Fuad F, Jones NS. Paroxysmal hemicrania and cluster headache: two discrete entities or is there an overlap? *Clin Otolaryngol Allied Sci.* 2002;**27**:472–479.

17. Sicuteri F, Raino L, Geppetti P. Substance P and endogenous opioids: how and where they could play a role in cluster headache. *Cephalalgia.* 1983;**3** (Suppl 1):143–145.

18. Otsuka F, Mizobuchi S, Ogura T, *et al.* Long-term effects of octreotide on pituitary gigantism: its analgesic action on cluster headache. *Endocr J.* 2004;**51**:449–452.

Corneal abrasion

LISA CALDER

■ Agents

- Topical NSAIDs
- Opioids

■ Evidence

Based upon their widespread effective use and reported results from meta-analysis of five RCTs, topical **NSAIDs** are the analgesic treatment of choice for traumatic corneal abrasions (CAs).[1] *Ketorolac* 0.5% and *indomethacin* 0.1% are the most studied agents, with significant efficacy compared with placebo.[2-7] Topical preparations of *diclofenac* (0.1%), *flurbiprofen* (0.03%), and *piroxicam* (0.5%) also reduce CA pain.[8-12] The only noted adverse effect in these studies of **NSAIDs** is transient (and minor) stinging. While data are limited, topical **NSAIDs** are probably safe in children and can be considered when no other alternatives are viable.[13]

There are no studies on the use of oral or parenteral **NSAIDs** in CA. However, there is intuitive basis for some benefit to their use, given the utility of topically administered **NSAIDs**.

Opioids have not been directly assessed as analgesics for CA. *Oxycodone* with *acetaminophen* (*paracetamol*) is useful as a rescue analgesic in patients failing topical **NSAIDs**; the primary utility of the **opioid** in this setting may be to aid in sleep.[11]

The ophthalmology literature makes frequent reference to the analgesic utility of bandage contact lenses in CA.[2,14,15] However, this approach is not recommended for ED use since **NSAIDs** work well and the contact lens approach is associated with potential infectious complications.[16]

Eye patching, long advocated for its theorized effects on patient comfort, lacks evidence basis for use in CA. A Cochrane review of nine RCTs addressing patching and ocular pain found no studies favoring patching, with two trials finding better pain control with *no* patching. Furthermore, the data (including pediatric studies) suggest that patching may in fact delay healing.[4,10,17–23]

There has been limited study of **cycloplegic** use in CA. An RCT showed no benefit as assessed by either pain score improvement or need for rescue oral analgesics.[8]

■ Summary and recommendations

First line: topical NSAID (e.g. ketorolac 0.5%, 1 drop QID)

Reasonable: oral opioids (e.g. 5–10 mg oxycodone PO q4–6 h)

Pregnancy: acetaminophen (1000 mg PO q4–6 h) with as-needed opioids (e.g. hydrocodone 5–10 mg PO q4–6 h)

Pediatric: topical NSAID (e.g. ketorolac 0.5%, 1 drop QID) or systemic NSAID (e.g. ibuprofen 10 mg/kg PO q4–6 h)

References

1. Calder LA, Balasubramanian S, Fergusson D. Topical nonsteroidal anti-inflammatory drugs for corneal abrasions: meta-analysis of randomized trials. *Acad Emerg Med*. 2005;**12**(5):467–473.
2. Donnenfeld ED, Selkin BA, Perry HD, *et al*. Controlled evaluation of a bandage contact lens and a topical nonsteroidal anti-inflammatory drug in treating traumatic corneal abrasions. *Ophthalmology*. 1995;**102**(6):979–984.
3. Goyal R, Shankar J, Fone DL, *et al*. Randomised controlled trial of ketorolac in the management of corneal abrasions. *Acta Ophthalmol Scand*. 2001;**79**(2):177–179.
4. Kaiser PK. A comparison of pressure patching versus no patching for corneal abrasions due to trauma or foreign body removal. Corneal Abrasion Patching Study Group. *Ophthalmology*. 1995;**102**(12):1936–1942.
5. Alberti MM, Bouat CG, Allaire CM, *et al*. Combined indomethacin/gentamicin eyedrops to reduce pain after traumatic corneal abrasion. *Eur J Ophthalmol*. 2001;**11**(3):233–239.

6. Patrone G, Sacca SC, Macri A, *et al.* Evaluation of the analgesic effect of 0.1% indomethacin solution on corneal abrasions. *Ophthalmologica.* 1999;**213** (6):350–354.

7. Solomon A, Halpert M, Frucht-Perry J. Comparison of topical indomethacin and eye patching for minor corneal trauma. *Ann Ophthalm.* 2000;**32**: 316–319.

8. Brahma AK, Shah S, Hillier VF, *et al.* Topical analgesia for superficial corneal injuries. *J Accid Emerg Med.* 1996;**13**(3):186–188.

9. Jayamanne DG, Fitt AW, Dayan M, *et al.* The effectiveness of topical diclofenac in relieving discomfort following traumatic corneal abrasions. *Eye.* 1997;**11**(Pt 1):79–83.

10. Le Sage N, Verreault R, Rochette L. Efficacy of eye patching for traumatic corneal abrasions: a controlled clinical trial. *Ann Emerg Med.* 2001;**38** (2):129–134.

11. Szucs PA, Nashed AH, Allegra JR, *et al.* Safety and efficacy of diclofenac ophthalmic solution in the treatment of corneal abrasions. *Ann Emerg Med.* 2000;**35**(2):131–137.

12. Vigasio F, Giroletti G. Piroxicam 0.5% topico e corpi estranei corneali. *Minerva Oftalmologica.* 1986;**28**(1):59–62.

13. Chung I, Buhr V. Topical ophthalmic drugs and the pediatric patient. *Optometry.* 2000;**71**(8):511–518.

14. Acheson JF, Joseph J, Spalton DJ. Use of soft contact lenses in an eye casualty department for the primary treatment of traumatic corneal abrasions. *Br J Ophthalmol.* 1987;**71**(4):285–289.

15. Salz JJ, Reader AL, 3rd, Schwartz LJ, *et al.* Treatment of corneal abrasions with soft contact lenses and topical diclofenac. *J Refract Corneal Surg.* 1994;**10** (6):640–646.

16. Vandorselaer T, Youssfi H, Caspers-Valu LE, *et al.* [Treatment of traumatic corneal abrasion with contact lens associated with topical nonsteroid anti-inflammatory agent (NSAID) and antibiotic: a safe, effective and comfortable solution.] *J Fr Ophtalmol.* 2001;**24**(10):1025–1033.

17. Turner A, Rabiu M. Patching for corneal abrasion. *Cochrane Database Syst Rev.* 2006(2):CD004764.

18. Hulbert MF. Efficacy of eyepad in corneal healing after corneal foreign body removal. *Lancet.* 1991;**337**(8742):643.

19. Kirkpatrick J, Hoh H, Cook S. No eye pad for corneal abrasion. *Eye.* 1993;**7** (pt 3):468–471.

20. Patterson J, Fetzer D, Krall J, et al. Eye patch treatment for the pain of corneal abrasion. *South Med J.* 1996;**89**(2):227 229.

21. Campanile TM, St Clair DA, Benaim M. The evaluation of eye patching in the treatment of traumatic corneal epithelial defects. *J Emerg Med.* 1997;**15**(6):769–774.

22. Arbour J. Should we patch corneal erosions? *Arch Ophthalm.* 1997;**115**(3):313–317.

23. Michael J, Hug D, Dowd M. Management of corneal abrasion in children: a randomized clinical trial. *Ann Emerg Med.* 2002;**40**(1):67–72.

Cystitis, urethritis, and prostatitis

BENJAMIN A. WHITE AND STEPHEN H. THOMAS

■ Agents

- Antibiotics
- Phenazopyridine
- Antispasmotics
- Petrolatum jelly

■ Evidence

The evidence addressing analgesia for the lower urinary tract is surprisingly sparse. When the search is limited to the infection-associated inflammatory pain most likely to be encountered in the ED, there are virtually no guiding RCT data. However, painful conditions of the genitourinary tract are quite commonly encountered. The variety of potential etiologies for pain prevent detailed consideration of some diagnoses. This chapter focuses on pain in the bladder, urethra, and prostate. Uterine pain is addressed in other chapters; pain from pelvic inflammatory disease is virtually unaddressed in the literature and is considered in the chapter on undifferentiated abdominal pain (p. 392).

Chronic conditions such as interstitial cystitis and chronic amicrobial prostatitis (male chronic inflammatory pelvic pain) are best treated with mild oral analgesics from the ED, with specific therapy left to the follow-up physicians. Treatment usually involves medications well outside the realm of acute care. Interstitial cystitis is treated with **heparinoids** (e.g. *pentosan polysulfate*), *botulinum toxin*, or intravesical *Bacillus Calmette-Guerin*.[1–3] There is some evidence for **NSAID** utility in prostatitis, but treatment for chronic prostatitis and male chronic inflammatory pelvic pain syndrome entails long-term therapy with drugs such as **alpha-blockers** and **immuno-modulators**.[4–7] The ED physician who is understandably reluctant to institute such agents may wish to prescribe, instead, an intermediate course of nonspecific chronic pain therapy (e.g. *gabapentin, amitriptyline*). Such an approach, as outlined in the chapter on chronic pain (p. 52), also has evidence basis in the realm of chronic genitourinary pain syndromes.[8,9]

The best mechanism for relieving pain from infectious urinary tract disease is administration of appropriate **antibiotics**.[10] **Antibiotics** form the mainstay of urethritis treatment, with pain relief expected within seven days of instituting treatment.[11] Only a few days of therapy are needed to achieve some degree of pain reduction. Multicenter data show that, regardless of whether the clinical picture is one of cystitis or urethritis, **antibiotics** begin to relieve pain and dysuria within 1.6 days.[12] Recommendations in this chapter assume that appropriate antibiotic therapy is provided.

The best-known urinary tract anesthetic for acute care use is *phenazopyridine*. This drug (available without a prescription in the USA) has been in use for nearly a century. *Phenazopyridine*'s very longevity may account for the paucity of trial data evaluating its efficacy. In fact, one of the only trials assessing *phenazopyridine* is a 30-year-old study that actually found it less useful than another agent – the now rarely used **antispasmotic** *flavoxate* – for relief of pain from prostatitis, urethritis, or cystitis.[13] Since there are no contemporary or high-quality data to guide therapeutic decisions, the decades of useful experience with *phenazopyridine* constitute the major supporting evidence for this drug's use. There is indirect evidence of the agent's utility for acute conditions. For example, *phenazopyridine* prevents cystitis-related dysautonomia in patients with spinal cord injury.[14]

Although clinicians seem to be unconcerned about the nonrobust strength of evidence demonstrating *phenazopyridine*'s efficacy, there is oft-discussed worry about the drug's successful pain relief masking ongoing urinary tract infection. Data show that worsening of infection and subsequent delayed patient presentation to organized healthcare is a significant issue with *phenazopyridine*'s over-the-counter use.[15,16] We agree with these concerns and believe *phenazopyridine* should be prescribed for only a few days (after which time **antibiotics** should suffice to improve infectious symptoms). It is fair to point out that the data-supported worries about *phenazopyridine*'s masking of infectious symptoms also constitute evidence of the drug's utility as a pain reliever. *Phenazopyridine* does not appear to have untoward effects on **antibiotic** efficacy, and the urinary tract anesthetic actually increases bioavailability of *ciprofloxacin* in the setting of cystitis.[17]

Phenazopyridine's urinary tract anesthetic effects do not extend to relief of pain caused by bladder distension, as shown in an RCT demonstrating the agent's failure to alleviate pain of bladder filling necessary for ultrasound-guided embryo transfer.[18]

The major disadvantages of *phenazopyridine* are the side effects (e.g. methemoglobinemia, hemolysis, skin discoloration), which can be particularly prominent in overdose or renal insufficiency (which can also be caused by *phenazopyridine*).[19,20] Urinary changes such as discoloration, while not constituting major problems, should be mentioned to patients in order to prevent unwarranted concern.

Ibuprofen does not reduce the dysuria or rectal pain associated with radiation therapy for prostatic cancer.[21] However, there is some evidence for occasional **NSAID** utility in relieving noninfectious chronic prostatitis.[22]

Given the absence of other evidence for **NSAIDs** or other analgesics, patients with refractory pain from infectious cystitis, urethritis, or prostatitis may require **opioids** for relief.

For the occasional patient with external (noninfectious) irritation causing urethritis, a small amount of a topical protective preparation may improve pain. The best example of such an approach is soap-induced urethral pain. In these cases, bathing can be rendered painless with the prebath application of a small amount of *petrolatum jelly*.[23]

■ Summary and recommendations

First line: phenazopyridine 200 mg PO TID (for two or three days only)

Reasonable: NSAIDs (e.g. ibuprofen 400–600 mg PO q6–8 h) if phenazopyridine is contraindicated or fails as monotherapy

Pregnancy: phenazopyridine (200 mg PO TID for two or three days) is probably safe in pregnancy in terms of the fetus, but the risk of masking ongoing or complicated infection is particularly worrisome in this population; if phenazopyridine is prescribed in pregnancy, early follow-up is advised

Pediatric: phenazopyridine 4 mg/kg PO TID (for two or three days only, if taken with an antibiotic)

Special case:
- *chemical or mechanical urethral irritation*: Depending on situation, topical petrolatum jelly may contribute to symptom relief. Phenazopyridine is also anecdotally useful for noninfectious causes of urinary tract pain.

References

1. Anderson VR, Perry CM. Pentosan polysulfate: a review of its use in the relief of bladder pain or discomfort in interstitial cystitis. *Drugs*. 2006;**66**(6):821–835.
2. Aghamir SM, Mohseni MG, Arasteh S. Intravesical Bacillus Calmette–Guerin for treatment of refractory interstitial cystitis. *Urol J*. 2007;**4**(1):18–23.
3. Cruz F, Dinis P. Resiniferatoxin and botulinum toxin type A for treatment of lower urinary tract symptoms. *Neurourol Urodynam*. 2007; **26**(6 Suppl): 920–927.
4. Djerklund Johansen TE, Weidner W. Understanding chronic pelvic pain syndrome. *Curr Opin Urol*. 2002;**12**(1):63–67.
5. Forrest JB, Nickel JC, Moldwin RM. Chronic prostatitis/chronic pelvic pain syndrome and male interstitial cystitis: enigmas and opportunities. *Urology*. 2007;**69**(4 Suppl):60–63.
6. Yang G, Wei Q, Li H, *et al*. The effect of alpha-adrenergic antagonists in chronic prostatitis/chronic pelvic pain syndrome: a meta-analysis of randomized controlled trials. *J Androl*. 2006;**27**(6):847–852.
7. Hua VN, Schaeffer AJ. Acute and chronic prostatitis. *Med Clin North Am*. 2004;**88**(2):483–494.
8. Sasaki K, Smith CP, Chuang YC, *et al*. Oral gabapentin (neurontin) treatment of refractory genitourinary tract pain. *Tech Urol*. 2001;**7**(1):47–49.
9. van Ophoven A, Hertle L. Long-term results of amitriptyline treatment for interstitial cystitis. *J Urol*. 2005;**174**(5):1837–1840.
10. Flottorp S, Oxman AD, Cooper JG, *et al*. [Guidelines for diagnosis and treatment of acute urinary tract problems in women.] *Tidsskr Nor Laegeforen*. 2000;**120**(15):1748–1753.

11. Asano H, Hibi H, Ohshima S, *et al*. [Treatment of chlamydial urethritis: studies on clinical effects of ofloxacin.] *Hinyokika Kiyo*. 1989;**35**(1):191–197.

12. Baerheim A, Digranes A, Hunskaar S. Equal symptomatic outcome after antibacterial treatment of acute lower urinary tract infection and the acute urethral syndrome in adult women. *Scand J Prim Health Care*. 1999;**17**(3):170–173.

13. Gould S. Urinary tract disorders. Clinical comparison of flavoxate and phenazopyridine. *Urology*. 1975;**5**(5):612–615.

14. Paola FA, Sales D, Garcia-Zozaya I. Phenazopyridine in the management of autonomic dysreflexia associated with urinary tract infection. *J Spinal Cord Med*. 2003;**26**(4):409–411.

15. Shi CW, Asch SM, Fielder E, *et al*. Consumer knowledge of over-the-counter phenazopyridine. *Ann Fam Med*. 2004;**2**(3):240–244.

16. Shi CW, Asch SM, Fielder E, *et al*. Usage patterns of over-the-counter phenazopyridine (pyridium). *J Gen Intern Med*. 2003;**18**(4):281–287.

17. Marcelin-Jimenez G, Angeles AP, Martinez-Rossier L, *et al*. Ciprofloxacin bioavailability is enhanced by oral co-administration with phenazopyridine: a pharmacokinetic study in a Mexican population. *Clin Drug Invest*. 2006;**26**(6):323–328.

18. Frishman GN, Allsworth JE, Gannon JB, *et al*. Use of phenazopyridine for reducing discomfort during embryo transfer. *Fertil Steril*. 2007;**87**(5):1010–1014.

19. Fincher ME, Campbell HT. Methemoglobinemia and hemolytic anemia after phenazopyridine hydrochloride (Pyridium) administration in end-stage renal disease. *South Med J*. 1989;**82**(3):372–374.

20. Onder AM, Espinoza V, Berho ME, *et al*. Acute renal failure due to phenazopyridine (Pyridium) overdose: case report and review of the literature. *Pediatr Nephrol*. 2006;**21**(11):1760–1764.

21. Coleman CN, Kelly L, Riese Daly N, *et al*. Phase III study of ibuprofen versus placebo for radiation-induced genitourinary side effects. *Int J Radiat Oncol Biol Phys*. 2002;**54**(1):191–194.

22. Vicari E, La Vignera S, Battiato C, *et al*. [Treatment with non-steroidal anti-inflammatory drugs in patients with amicrobial chronic prostato-vesiculitis: transrectal ultrasound and seminal findings.] *Minerva Urol Nefrol*. 2005;**57**(1):53–59.

23. Okeke LI. Soap induced urethral pain in boys. *West Afr J Med*. 2004;**23**(1):48–49.

Dysmenorrhea

BENJAMIN A. WHITE AND STEPHEN H. THOMAS

■ Agents

- Acetaminophen
- Caffeine
- NSAIDs

■ Evidence

This chapter addresses relief of abdominal cramping and related symptoms (e.g. pelvic pain, backache) associated with the menstrual cycle. Other painful conditions that can be associated with menstruation (e.g. cyclic mastalgia) are addressed elsewhere in this text or tend to be treated in similar fashion as nonmenstrual occurrences (e.g. **triptans** for menstrual migraines) [1] This chapter focuses on analgesic control of dysmenorrhea symptoms, rather than hormonal regulation of the ovulatory cycle (e.g. with **oral contraceptives**). Hormonal therapy may be needed to control dysmenorrhea in the 10–20% of patients unable to be managed by the analgesics discussed here.

Placebo-controlled trial evidence demonstrates some utility of *acetaminophen* (*paracetamol*) for relieving dysmenorrhea, but the optimal approach when using this agent is to combine it with *caffeine*. A large RCT with crossover design comparing monotherapy with either *acetaminophen* (1 g PO) or *caffeine* (130 mg PO) or combination therapy with both agents showed significantly better relief of dysmenorrhea-associated abdominal cramping and backache with the combination.[2]

Prostaglandin inhibition by **NSAIDs** is responsible for their decades of successful use as the mainstay of dysmenorrhea treatment.[3–7] An RCT in patients undergoing fractional curettage demonstrated the potent analgesic effects of **NSAIDs** on uterine pain. When administered a few hours before the procedure, a dose of *mefenamic acid* (500 mg PO) provided equal pain relief to that achieved with paracervical block.[8] Although *mefenamic acid* is often mentioned in the dysmenorrhea literature, and this agent is indeed effective, there seems little justification for selecting this drug over other **NSAIDs**. Cochrane review of RCTs confirmed substantial analgesic effect of many **NSAIDs** in dysmenorrhea.[9] Available data indicate, for instance, that commonly used **NSAIDs** (e.g. *diclofenac* 12.5–25 mg PO) effectively relieve mild-to-moderate dysmenorrhea pain.[10]

Because of the need for chronic use, the **COX-2 selective NSAIDs** are sometimes recommended as a treatment for dysmenorrhea.[11–13] Data show that *valdecoxib*, administered in a single dose of 40 mg PO, provides dysmenorrhea pain relief within 30 min that lasts for up to 24 h.[14] A dosage regimen of 20–40 mg *valdecoxib* BID is equally effective as BID *naprosyn sodium* (550 mg PO BID).[15] The newer **COX-2 selective NSAID** *lumaricoxib*, 400 mg PO QD, provides equally effective dysmenorrhea relief to that achieved with other **NSAIDs**.[16] Similar dysmenorrhea relief results are seen with another **COX-2 selective NSAID**, *etoricoxib*.[17] The risks and benefits of the **COX-2 selective NSAIDs** must be weighed when considering this class; further information is outlined in the Arthritis chapter (p. 94).

The novel analgesic *flupirtine* is suggested by some to have utility in dysmenorrhea, but this centrally acting agent is not recommended owing to limited evidence and frequent side effects.[18]

■ Summary and recommendations

First line: NSAID (e.g. ibuprofen 400–800 mg PO q4–6 h, maximum 2400 mg/day)

Reasonable: combination therapy with acetaminophen (1000 mg PO) and caffeine (130–300 mg PO); repeat dosing q6–8 h (maximum daily caffeine dose 1000 mg)

Pregnancy: acetaminophen (1000 mg PO q4–6 h), with caffeine (130–300 mg q6–8 h with maximum daily caffeine dose 1000 mg) if acetaminophen alone provides insufficient pain relief

Pediatric: ibuprofen (10 mg/kg PO q6–8 h)

Special case:

- *refractory pain*: opioids (e.g. morphine initial dose 4–6 mg IV, then titrate) in the ED, followed by outpatient referral for consideration of instituting hormonal therapy

References

1. Allais G, Acuto G, Cabarrocas X, *et al*. Efficacy and tolerability of almotriptan versus zolmitriptan for the acute treatment of menstrual migraine. *Neurol Sci.* 2006;**27**(Suppl 2):S193–S197.

2. Ali Z, Burnett I, Eccles R, *et al*. Efficacy of a paracetamol and caffeine combination in the treatment of the key symptoms of primary dysmenorrhoea. *Curr Med Res Opin.* 2007;**23**(4):841–851.

3. Brogden RN, Heel RC, Speight TM, *et al*. Naproxen up to date: a review of its pharmacological properties and therapeutic efficacy and use in rheumatic diseases and pain states. *Drugs.* 1979;**18**(4):241–277.

4. Brooks P. Use and benefits of nonsteroidal anti-inflammatory drugs. *Am J Med.* 1998;**104**(Suppl 3A):9S–13S; discussion 21S–22S.

5. Budoff PW. Antiprostaglandins for primary dysmenorrhea. *JAMA.* 1981;**246** (22):2576–2577.

6. Budoff PW. Mefenamic acid for dysmenorrhea in patients with intrauterine devices. *JAMA.* 1979;**242**(7):616–617.

7. Budoff PW. Use of mefenamic acid in the treatment of primary dysmenorrhea. *JAMA.* 1979;**241**(25):2713–2716.

8. Buppasiri P, Tangmanowutikul S, Yoosuk W. Randomized controlled trial of mefenamic acid vs paracervical block for relief of pain for outpatient uterine curettage. *J Med Assoc Thai.* 2005;**88**(7):881–885.

9. Marjoribanks J, Proctor ML, Farquhar C. Nonsteroidal anti-inflammatory drugs for primary dysmenorrhoea. *Cochrane Database Syst Rev.* 2003(4): CD001751.

10. Moore N. Diclofenac potassium 12.5 mg tablets for mild to moderate pain and fever: a review of its pharmacology, clinical efficacy and safety. *Clin Drug Invest.* 2007;**27**(3):163–195.

11. Anonymous. [New indication for selective COX-2 inhibitors. Now also approve for acute pain.] *MMW Fortschr Med.* 2002;**144**(10):62.

12. Fine PG. The role of rofecoxib, a cyclooxygenase-2-specific inhibitor, for the treatment of non-cancer pain: a review. *J Pain.* 2002;**3**(4):272–283.

13. Martina SD, Vesta KS, Ripley TL. Etoricoxib: a highly selective COX-2 inhibitor. *Ann Pharmacother.* 2005;**39**(5):854–862.

14. Alsalameh S, Burian M, Mahr G, *et al.* Review article: the pharmacological properties and clinical use of valdecoxib, a new cyclo-oxygenase-2-selective inhibitor. *Aliment Pharmacol Ther.* 2003;**17**(4):489–501.

15. Fenton C, Keating GM, Wagstaff AJ. Valdecoxib: a review of its use in the management of osteoarthritis, rheumatoid arthritis, dysmenorrhoea and acute pain. *Drugs.* 2004;**64**(11):1231–1261.

16. Bannwarth B, Berenbaum F. Clinical pharmacology of lumiracoxib, a second-generation cyclooxygenase 2 selective inhibitor. *Expert Opin Invest Drugs.* 2005;**14**(4):521–533.

17. Cochrane DJ, Jarvis B, Keating GM. Etoricoxib. *Drugs.* 2002;**62**(18):2637–2651; discussion 2652–2653.

18. Friedel HA, Fitton A. Flupirtine. A review of its pharmacological properties, and therapeutic efficacy in pain states. *Drugs.* 1993;**45**(4):548–569.

Endometriosis

JOSHUA H. TAMAYO-SARVER AND RITA K. CYDULKA

■ Agents

- NSAIDs
- Combined oral contraceptive pills
- Medroxyprogesterone
- Danazol
- Gonadotropin-releasing hormone (GnRH) agonists

■ Evidence

NSAIDs are widely considered first-line therapy for the pain associated with endometriosis, although there is little more than anecdotal evidence supporting their use.[1-6] In fact, only one RCT is identified in a 2005 Cochrane review.[2] The study, which assessed utility of *naproxen* (275 mg PO QID) for endometriosis, found that the **NSAID** offered no advantage over placebo.[7] Some potential utility for **NSAIDs** in endometriosis is supported by another trial, which found clinical relief for women with the condition who took the **COX-2 selective NSAID** *rofecoxib* (25 mg PO QD).[8]

When **NSAIDs** are contraindicated or fail (and assuming the endometriosis diagnosis is confirmed), the remaining therapies fall under the general category of endocrine agents with antiovulatory activity. **Combined oral contraceptive pills (COCPs)** are generally recommended as the second-line therapy for endometriosis pain.[1,3-7] The best evidence for the **COCPs** in endometriosis is found in a study of women receiving monophasic *ethinyl estradiol/desogestrel* (0.02/0.15 mg PO daily) for six months; subjects on this regimen reported improvement in dysmenorrhea, dyspareunia, and nonspecific pelvic pain.[9] While the evidence is imperfect, a 2007 Cochrane review concluded that **COCPs** are at least as effective as **gonadotropin-releasing hormone (GnRH) agonists**.[10]

Medroxyprogesterone acetate (100mg PO daily) is comparable to the **androgen** *danazol* (600 mg PO daily), with both agents reducing pain scores by 50–74% compared with placebo.[11] Similarly, a depot preparation of *medroxyprogesterone acetate* (150 mg IM q3 months) is comparable to *ethinyl estradiol/desogestrel* (0.02/0.15 mg PO daily) plus *danazol* (50 mg PO daily while taking the oral contraceptive pills).[12] An SC form of depot *medroxyprogesterone* appears to relieve endometriosis as effectively as the proven approach of the **GnRH agonist** *leuprolide acetate* (3.75–11.25 mg IM q1–3 months).[13]

Other endocrine approaches, including the synthetic steroid *gestrinone* and a *levonorgestrel*-releasing intrauterine device, are efficacious in the outpatient setting but have limited ED utility unless they are prescribed in close cooperation with follow-up providers. Cochrane review has shown that there is generally equivalent pain relief achieved with multiple endocrine therapies for endometriosis.[10] The myriad menopausal, androgenic, and hepatic side effects from some of the endocrine agents (e.g. *danazol*) used to treat endometriosis should serve to underline the importance of ED physician communication and follow-up arrangements with longitudinal care providers.[14]

■ Summary and recommendations

First line: NSAID (e.g. ibuprofen 600–800 mg PO TID)

Reasonable: medroxyprogesterone (100 mg PO QD *or* 150 mg depot IM q3 months)

Pediatric: NSAID (e.g. ibuprofen 600–800 mg PO TID)

Special case:
■ *failure of initial therapies and in close consultation with gynecologist:* danazol (600 mg PO QD) or leuprolide acetate (3.75 mg IM monthly)

References

1. Jackson B, Telner DE. Managing the misplaced: approach to endometriosis. *Can Fam Physician*. 2006;**52**(11):1420–1424.
2. Allen C, Hopewell S, Prentice A. Non-steroidal anti-inflammatory drugs for pain in women with endometriosis. *Cochrane Database Syst Rev*. 2005(4):CD004753.

3. Olive DL, Lindheim SR, Pritts EA. New medical treatments for endometriosis. *Best Pract Res Clin Obstet Gynaecol*. 2004;**18**(2):319–328.

4. Olive DL, Pritts EA. The treatment of endometriosis: a review of the evidence. *Ann N Y Acad Sci*. 2002;**955**:360–372; discussions 389–393, 396–406.

5. Olive DL, Pritts EA. Treatment of endometriosis. *N Engl J Med*. 2001;**345** (4):266–275.

6. Valle RF. Endometriosis: current concepts and therapy. *Int J Gynaecol Obstet*. 2002;**78**(2):107–119.

7. Kauppila A, Ronnberg L. Naproxen sodium in dysmenorrhea secondary to endometriosis. *Obstet Gynecol*. 1985;**65**(3):379–383.

8. Cobellis L, Razzi S, De Simone S, et al. The treatment with a COX-2 specific inhibitor is effective in the management of pain related to endometriosis. *Eur J Obstet Gynecol Reprod Biol*. 2004;**116**(1):100–102.

9. Vercellini P, Trespidi L, Colombo A, et al. A gonadotropin-releasing hormone agonist versus a low-dose oral contraceptive for pelvic pain associated with endometriosis. *Fertil Steril*. 1993;**60**(1):75–79.

10. Davis L, Kennedy S, Moore J, et al. Modern combined oral contraceptives for pain associated with endometriosis. *Cochrane Database Syst Rev*. 2007(3): CD001019.

11. Telimaa S, Puolakka J, Ronnberg L, et al. Placebo-controlled comparison of danazol and high-dose medroxyprogesterone acetate in the treatment of endometriosis. *Gynecol Endocrinol*. 1987;**1**(1):13–23.

12. Vercellini P, De Giorgi O, Oldani S, et al. Depot medroxyprogesterone acetate versus an oral contraceptive combined with very-low-dose danazol for long-term treatment of pelvic pain associated with endometriosis. *Am J Obstet Gynecol*. 1996;**175**(2):396–401.

13. Schlaff WD, Carson SA, Luciano A, et al. Subcutaneous injection of depot medroxyprogesterone acetate compared with leuprolide acetate in the treatment of endometriosis-associated pain. *Fertil Steril*. 2006;**85**(2):314–325.

14. Selak V, Farquhar C, Prentice A, et al. Danazol for pelvic pain associated with endometriosis. *Cochrane Database Syst Rev*. 2001(4):CD000068.

Esophageal spasm

KALANI OLMSTED AND DEBORAH B. DIERCKS

■ Agents

- Proton pump inhibitors
- Nitrates
- Anticholinergic agents
- Calcium channel blockers
- Antidepressants: tricyclics, trazadone, SSRIs

■ Evidence

Proton pump inhibitors (**PPIs**) are recommended as a first-line therapy when chest pain is thought to be caused by esophageal spasm. This is because gastroesophageal reflux (GERD) causes similar symptoms, and GERD is much more common than esophageal spasm.[1] The diagnosis is complicated by the complexity of esophageal pain pathways. Central convergence of pain blurs the distinction between reflux pain and discomfort from esophageal spasm (as well as other disorders).[1,2] The case for early use of **PPIs** in suspected esophageal spasm is strengthened by the fact that acid reflux can actually cause spasm.[1]

Both long- and short-acting **nitrates** have been shown to provide some relief of pain caused by esophageal spasm.[3,4] In the ED treatment of patients presenting with chest pain, it is reasonable to try sublingual *nitroglycerin* (*glyceryl trinitrate*) early. Through its mechanism of smooth muscle relaxation (at both vascular and esophageal sites) *nitroglycerin* can potentially improve symptoms in cardiac chest pain, GERD, or esophageal spasm.[3,5] There have, however, been only small studies (and no controlled trials) of **nitrates** in patients with chest pain of esophageal origin. While amplitude, frequency, and duration of esophageal contractions are decreased with **nitrates**, clinical pain reduction seems to be inconsistent and unpredictable.[1,5]

Calcium channel blockers decrease the amplitude and duration of esophageal spasms, but their use does not consistently result in better analgesia than achieved with placebo.[6] There are relatively few studies, and all of the trials are limited by low numbers. The agents that have been assessed for utility in esophageal spasm are *nifedipine*, *verapamil*, and *diltiazem*. Two studies, conducted in patients with nutcracker esophagus, found that *diltiazem* (administered in a variety of regimens ranging upwards from 90 mg QID) decreased mean chest pain scores.[6,7] A small uncontrolled trial found that *nifedipine* (10 mg PO) reduced esophageal pain acutely.[8] Other studies, following patients for more extended periods of time, showed little or no clinical benefit.[5,8] Inconsistent **calcium channel blocker** pain relief for esophageal spasm is probably related to the absence of correlation between reduction of esophageal contraction amplitude and pain improvement.[9]

Anticholinergic agents such as *atropine* (6–12 µg/kg IV), *hyoscyamine* (0.6mg PO), or *propantheline bromide* (30 mg PO) decrease peristaltic contractions and reduce esophageal sphincter tone.[5,10] Despite these promising physiologic findings, and the frequent mention of **anticholinergic agents** as potentially useful in the treatment of esophageal motility disorders, there have been no clinical trials of drugs in this class for esophageal spasm pain.[5,9] Given the absence of supporting evidence for analgesia, and the known unreliability of esophageal muscular tone as an indicator of clinical pain relief in esophageal spasm, **anticholinergics** cannot be recommended for routine use in acute treatment of esophageal spasm pain.

There is evidence supporting the use of **antidepressants** such as **tricyclics**, *trazodone*, and **SSRIs** for treating chest pain caused by esophageal spasm.[5,9] Compared with the relatively new **SSRI** agents, **tricyclic** drugs and *trazodone* (which has a slightly more favorable safety profile) are more extensively studied for esophageal spasm pain. Early data show *sertraline* decreases frequency of chest pain episodes.[11,12] The **tricyclic** drugs seem to work somewhat better than *trazodone*; useful ones include *amitripyline*, *nortriptyline*, *imipramine*, and desipramine.[9,13]

The mechanism by which **antidepressants** relieve chest pain of esophageal origin is poorly understood. One theory, based on the idea that pain is caused more by hyperalgesia than spasm itself, is that **antidepressants** work via central modulation of pain.[14] Another putative mechanism for the effectiveness of **antidepressants** is related to the association between noncardiac chest pain and the presence of psychiatric disorders such as anxiety and depression.[9] Regardless of their possible utility in the long term, **antidepressants** are not likely to be of help in the acute management of esophageal spasm pain in the ED. In situations where patients have recurrent ED visits for presumed esophageal spasm pain, and where initial therapeutic approaches (e.g. **PPIs**) fail, it may be reasonable for the acute care provider to institute a trial of an **SSRI**, if the patient has a primary care physician to manage the regimen long term.

■ Summary and recommendations

First line:
- nitroglycerin 0.4 mg SL
- PPI (e.g. omeprazole 20 mg PO QD)

Reasonable: nifedipine 10 mg PO TID (other calcium channel blockers are likely equally effective)

Pregnancy: PPI (e.g. omeprazole 20 mg PO QD)

Pediatric: omeprazole 20 mg PO QD if weight > 20 kg (10 mg PO QD if weight < 20 kg and age > 2 years)

Special cases:
- *possible GERD contributing to spasm pain:* antacids (e.g. magnesium/ aluminum salts, 20 mL PO between meals and HS)
- *for patients with recurrent ED visits and good follow-up*: trazodone 50 mg PO qHS (can be titrated upwards to 400 mg/day or 6 mg/kg per day)

References

1. Tutuian R, Castell DO. Review article: oesophageal spasm – diagnosis and management. *Aliment Pharmacol Ther*. 2006;**23**(10):1393–1402.
2. Lynn RB. Mechanisms of esophageal pain. *Am J Med*. 1992;**92**(5A):11S-19S.

3. Orlando RC, Bozymski EM. Clinical and manometric effects of nitroglycerin in diffuse esophageal spasm. *N Engl J Med*. 1973;**289**(1):23–25.

4. Swamy N. Esophageal spasm: clinical and manometric response to nitroglycerine and long acting nitrites. *Gastroenterology*. 1977;**72**(1):23–27.

5. Achem SR, Kolts BE. Current medical therapy for esophageal motility disorders. *Am J Med*. 1992;**92**(5A):98S–105S.

6. Richter JE, Spurling TJ, Cordova CM, *et al*. Effects of oral calcium blocker, diltiazem, on esophageal contractions. Studies in volunteers and patients with nutcracker esophagus. *Dig Dis Sci*. 1984;**29**(7):649–656.

7. Cattau EL, Jr., Castell DO, Johnson DA, *et al*. Diltiazem therapy for symptoms associated with nutcracker esophagus. *Am J Gastroenterol*. 1991;**86** (3):272–276.

8. Blackwell JN, Holt S, Heading RC. Effect of nifedipine on oesophageal motility and gastric emptying. *Digestion*. 1981;**21**(1):50–56.

9. Schmulson MJ, Valdovinos MA. Current and future treatment of chest pain of presumed esophageal origin. *Gastroenterol Clin North Am*. 2004;**33** (1):93–105.

10. Dodds WJ, Dent J, Hogan WJ, *et al*. Effect of atropine on esophageal motor function in humans. *Am J Physiol*. 1981;**240**(4):G290–G296.

11. Clouse RE, Lustman P, Eckert T, *et al*. Low-dose trazodone for symptomatic patients with esophageal contraction abnormalities: a double-blind, placebo-controlled trial. *Gastroenterology*. 1987;**92**(4):1027–1036.

12. Handa M, Mine K, Yamamoto H, *et al*. Antidepressant treatment of patients with diffuse esophageal spasm: a psychosomatic approach. *J Clin Gastroenterol*. 1999;**28**(3):228–232.

13. Cannon R, Quyyumi A, Mincemoyer R, *et al*. Imipramine in patients with chest pain despite normal coronary angiograms. *N Engl J Med*. 1994;**330** (20):1411–1417.

14. Rao SS, Hayek B, Summers RW. Functional chest pain of esophageal origin: hyperalgesia or motor dysfunction. *Am J Gastroenterol*. 2001;**96**(9):2584–2589.

Fibromyalgia

MICHAEL WALTA AND STEPHEN H. THOMAS

■ Agents

- Antidepressants
- Anticonvulsants
- Opioids
- Acetaminophen
- Ondansetron
- Benzodiazepines
- NSAIDs
- Steroids
- Local anesthetics

■ Evidence

Fibromyalgia is marked by high interpatient variability in both clinical course and efficacy of particular therapies. A large part of this variability results from the somatization, which makes up a significant portion of "fibromyalgia pain" seen in the acute care setting. Although this chapter outlines some worthy trials assessing fibromyalgia treatment, the acute care provider considering prescribing such therapy must integrate any acute intervention into the patient's longitudinal care plan. Initiating new fibromyalgia drugs – even if evidenced-based logic is applied – is problematic and should not be embarked upon unless there is appropriate communication with the physician who will guide long-term care. If new drugs *are* initiated, the need to titrate dosing upwards over days or weeks usually means that neither the acute care provider nor the patient should rely upon rapid symptom relief. In short, the special situation presented by patients with fibromyalgia is such that the acute care provider should be loathe to change a patient's pain management plan, unless such a change is accompanied by communication with the follow-up provider.

Fibromyalgia pain does not result from peripheral nociceptor stimulation but instead arises from deficient CNS processing and modulation of pain signals. Consequently, centrally acting medications form the mainstay of the management of chronic fibromyalgia pain.[1] Fortunately, management decisions in this challenging disease can be informed by results from a number of studies assessing myriad analgesic approaches.

Tricyclic antidepressants (TCAs) and related drugs have some efficacy when compared with placebo in clinical trials. The best evidence exists for *cyclobenzaprine* (30–50 mg/day), which in five clinical trials showed a 20% response rate (i.e. need to treat 4.8 patients to achieve significant pain relief in a single subject).[2] Several studies have demonstrated that low-dose *amitriptyline* (25–50 mg/day) produces significant pain score reductions compared with placebo controls, in 25–45% of patients.[3-5] Utility of **TCAs** is limited by a high (> 50%) rate of nonresponse to both *cyclobenzaprine* and *amitriptyline*. Furthermore, the side effect profile of **TCAs** (e.g. drowsiness, dry mouth, constipation, edema, weight gain) in fibromyalgia patients contributes to rates of medication self-discontinuation that approach 50% in the first 12 months of therapy.[6,7]

There is mixed evidence regarding **antidepressants** other than **TCAs** for fibromyalgia pain relief. *Fluoxetine* and *duloxetine* are the most extensively studied **SSRIs**. One multicenter trial found no pain relief with *duloxetine* compared with placebo, but another placebo-controlled trial found modest pain score reductions.[8,9] Considering the available data, it seems likely that there is some role for *duloxetine* (60 mg QD, titrated to 60 mg PO BID) in fibromyalgia.[10]

Fluoxetine outperforms placebo in RCTs but only when given in a high-dose (80 mg/day) regimen.[11,12] However, one trial suggests that adding low-dose *fluoxetine* (20 mg/day) to a **TCA** (*amitriptyline* 25mg/day) yields better pain relief than that which is achieved with **TCA** monotherapy.[13] Other **antidepressants** (e.g. *desipramine*, *citalopram*, *venlafaxine*, *milnacipran*, *bupropion*) have been studied for treating fibromyalgia pain, but there is currently no basis for recommending acute care use of these drugs.[14-17]

In addition to **TCAs** and other **antidepressants**, the other commonly seen approach to treating fibromyalgia pain is the use of **anticonvulsants**.

A multicenter placebo-controlled trial supported the use of *pregabalin* (150–450 mg/day), though it appears that higher doses (450 mg/day) were required to achieve a clinically significant response of at least 50% reduction in pain; this was achieved in 29% of patients receiving *pregabalin* 450 mg/day compared with 13% receiving placebo.[18] Although *gabapentin* and other **anticonvulsants** (e.g. *carbamazepine*, *phenytoin*) are sometimes used in fibromyalgia, there is no evidence supporting their efficacy.[19]

Few studies specifically examine the use of **opioids** for the treatment of acute fibromyalgia pain. However, there is general consensus on **opioids'** efficacy for the treatment of chronic noncancer pain, of which fibromyalgia is considered a subset.[20] In this nonspecific pain population, the acute care clinician can expect a 30% reduction in non-nociceptive pain with commencement of *morphine* (15–240 mg/day PO), *oxycodone* (10–120 mg/day), or *codeine* (20–180 mg/day); IV **opioids** have similar efficacy.[20–23] Patients in this population who fail to respond to IV **opioids** will not generally respond to equianalgesic doses of oral **opioids**.[21] It is noteworthy that there are addiction and long-term dependence issues that should make the ED physician reluctant to institute therapy with **opioids** or **benzodiazepines** in the population with fibromyalgia.

Several fibromyalgia review articles advocate use of *tramadol*, and the overall evidence supporting this drug's efficacy in fibromyalgia pain is, on balance, good.[20,24,25] One small (*n* = 12) placebo-controlled crossover RCT demonstrated no efficacy of *tramadol* (100 mg IV).[26] A larger (*n* = 100) placebo-controlled study of oral *tramadol* (150–600 mg/day) found clinically significant pain reduction.[27] A placebo-controlled trial of combination therapy with *tramadol* (75–300 mg/day) plus *acetaminophen* (1300–4000 mg/day) showed significant, though modest, outperformance compared with placebo (pain reduction of 19 mm versus 7 mm on a 100 mm scale).[28] Another large placebo-controlled study demonstrated that patients taking oral *tramadol* plus *acetaminophen* achieved significant improvement in both pain and quality of life indices compared with placebo.[29]

In fibromyalgia patients taking long-term **opioids**, a methodologically rigorous study showed that administration of the non-ergot **dopamine**

agonist *pramipexole* (4.5 mg/day) significantly reduced pain (42% of subjects achieving at least 50% pain reduction) and improved myriad quality-of-life indices.[30]

Acetaminophen (*paracetamol*; 2000–4000 mg/day) monotherapy is no more effective than placebo.[25] In a double-blind crossover study comparing *acetaminophen* with *ondansetron* (4 mg/day PO), the selective **serotonin blocker** achieved significantly greater pain score reductions.[31]

The **benzodiazepines** are also associated with mixed results in fibromyalgia trials. *Alprazolam* (0.5–3.0 mg/day PO), either as monotherapy or in combination with the **NSAID ibuprofen** (1600–2400 mg/day), was associated with significant pain score reductions as assessed in a double-blind placebo-controlled trial.[32] Dual therapy with the **benzodiazepine**-derivative *bromazepam* (3 mg/day PO) plus the **NSAID** *tenoxicam* (20 mg/day PO) was associated with no improvement over placebo in a trial of 164 patients.[33]

Given the lack of inflammatory pathophysiology in fibromyalgia, it is not surprising that no data support use of **corticosteroids** or **NSAIDs** in treating fibromyalgia pain. Both *prednisone* (20 mg/day) and **NSAIDs** such as *ibuprofen* (1600–2400 mg/day) and *naproxen* (1000 mg/day) were ineffective in placebo-controlled studies of fibromyalgia pain.[34,35]

Local anesthetics have shown mixed results in fibromyalgia trials. *Lidocaine* (4% solution) administered as a topical sphenopalatine block achieved no efficacy compared with placebo.[36] Investigators in an uncontrolled small trial ($n = 10$) employing injection of tender points with *lidocaine* (0.5–1.0 mL of 0.5–1% solution) found clinically significant pain score reductions at the time of injection and at 7 and 30 days afterwards.[37]

The incomplete success of the preceding approaches has prompted investigation of novel therapies for fibromyalgia pain. A small uncontrolled study showed pain score reduction with SC *gamma-hydroxybutyrate* (2.25 g HS and 4 h later).[38] Placebo-controlled double-blind trials of the biological cofactor *S-adenosylmethionine* showed significant pain relief associated with oral dosing (400–800 mg/day), but no benefit with IV dosing (400 mg/day).[39,40] Neither *malic acid* nor *calcitonin* provide better pain relief than that achieved with placebo.[41,42]

■ Summary and recommendations

First line:

- cyclobenzaprine (10 mg PO TID) *or*
- tramadol (25 mg PO daily, titrated up to 25 mg four times daily) plus acetaminophen (1000 mg q 6 h)

Reasonable:

- amitriptyline (25–50 mg PO QD)
- pregabalin (150 mg/day PO divided BID–TID; may increase to 450 mg/day PO divided BID–TID)
- pramipexole (0.125 mg PO TID)
- alprazolam (0.5 mg PO QD)

Pregnancy: ondansetron (4 mg PO QD–TID)

Pediatric:

- ondansetron (4 mg PO TID; lower doses if age < 4 years)
- low-dose TCA such as amitriptyline (1 mg/kg PO divided TID has been recommended but there is limited supporting evidence; particular caution is warranted in patients under 12 years)
- local anesthetic injection

Special cases:

- *patient with refractory pain and no non-opioid options*: trial of IV opioids (e.g. morphine initial dose 4–6 mg IV, then titrate) with outpatient opioids (e.g. oxycodone 5–10 mg PO q4–6 h) prescribed *if* there is response to IV therapy
- *patients already on therapy*: most patients have tried (many) therapeutic approaches before presenting to acute care providers; in many cases, the drugs patients are already taking may be dose escalated to the maxima outlined in this chapter
- *patients starting on a new drug*: optimal fibromyalgia patient care requires a long-term plan; acute care providers instituting a new agent can, in consultation with follow-up providers where possible, plan for dose escalation of new agents (e.g. tramadol, pregabalin) for which the initial dose is much lower than the maximum (and more effective) dose

References

1. Maizels M, McCarberg B. Antidepressants and antiepileptic drugs for chronic non-cancer pain. *Am Fam Physician*. 2005;**71**(3):483–490.

2. Tofferi JK, Jackson JL, O'Malley PG. Treatment of fibromyalgia with cyclobenzaprine: a meta-analysis. *Arthritis Rheum*. 2004;**51**(1):9–13.

3. Heymann RE, Helfenstein M, Feldman D. A double-blind, randomized, controlled study of amitriptyline, nortriptyline and placebo in patients with fibromyalgia. An analysis of outcome measures. *Clin Exp Rheumatol*. 2001;**19**(6):697–702.

4. Bennett RM. Antidepressants do not have better results than placebo in the treatment of fibromyalgia in Brazil. *Curr Rheumatol Rep*. 2002;**4**(4):284–285.

5. Carette S, McCain GA, Bell DA, *et al*. Evaluation of amitriptyline in primary fibrositis. A double-blind, placebo-controlled study. *Arthritis Rheum*. 1986;**29**(5):655–659.

6. Arnold LM, Keck PE, Jr., Welge JA. Antidepressant treatment of fibromyalgia. A meta-analysis and review. *Psychosomatics*. 2000;**41**(2):104–113.

7. O'Malley PG, Balden E, Tomkins G, *et al*. Treatment of fibromyalgia with antidepressants: a meta-analysis. *J Gen Intern Med*. 2000;**15**(9):659–666.

8. Arnold LM, Lu Y, Crofford LJ, *et al*. A double-blind, multicenter trial comparing duloxetine with placebo in the treatment of fibromyalgia patients with or without major depressive disorder. *Arthritis Rheum*. 2004;**50**(9):2974–2984.

9. Arnold LM, Rosen A, Pritchett YL, *et al*. A randomized, double-blind, placebo-controlled trial of duloxetine in the treatment of women with fibromyalgia with or without major depressive disorder. *Pain*. 2005;**119**(1–3):5–15.

10. Goldstein DJ, Lu Y, Detke MJ, *et al*. Duloxetine vs. placebo in patients with painful diabetic neuropathy. *Pain*. 2005;**116**(1–2):109–118.

11. Arnold LM, Hess EV, Hudson JI, *et al*. A randomized, placebo-controlled, double-blind, flexible-dose study of fluoxetine in the treatment of women with fibromyalgia. *Am J Med*. 2002;**112**(3):191–197.

12. Wolfe F, Cathey MA, Hawley DJ. A double-blind placebo controlled trial of fluoxetine in fibromyalgia. *Scand J Rheumatol*. 1994;**23**(5):255–259.

13. Goldenberg D, Mayskiy M, Mossey C, *et al*. A randomized, double-blind crossover trial of fluoxetine and amitriptyline in the treatment of fibromyalgia. *Arthritis Rheum*. 1996;**39**(11):1852–1859.

14. Anderberg UM, Marteinsdottir I, von Knorring L. Citalopram in patients with fibromyalgia: a randomized, double-blind, placebo-controlled study. *Eur J Pain*. 2000;**4**(1):27–35.

15. Sayar K, Aksu G, Ak I, *et al.* Venlafaxine treatment of fibromyalgia. *Ann Pharmacother.* 2003;**37**(11):1561–1565.

16. Vitton O, Gendreau M, Gendreau J, *et al.* A double-blind placebo-controlled trial of milnacipran in the treatment of fibromyalgia. *Hum Psychopharmacol.* 2004;**19**(Suppl 1):S27–S35.

17. Clayton AH, Kaltsounis-Puckett J. Combination therapy in the treatment of major depressive disorder complicated by fibromyalgia and menopause. *Psychosomatics.* 2002;**43**(6):491–493.

18. Crofford LJ, Rowbotham MC, Mease PJ, *et al.* Pregabalin for the treatment of fibromyalgia syndrome: results of a randomized, double-blind, placebo-controlled trial. *Arthritis Rheum.* 2005;**52**(4):1264–1273.

19. Lindner V, Deuschl G. [Antidepressants and anticonvulsive agents. Practical utility profile in pain therapy.] *Schmerz.* 2004;**18**(1):53–60.

20. Furlan AD, Sandoval JA, Mailis-Gagnon A, *et al.* Opioids for chronic non-cancer pain: a meta-analysis of effectiveness and side effects. *CMAJ.* 2006;**174**(11):1589–1594.

21. Kalso E, Edwards JE, Moore RA, *et al.* Opioids in chronic non-cancer pain: systematic review of efficacy and safety. *Pain.* 2004;**112**(3):372–380.

22. Attal N, Guirimand F, Brasseur L, *et al.* Effects of IV morphine in central pain: a randomized placebo-controlled study. *Neurology.* 2002;**58**(4):554–563.

23. Dellemijn PL, Vanneste JA. Randomised double-blind active-placebo-controlled crossover trial of intravenous fentanyl in neuropathic pain. *Lancet.* 1997;**349**(9054):753–758.

24. Leventhal LJ. Management of fibromyalgia. *Ann Intern Med.* 1999;**131**(11):850–858.

25. Schug SA. Combination analgesia in 2005 – a rational approach: focus on paracetamol–tramadol. *Clin Rheumatol.* 2006;**25**(Suppl 1):16–21.

26. Biasi G, Manca S, Manganelli S, *et al.* Tramadol in the fibromyalgia syndrome: a controlled clinical trial versus placebo. *Int J Clin Pharmacol Res.* 1998;**18**(1):13–19.

27. Russell IJ, Kamin M. Efficacy of Ultram (tramadol HCl) treatment of fibromyalgia syndrome: preliminary analysis of a multicenter, randomized, placebo-controlled study. *Arthritis Rheum.* 1997;**40**(9):S117.

28. Bennett RM, Kamin M, Karim R, *et al.* Tramadol and acetaminophen combination tablets in the treatment of fibromyalgia pain: a double-blind, randomized, placebo-controlled study. *Am J Med.* 2003;**114**(7):537–545.

29. Bennett RM, Schein J, Kosinski MR, *et al.* Impact of fibromyalgia pain on health-related quality of life before and after treatment with tramadol/acetaminophen. *Arthritis Rheum.* 2005;**53**(4):519–527.

30. Holman AJ, Myers RR. A randomized, double-blind, placebo-controlled trial of pramipexole, a dopamine agonist, in patients with fibromyalgia receiving concomitant medications. *Arthritis Rheum.* 2005;**52**(8):2495–2505.

31. Hrycaj P, Stratz T, Mennet P, *et al.* Pathogenetic aspects of responsiveness to ondansetron (5 hydroxytryptamine type 3 receptor antagonist) in patients with primary fibromyalgia syndrome: a preliminary study. *J Rheumatol.* 1996;**23**(8):1418–1423.

32. Russell IJ, Fletcher EM, Michalek JE, *et al.* Treatment of primary fibrositis/fibromyalgia syndrome with ibuprofen and alprazolam. A double-blind, placebo-controlled study. *Arthritis Rheum.* 1991;**34**(5):552–560.

33. Quijada-Carrera J, Valenzuela-Castano A, Povedano-Gomez J, *et al.* Comparison of tenoxicam and bromazepan in the treatment of fibromyalgia: a randomized, double-blind, placebo-controlled trial. *Pain.* 1996;**65**(2–3):221–225.

34. Goldenberg DL, Burckhardt C, Crofford L. Management of fibromyalgia syndrome. *JAMA.* 2004;**292**(19):2388–2395.

35. Clark S, Tindall E, Bennett RM. A double blind crossover trial of prednisone versus placebo in the treatment of fibrositis. *J Rheumatol.* 1985;**12**(5):980–983.

36. Scudds RA, Janzen V, Delaney G, *et al.* The use of topical 4% lidocaine in spheno-palatine ganglion blocks for the treatment of chronic muscle pain syndromes: a randomized, controlled trial. *Pain* 1995;**62**(1):69–77.

37. Bennett MI, Tai YM. Intravenous lignocaine in the management of primary fibromyalgia syndrome. *Int J Clin Pharmacol Res.* 1995;**15**(3):115–119.

38. Scharf MB, Hauck M, Stover R, *et al.* Effect of gamma-hydroxybutyrate on pain, fatigue, and the alpha sleep anomaly in patients with fibromyalgia. Preliminary report. *J Rheumatol.* 1998;**25**(10):1986–1990.

39. Jacobsen S, Danneskiold-Samsoe B, Andersen RB. Oral *S*-adenosylmethionine in primary fibromyalgia. Double-blind clinical evaluation. *Scand J Rheumatol.* 1991;**20**(4):294–302.

40. Volkmann H, Norregaard J, Jacobsen S, *et al.* Double-blind, placebo-controlled cross-over study of intravenous *S*-adenosyl-ʟ-methionine in patients with fibromyalgia. *Scand J Rheumatol.* 1997;**26**(3):206–211.

41. Russell IJ, Michalek JE, Flechas JD, *et al.* Treatment of fibromyalgia syndrome with Super Malic: a randomized, double blind, placebo controlled, crossover pilot study. *J Rheumatol.* 1995;**22**(5):953–958.

42. Bessette L, Carette S, Fossel AH, *et al.* A placebo controlled crossover trial of subcutaneous salmon calcitonin in the treatment of patients with fibromyalgia. *Scand J Rheumatol.* 1998;**27**(2):112–116.

Gastritis and peptic ulcer disease

MEGAN L. FIX AND STEPHEN H. THOMAS

■ Agents

- Antacids
- Belladonna alkaloids plus phenobarbital
- Viscous lidocaine
- H2-receptor antagonists
- Proton pump inhibitors
- Sucralfate
- Prokinetics

■ Evidence

This chapter groups the clinically distinct, but similarly treated, entities of gastritis and peptic ulcer disease (GPUD). While some patients with endoscopically confirmed ulcers or gastritis present to the ED with refractory pain, in most cases it is not easy to distinguish between the various GI causes of epigastric pain. In fact, endoscopy trials show that neither clinical gestalt nor multivariate modeling (using ED-available information) can reliably distinguish between organic and functional dyspepsia.[1] Consequently, even in those ED cases for which a GI origin for epigastric pain can be assumed, diagnostic uncertainty is common. Clinicians treating epigastric pain may find useful information in some other chapters (e.g. those on biliary tract pain or gastroesophageal reflux disease [GERD]).

The diagnostic imprecisions of the ED population prompt additional caveats. First, acute care clinicians trying to apply the literature on epigastric pain therapy should keep in mind that the typical clinical study subject is one in whom there is an endoscopically characterized diagnosis – a luxury the acute care provider must often do without. Second, the interpretation of dyspepsia studies is influenced by the fact that only since the mid-1990s has there been a full appreciation of the role of *Helicobacter pylori* in GPUD cure and symptom relief; a study's publication year, therefore, has added relevance.

This chapter focuses on patients with organic disease, with some concluding notes on the challenging management of functional dyspepsia. Although this discussion does not include non-GI causes of epigastric pain, we warn and strongly advise against incorporating pain response to "GI" therapy into acute care diagnosis. Just as relief with *nitroglycerin* (*glyceryl trinitrate*) is unreliably indicative of a cardiac pain etiology, symptomatic improvement after GI-directed medications should not impact the ED diagnostic process.[2-5] Specifically, a common error in the diagnosis of ischemic coronary syndromes is to assume one is dealing with GERD or peptic ulcer disease because the patient responds to GI therapy. Acute coronary syndromes, and inferior wall disease in particular, can be frequently accompanied by indigestion or heartburn sensation.

The most basic treatment for patients with GPUD is administration of **antacids**. These agents (e.g. *magnesium hydroxide*, *aluminum hydroxide*) are usually given in liquid form in the ED. Many commercial preparations include the anti-gas agent *simethicone*. There is little difference between various **antacid** preparations, and there is no strong evidence supporting liquid over tablet formulations. Some data suggest that a combination-type **antacid** (e.g. with *alum earth*, *aluminum hydroxide*, and *magnesium hydroxide*) relieves symptoms better than a single-component approach, but the existing literature is insufficiently convincing to recommend one specific approach.[6] The probable benefit of the combined tablet is to avoid the diarrhea caused by *magnesium* preparations alone or the constipation caused by the *aluminum* tablets alone. A typical regimen for GPUD entails doses of 15–30 mL, 1 and 3 h after meals and at bedtime. Alternatively, two antacid tablets may be taken between meals and at bedtime.

As is the case with GERD, the most useful role of **antacids** in GPUD will usually be as an adjunct for occasional symptomatic relief. Most **antacids** are safe in pregnancy, but agents in this class can interfere with iron absorption. Therefore, pregnant patients should maximize time intervals between ingestion of **antacids** and prenatal vitamins and iron supplements.[7]

In the ED, liquid **antacids** are often combined with other agents to form a "**GI cocktail**." In spite of – or perhaps because of – the widespread use of the

GI cocktail, there is variance as to which agents are added to the **antacid** base. The RCTs addressing composition of a **GI cocktail** provide some guidance, but results are inconsistent. The most common additives to **antacids** are *viscous lidocaine* and an elixir combination of **anticholinergics** (*belladonna: atropine*, *hyoscyamine*, and *scopolamine* [*hyoscine*]) and *phenobarbital*. An older RCT found significant benefit from adding *viscous lidocaine* (15 mL of a 2% preparation) to the **antacid** base.[8] Noncontrolled trial data find no benefit in substituting *benzocaine* for *lidocaine* in a **GI cocktail**, with both preparations providing significant pain relief.[9] A more recent, more methodologically robust, study found that addition of viscous *lidocaine*, elixir of **anticholinergics** plus *phenobarbital*, or both, resulted in no incremental analgesic effect over that achieved with **antacids** alone.[10] No other high-grade trials assessing the composition of a **GI cocktail** are found, so there is a relative paucity of evidence. There is anecdotal experience of **GI cocktail** efficacy, even if pain relief is achieved by mechanisms other than direct topical activity. Also, the relative risk of supplementing **antacids** to formulate a **GI cocktail** is low. Therefore, we believe that the **antacid**-only approach is appropriate, but that it is also reasonable to administer a **GI cocktail**, particularly if patients report success with previous use of a mixture. We again remind the reader that positive response to a **GI cocktail** does not provide negative evidence against ischemic coronary disease. Analgesia after GI medications is obviously a good thing, but not a finding with diagnostic utility.

The long history of **bismuth salt** use for dyspepsia is supported by literature suggesting some potential ED role for these agents. A typical trial finds that administration of *colloidal bismuth subcitrate* provides significant pain relief in just over half of patients with either gastritis or duodenitis.[11] Other trial data confirm that, for patients with biopsy-demonstrated gastritis (but not for those with negative biopsies), *bismuth subcitrate* provides significant pain relief, hastens healing, and reduces need for **antacids**.[12] Other **bismuth salts** (e.g. *bismuth aluminate*) have also been shown to be reliable, if partial, relievers of gastritis pain.[13] The consistent, though incomplete, degree of GPUD pain relief provided by **bismuth salts** translates into a role for these agents as occasional agents for breakthrough pain.

The importance of *H. pylori* means that there may be a role for **antibiotics** in control of GPUD symptoms. The link between *H. pylori* presence and (non-GERD) dyspepsia symptoms is reasonably well characterized. Furthermore, there is evidence that eradication of *H. pylori* is associated with symptomatic relief (except in those with chronic dyspepsia).[14] In fact, studies of patients with epigastric pain have shown occasional symptomatic relief from bacterial eradication even in patients lacking ulceration.[15] A comprehensive overview of the literature addressing *H. pylori* eradication and dyspepsia is beyond this chapter's scope, but the topic warrants mention given the strong association of *H. pylori* with both gastric (70%) and duodenal (95%) ulcers. For the acute care provider, it is reasonable to consider institution of eradication therapy in patients with high likelihood of *H. pylori*. At minimum, the topic should be discussed with patients and follow-up arranged for appropriate diagnostic testing. For those patients where ED providers will initiate eradication therapy, Cochrane review has shown equal relief of symptoms (and eradication of *H. pylori*) with a seven day course as with a 14 day course of PO therapy as follows: *pantoprazole* (40 mg BID), *clarithromycin* (500 mg BID), and *metronidazole* (500 mg BID).[14,16]

The reason that agents such as **antacids** and **bismuth salts** are reserved for occasional symptomatic relief is that more consistent success is achieved with newer agents such as the **proton pump inhibitors** (**PPIs**). The many **PPIs** available for acid suppression and GPUD relief are probably similar in terms of their excellent efficacy – any of the **PPIs** will be effective in most patients.[17,18] Some data suggest that the newer agents may have higher efficacy (e.g. faster onset of pain relief).[19,20] An example meta-analysis assessing peptic ulcer relief found *pantoprazole* (40 mg daily) provided slightly better analgesic effect than *omeprazole* (20 mg daily). However, the review's authors considered that the difference was more likely related to dosage (40 mg versus 20 mg) rather than agent.[18] We find this argument plausible and recommend increasing a **PPI** to agent-specific ceiling levels if incomplete response is obtained with submaximal dosing. The evidence of **PPIs**' efficacy supports a presumed hyperacid secretion etiology for both duodenal ulceration and alcohol-induced gastritis. (Alcohol cessation is also recommended as a means of providing partial or complete symptom relief for some patients with GPUD.)

The following chapter (on GERD) outlines some potential age-specific preferences for certain **PPIs**, but there is limited evidence on the topic as relates to GPUD. The various available **PPIs** do come in different formulations, but the clinical significance of different formulations is yet to be fully elucidated.[21]

Overviews of the **PPIs** note that these agents are effective in many patients who are poorly responsive to **H2-receptor antagonists**.[22] The **PPIs** also relieve symptoms better than does the gastroprotective agent *sucralfate*. Data from a RCT comparing *omeprazole* (40 mg PO QD) and *sucralfate* (2 g PO BID) indicated superior symptom relief with omeprazole after a two week follow-up assessment; the **PPI** also reduced symptom recurrence.[23] The improvements in both symptom reduction and relapse rates with the PPI contributed to conclusions that primary use of this class is cost effective.[22] Finally, the **PPIs** are preferable to the **H2-receptor antagonists** for combination with **antibiotics** to achieve GPUD symptom relief (and cure) via eradication of *H. pylori*.[24]

Although not as effective as the **PPIs**, *sucralfate* (1 g PO TID, or 1 g PO before meals and at bedtime) has efficacy that is good and approximately equal to that of the **H2-receptor antagonists**. Data from RCTs show that *sucralfate* use provides ulcer pain relief in the same proportion of patients (nearly 80%) as **H2-receptor antagonists** such as *ranitidine* (150 mg PO BID).[25,26] Compared with **H2-receptor antagonists**, *sucralfate* does appear to be associated with slightly more side effects (particularly constipation), and *sucralfate*'s effect on absorption of other medications may be a consideration in some patients.[26]

Sucralfate's efficacy appears to be unrelated to its formulation. For relief of gastritis symptoms, a BID regimen of *sucralfate* gel is as effective as the standard QID regimen of *sucralfate* suspension.[27]

For acid-related pain, the inferiority of **H2-receptor antagonists** to **PPIs** may be because the former agents block only one gastric parietal cell acid secretion mechanism (i.e. the histaminic). Compared with *sucralfate*, the **H2-receptor antagonist ranitidine** (150 mg PO BID) provides similar pain relief, with potentially better early symptom relief (i.e. improvement during the initial weeks of follow-up).[25] Trials have found that **H2-receptor**

antagonists provide significant pain relief from gastritis within a few days of instituting therapy, and that side effect rates are low (and more favorable than seen with *sucralfate*).[26,28]

After **antacids** and *sucralfate*, **H2-receptor antagonists** such as *ranitidine* from the second tier for GERD treatment during pregnancy.[29,30] The fetal safety of the **H2-receptor antagonists** for GERD is logically extended to the use of these agents in GPUD.

Since altered gastroduodenal motility is a postulated occasional cause of gastritis, the **prokinetic** drugs have been employed to treat GPUD.[31] These are used less frequently than other therapies mentioned in this chapter, but they may be a reasonable choice for relief of nonspecific dyspepsia, especially if *H. pylori* status is negative or unknown.[32,33] **Prokinetic** drugs are also recommended as a first-line alternative to **H2-receptor antagonists** in elderly patients with dyspepsia that is nonspecific or not yet endoscopically investigated.[33,34]

Trial data suggest that, for patients with nonspecific dyspepsia, the **prokinetic** *cisapride* (10 mg PO BID) slightly outperforms the **H2-receptor antagonist** *ranitidine* (150 mg PO BID) in terms of symptom relief and relapse.[33] Data from an RCT of patients with gastritis suggest that newer **prokinetics** such as *clebopride* are significantly more effective than older agents such as *domperidone*.[35] Data from one trial in patients with antral gastritis indicated that addition of the **prokinetic** *cisapride* (10 mg PO QID) augmented relief afforded by the **H2-receptor antagonist** *famotidine* (40 mg PO QD).[36] Though some newer **H2-receptor antagonists** (e.g. *nizatidine*) have **prokinetic**-like characteristics, data suggest that these characteristics are not responsible for any significant benefit.[37] **Prokinetics** may occasionally cause unwanted CNS or cardiac side effects.

This chapter is not intended to address functional dyspepsia in detail, but the therapies mentioned for GPUD (particularly **PPIs**, **H2-receptor antagonists**) may be tried for patients with this chronic disorder.[38,39] Unfortunately, treatments useful for GPUD are often unhelpful in relieving functional dyspepsia, and those that are helpful are often only marginally so.[40] Available meta-analysis data suggest that **PPIs** are preferred for functional dyspepsia similar to GPUD-like pain.[38] For patients with non-ulcer dyspepsia, two trials (one of which enrolled only *H. pylori*-negative subjects) concluded that *sucralfate* was more effective than *ranitidine*.[41,42] Cochrane review of non-ulcer dyspepsia pain relief concluded that **antacids**, **bismuth salts**, and *sucralfate* are no better than placebo; the same review labels as methodologically suspect studies suggesting benefits from **H2-receptor antagonists**.[39,43]

The future for functional dyspepsia management is not promising. Placebo-controlled trials demonstrate that the disorder is refractory even to the latest gastroprotective agents (e.g. *rebamipide*).[44] Even the eradication of *H. pylori* does not reliably improve functional dyspepsia. While Cochrane review has suggested a possible role for *H. pylori* eradication in functional dyspepsia, a typical RCT in *H. pylori*-positive functional dyspeptics revealed no symptomatic improvement even when follow-up assessment (after *omeprazole* plus **antibiotics**) confirmed bacterial eradication and resolution of gastric inflammation.[45,46] The treatment of non-ulcer dyspepsia is most likely to be effective when psychological approaches (and medications) are considered in addition to prescription of GI-active agents.[47]

■ Summary and recommendations

First line: pantoprazole 40 mg PO once daily

Reasonable (*none of the following agents are as effective as PPIs, but all provide some symptom relief*):
- antacids (e.g. aluminum/magnesium salts, 2–4 teaspoons or 2–4 tablets PO, between meals and HS)
- H2-receptor antagonist (e.g. ranitidine 150 mg PO BID or 300 mg HS)
- sucralfate 1 g PO QID (before meals and HS)
- cisapride (10 mg PO BID)

Pediatric:
- sucralfate 500 mg PO QID (before meals and HS)
- children at least 1 year of age: lansoprazole (initial dose, administered in the morning, of 15 mg/day PO if < 30 kg, 30 mg/day PO if at least 30 kg)
- children at least 12 years of age: antacid preparation at adult dose (e.g. aluminum/magnesium salts, 2–4 teaspoons or 2–4 tablets PO, between meals and HS)

Pregnancy:

- H2-receptor antagonist (e.g. ranitidine 150 mg PO BID) and sucralfate (1 g PO QID) are recommended since they are both pregnancy Category B
- antacids taken with time spacing from prenatal vitamins and iron (e.g. aluminum/magnesium salts, 2–4 teaspoons or 2–4 tablets PO, between meals and HS)

Special cases:

- *patients requiring on-demand relief for occasional pain:* pantoprazole 20 mg PO QD
- *patients on chronic therapy (e.g. a PPI) with intermittent need for break-through pain:* bismuth salts or antacids (e.g. aluminum/magnesium salts, 2–4 teaspoons or 2–4 tablets PO, between meals and HS)
- *elderly patients or others with noncharacterized dyspepsia*: a trial of cis-apride (10 mg PO BID) is reasonable and can be added to existing therapy with PPIs or H2-receptor antagonists
- *breastfeeding patients requiring systemic therapy:* ranitidine 150 mg PO BID
- *functional dyspepsia*: PPIs as first line; H2-receptor antagonists (e.g. rani-tidine 150 mg PO BID) or, if symptoms are not ulcer-like, sucralfate (1 g PO QID) as second line
- H. pylori *eradication regimen (7-day course)*: pantoprazole (40 mg PO BID), clarithromycin (500 mg PO BID), and metronidazole (500 mg PO BID)

References

1. Moayyedi P, Talley NJ, Fennerty MB, *et al.* Can the clinical history distinguish between organic and functional dyspepsia? *JAMA.* 2006;**295**(13):1566–1576.
2. Servi RJ, Skiendzielewski JJ. Relief of myocardial ischemia pain with a gastro-intestinal cocktail. *Am J Emerg Med.* 1985;**3**(3):208–209.
3. Diercks DB, Boghos E, Guzman H, *et al.* Changes in the numeric descriptive scale for pain after sublingual nitroglycerin do not predict cardiac etiology of chest pain. *Ann Emerg Med.* 2005;**45**(6):581–585.
4. Dickinson MW. The "GI cocktail" in the evaluation of chest pain in the emer-gency department. *J Emerg Med.* 1996;**14**(2):245–246.

5. Wrenn K, Slovis CM, Gongaware J. Using the "GI cocktail": a descriptive study. *Ann Emerg Med.* 1995;**26**(6):687–690.

6. Lichtenstein H. [Antacid therapy of upper abdominal symptoms. Double-blind study on the effect and tolerance of 2 antacids in gastritis, esophagitis and functional upper abdominal symptoms.] *Fortschr Med.* 1991;**109**(26):528–532.

7. Cappell MS. Gastric and duodenal ulcers during pregnancy. *Gastroenterol Clin North Am.* 2003;**32**(1):263–308.

8. Welling LR, Watson WA. The emergency department treatment of dyspepsia with antacids and oral lidocaine. *Ann Emerg Med.* 1990;**19**(7):785–788.

9. Vilke GM, Jin A, Davis DP, *et al.* Prospective randomized study of viscous lidocaine versus benzocaine in a GI cocktail for dyspepsia. *J Emerg Med.* 2004;**27**(1):7–9.

10. Berman DA, Porter RS, Graber M. The GI cocktail is no more effective than plain liquid antacid: a randomized, double blind clinical trial. *J Emerg Med.* 2003;**25**(3):239–244.

11. Khanna MU, Abraham P, Nair NG, *et al.* Colloidal bismuth subcitrate in non-ulcer dyspepsia. *J Postgrad Med.* 1992;**38**(3):106–108.

12. Kang JY, Tay HH, Wee A, *et al.* Effect of colloidal bismuth subcitrate on symptoms and gastric histology in non-ulcer dyspepsia. A double blind placebo controlled study. *Gut.* 1990;**31**(4):476–480.

13. Stanescu A, Malfertheiner P, Mayer D, *et al.* [Bismuth aluminate in gastroenterology. Therapeutic effects in chronic erosive *Campylobacter pylori*-associated gastritis.] *Fortschr Med.* 1989;**107**(29):623–626.

14. Dammann HG, Folsch UR, Hahn EG, *et al.* Eradication of *H. pylori* with pantoprazole, clarithromycin, and metronidazole in duodenal ulcer patients: a head-to-head comparison between two regimens of different duration. *Helicobacter.* 2000;**5**(1):41–51.

15. Bruley Des Varannes S, Flejou JF, Colin R, *et al.* There are some benefits for eradicating *Helicobacter pylori* in patients with non-ulcer dyspepsia. *Aliment Pharmacol Ther.* 2001;**15**(8):1177–1185.

16. Ford AC, Delaney BC, Forman D, *et al.* Eradication therapy for peptic ulcer disease in *Helicobacter pylori* positive patients. *Cochrane Database Syst Rev.* 2006(2):CD003840.

17. Wang X, Fang JY, Lu R, *et al.* A meta-analysis: comparison of esomeprazole and other proton pump inhibitors in eradicating *Helicobacter pylori*. *Digestion.* 2006;**73**(2–3):178–186.

18. Klok RM, Postma MJ, van Hout BA, *et al.* Meta-analysis: comparing the efficacy of proton pump inhibitors in short-term use. *Aliment Pharmacol Ther.* 2003;**17**(10):1237–1245.

19. Florent C. Progress with proton pump inhibitors in acid peptic disease: treatment of duodenal and gastric ulcer. *Clin Ther.* 1993;**15**(Suppl B): 14–21.

20. Matheson AJ, Jarvis B. Lansoprazole: an update of its place in the management of acid-related disorders. *Drugs.* 2001;**61**(12):1801–1833.

21. Devlin JW, Welage LS, Olsen KM. Proton pump inhibitor formulary considerations in the acutely ill. Part 2: Clinical efficacy, safety, and economics. *Ann Pharmacother.* 2005;**39**(11):1844–1851.

22. Barradell LB, McTavish D. Omeprazole: a pharmacoeconomic evaluation of its use in duodenal ulcer and reflux oesophagitis. *Pharmacoeconomics.* 1993;**3**(6):482–510.

23. Sorensen HT, Rasmussen HH, Balslev I, *et al.* Effect of omeprazole and sucralfate on prepyloric gastric ulcer. A double blind comparative trial and one year follow up. *Gut.* 1994;**35**(6):837–840.

24. Gisbert JP, Khorrami S, Calvet X, *et al.* Meta-analysis: proton pump inhibitors vs. H_2-receptor antagonists: their efficacy with antibiotics in *Helicobacter pylori* eradication. *Aliment Pharmacol Ther.* 2003;**18**(8):757–766.

25. Guslandi M. Comparison of sucralfate and ranitidine in the treatment of chronic nonerosive gastritis. A randomized, multicenter trial. *Am J Med.* 1989;**86**(6A):45–48.

26. Rey JF, Legras B, Verdier A, *et al.* Comparative study of sucralfate versus cimetidine in the treatment of acute gastroduodenal ulcer. Randomized trial with 667 patients. *Am J Med.* 1989;**86**(6A):116–121.

27. Guslandi M, Ferrero S, Fusillo M. Sucralfate gel for symptomatic chronic gastritis: multicentre comparative trial versus sucralfate suspension. *Ital J Gastroenterol.* 1994;**26**(9):442–445.

28. Miwa T, Miyoshi A. Famotidine in the treatment of gastritis. *Scand J Gastroenterol Suppl.* 1987;**134**:46–50.

29. Richter JE. Gastroesophageal reflux disease during pregnancy. *Gastroenterol Clin North Am.* 2003;**32**(1):235–261.

30. Richter JE. Review article: the management of heartburn in pregnancy. *Aliment Pharmacol Ther.* 2005;**22**(9):749–757.

31. Bazaldua OV, Schneider FD. Evaluation and management of dyspepsia. *Am Fam Physician.* 1999;**60**(6):1773–1784, 1787–1788.

32. Bodger K, Daly MJ, Heatley RV. Prescribing patterns for dyspepsia in primary care: a prospective study of selected general practitioners. *Aliment Pharmacol Ther.* 1996;**10**(6):889–895.

33. Quartero AO, Numans ME, de Melker RA, *et al.* Dyspepsia in primary care: acid suppression as effective as prokinetic therapy. A randomized clinical trial. *Scand J Gastroenterol.* 2001;**36**(9):942–947.

34. Pound SE, Heading RC. Diagnosis and treatment of dyspepsia in the elderly. *Drugs Aging.* 1995;**7**(5):347–354.

35. Angelini G, Castagnini A, Rizzoli R, *et al.* Treatment of reflux gastritis: double blind comparison between clebopride and domperidone. A preliminary report. *Ital J Gastroenterol.* 1990;**22**(1):24–27.

36. Dallera F, Scanzi G, Gendarini A. [Prokinetic activity and antral inflammation. Usefulness of cisapride combined with H2 antagonists in gastritis.] *Clin Ter.* 1994;**144**(1):23–26.

37. Koskenpato J, Punkkinen JM, Kairemo K, *et al.* Nizatidine and gastric emptying in functional dyspepsia. *Dig Dis Sci.* 2008;**53**(2):352–357.

38. Wang WH, Huang JQ, Zheng GF, *et al.* Effects of proton-pump inhibitors on functional dyspepsia: a meta-analysis of randomized placebo-controlled trials. *Clin Gastroenterol Hepatol.* 2007;**5**(2):178–185; quiz 140.

39. Moayyedi P, Soo S, Deeks J, *et al.* Pharmacological interventions for non-ulcer dyspepsia. *Cochrane Database Syst Rev.* 2006(4):CD001960.

40. Bytzer P, Talley NJ. Current indications for acid suppressants in dyspepsia. *Best Pract Res Clin Gastroenterol.* 2001;**15**(3):385–400.

41. Dhali GK, Garg PK, Sharma MP. Role of anti-*Helicobacter pylori* treatment in *H. pylori*-positive and cytoprotective drugs in *H. pylori*-negative, non-ulcer dyspepsia: results of a randomized, double-blind, controlled trial in Asian Indians. *J Gastroenterol Hepatol.* 1999;**14**(6):523–528.

42. Misra SP, Dwivedi M, Misra V, *et al.* Sucralfate versus ranitidine in non-ulcer dyspepsia: results of a prospective, randomized, open, controlled trial. *Indian J Gastroenterol.* 1992;**11**(1):7–8.

43. Moayyedi P, Soo S, Deeks J, *et al.* Systematic review: Antacids, H_2-receptor antagonists, prokinetics, bismuth and sucralfate therapy for non-ulcer dyspepsia. *Aliment Pharmacol Ther.* 2003;**17**(10):1215–1227.

44. Miwa H, Osada T, Nagahara A, *et al.* Effect of a gastro-protective agent, rebamipide, on symptom improvement in patients with functional dyspepsia: a double-blind placebo-controlled study in Japan. *J Gastroenterol Hepatol.* 2006;**21**(12):1826–1831.

45. Ashorn M, Rago T, Kokkonen J, *et al.* Symptomatic response to *Helicobacter pylori* eradication in children with recurrent abdominal pain: double blind randomized placebo-controlled trial. *J Clin Gastroenterol.* 2004;**38**(8):646–650.

46. Moayyedi P, Soo S, Deeks J, *et al.* Eradication of *Helicobacter pylori* for non-ulcer dyspepsia. *Cochrane Database Syst Rev.* 2006(2):CD002096.

47. Dickerson LM, King DE. Evaluation and management of nonulcer dyspepsia. *Am Fam Physician.* 2004;**70**(1):107–114.

Gastroesophageal reflux disease

KALANI OLMSTED AND DEBORAH B. DIERCKS

■ Agents

- Morphine
- Antacids
- Proton pump inhibitors
- H2-Receptor antagonists
- Sucralfate
- Prokinetic drugs

■ Evidence

The etiology of chest pain is often unclear upon initial patient evaluation. Given this lack of clarity, and the fact that acute coronary syndromes claim a prominent position in the differential diagnosis, **opioids** such as *morphine* are often used early in patients subsequently diagnosed with gastroesophageal reflux disease (GERD). In fact, *morphine* effectively relieves GERD pain by decreasing the rate of transient lower esophageal sphincter relaxations and by increasing tone – and thus decreasing volume – in the proximal stomach.[1,2]

Antacids (e.g. *aluminum hydroxide, magnesium hydroxide, calcium carbonate*) provide GERD relief by buffering the refluxed gastric contents.[3,4] **Antacids** are readily available, relatively safe, and fast acting. Although they tend to be insufficient as monotherapy, **antacids** represent a viable option for occasional symptom relief, especially when employed in an adjunctive role.[3,5]

Antacids constitute first-line GERD therapy in pregnancy.[6] Most **antacids** are safe in pregnancy, but agents in this class can interfere with iron absorption and so must be taken at times distant from ingestion of prenatal vitamins and iron supplements.[7]

Proton pump inhibitors (**PPIs**) are a first-line treatment for noncardiac chest pain, and for GERD in particular[3,5,8–10] All **PPIs** effectively inhibit gastric acid secretion mediated by a variety of stimuli, and double-blind trials have demonstrated significant improvement in GERD pain relief with **PPIs** compared with **H2-receptor antagonists**.[11]

While the evidence does not indicate a marked superiority of one particular **PPI**, the literature provides some guidance in selecting among available agents. Double-blind trials have demonstrated increased efficacy of newer agents such as *esomeprazole* (40 mg PO once daily) compared with the older **PPI** *omeprazole* (20 mg PO).[12] Another relatively new **PPI**, *pantoprazole*, has also been shown to have advantages over *omeprazole*. A multicenter RCT comparing *pantoprazole* (40 mg PO daily) with *omeprazole* (20 mg PO daily) showed that the former was associated with significantly (by two days) faster achievement of both GERD pain relief and secondary quality-of-life indicators.[13] Another multicenter RCT comparing QD 40 mg PO doses of *pantoprazole* and *esomeprazole* found similar overall efficacy, but again showed *pantoprazole* use was associated with faster onset of 50% pain reduction for both daytime and nighttime pain (3.7 days versus 5.9 days for daytime pain, 1.7 versus 3.5 days for nighttime pain).[14] A trial assessing 20 mg QD doses of *pantoprazole* PO and *esomeprazole* PO suggested that GERD symptom relief is similar in the two groups.[15] This study found significant pain relief within two days for both approaches, but sustained GERD pain relief was seen faster with *pantoprazole* (10 days versus 13 days).[15] One evidence review of the comparative efficacy of the **PPIs** suggested that the incremental gains suggested by studies of newer agents are actually a result of higher relative dosing, rather than intrinsic efficacy advantages.[16] Given the usual 40 mg dosage for newer **PPIs** in trials, compared with 20 mg of older agents, the argument that efficacy is dose based (rather than generation based) has plausibility.

There may be some age-specific preferences for certain **PPIs**. A study in adolescents 12–16 years of age found equivalence between two doses (20 mg PO or 40 mg PO) of *pantoprazole*.[17] The agent *lansoprazole* has been used in children as young as 1 year of age. Expert reviewers have suggested that the preferred approach for geriatric GERD is **PPIs** in general, and *pantoprazole* in particular.[18]

In general, **PPIs** for GERD are administered in "double" doses equaling twice the amount used for ulcer pain (e.g. 40 mg of *pantoprazole* or *esomeprazole*);

this high-dose therapy is continued for two to four weeks.[5,19,20] However, for on-demand relief of mild GERD pain, RCT data have indicated that *pantoprazole* can be administered in a lower dose of 20 mg PO without loss of efficacy, compared with the 40 mg oral dose.[21] Similarly, RCT data for prevention of nighttime GERD symptoms, have demonstrated that 20 mg PO *esomeprazole* is as effective as a 40 mg dose of the same medication (about 50% have resolution of symptoms).[22]

Although pain relief can be seen in as little as two days in patients who are likely to be helped by **PPIs**, a month should be allowed for a full response.[5]

PPIs are a third-tier choice (after **antacids**, *sucralfate*, and *ranitidine*) for GERD during pregnancy.

Meta-analysis finds **PPIs** are ineffective for GERD-associated laryngitis pain.[23]

H2-receptor antagonists such as *ranitidine* (150 mg PO as needed for GERD pain) have been shown in double-blinded trials to achieve better on-demand pain relief than **antacids**.[24] Since **H2-receptor antagonists** block only one gastric parietal cell acid secretion mechanism (i.e. the histaminic), they are less useful than **PPIs** for GERD.[3,5,20,25] The **H2-receptor antagonists** are, however, useful adjuncts for nocturnal pain relief in patients with incomplete symptomatic response to **PPIs**.[3,26]

H2-receptor antagonists, specifically *ranitidine* (pregnancy category B, also safe in breastfeeding) constitute the second tier (after **antacids** and *sucralfate*) in the treatment of GERD during pregnancy.[6,27]

Sucralfate forms a protective barrier by binding to injured gastroesophageal mucosa. Its negligible systemic absorption translates into particular utility of as first-line therapy for mild-to-moderate GERD during pregnancy (it is Pregnancy Category B).[3,6,7]

Prokinetic drugs such as *metoclopramide* and *cisapride* are postulated to relieve GERD by increasing resting lower esophageal sphincter tone and increasing gastric emptying. Data from an RCT showed that *cisapride* (20 mg PO twice daily) significantly reduced GERD pain.[28] Though most acute care providers commonly use *metoclopramide* with minimal adverse effect, there are reports of **prokinetic** drugs causing CNS (e.g. with *metoclopramide*) or cardiac (e.g. with *cisapride*) toxicity. Furthermore, RCTs show that the addition of *metoclopramide* to **H2-receptor antagonists** or **PPIs**

adds no efficacy and incurs substantial risk of additional side effects.[3,29,30] In fact, a 2006 meta-analysis of *metoclopramide* for pediatric GERD treatment was aborted owing to lack of any conclusive evidence; the authors recommend that *metoclopramide* be used with caution given growing recognition of its adverse effects in the pediatric population.[31] The novel prokinetic agent *itopride* has promising preliminary results in an open-label GERD trial, but recommendation for its acute care use must await further data.[32]

Nitrates and **calcium channel blockers** may have a role in pain caused by esophageal spasm, but there is little or no evidence supporting their use in GERD.[33]

■ Summary and recommendations

First line: pantoprazole 40 mg PO QD

Reasonable:

- antacids (e.g. aluminum/magnesium salts, 2–4 teaspoons or 2–4 tablets PO, between meals and HS)
- H2-receptor antagonists (e.g. ranitidine 150 mg PO BID or 300 mg PO HS)
- sucralfate 1 g PO QID (before meals and HS)

Pediatric:

- sucralfate 500 mg PO QID (before meals and HS)
- children at least 1 year of age: lansoprazole (morning dose of 15 mg/day PO if <30 kg; 30 mg/day PO if at least 30 kg)
- children at least 12 years of age: antacid preparation at adult dose (e.g. aluminum/magnesium salts, 2–4 teaspoons or 2–4 tablets PO, between meals and HS)

Pregnancy:

- H2-receptor antagonists (e.g. ranitidine 150–300 mg PO BID) or sucralfate (1 g PO QID)
- antacids taken with time spacing from prenatal vitamins and iron (e.g. aluminum/magnesium salts, 2–4 teaspoons or 2–4 tablets PO, between meals and HS)

Special cases:

■ *patients requiring on-demand relief for occasional GERD pain*: pantoprazole 20 mg PO QD

■ *patients on chronic therapy (e.g. a PPI) with intermittent need for breakthrough pain relief*: antacids (e.g. aluminum/magnesium salts, 2–4 teaspoons or 2–4 tablets PO, between meals and HS)

■ *breastfeeding patients requiring systemic therapy*: ranitidine 150 mg PO BID

References

1. Penagini R, Bianchi PA. Effect of morphine on gastroesophageal reflux and transient lower esophageal sphincter relaxation. *Gastroenterology.* 1997;**113**(2):409–414.

2. Penagini R, Allocca M, Cantu P, *et al.* Relationship between motor function of the proximal stomach and transient lower oesophageal sphincter relaxation after morphine. *Gut.* 2004;**53**(9):1227–1231.

3. Cappell MS. Clinical presentation, diagnosis, and management of gastroesophageal reflux disease. *Med Clin North Am.* 2005;**89**(2):243–291.

4. Fass R, Bautista J, Janarthanan S. Treatment of gastroesophageal reflux disease. *Clin Cornerstone.* 2003;**5**(4):18–29; discussion 30–31.

5. Eslick GD, Fass R. Noncardiac chest pain: evaluation and treatment. *Gastroenterol Clin North Am.* 2003;**32**(2):531–552.

6. Richter JE. Gastroesophageal reflux disease during pregnancy. *Gastroenterol Clin North Am.* 2003;**32**(1):235–261.

7. Cappell MS. Gastric and duodenal ulcers during pregnancy. *Gastroenterol Clin North Am.* 2003;**32**(1):263–308.

8. Achem SR, Kolts BE, MacMath T, *et al.* Effects of omeprazole versus placebo in treatment of noncardiac chest pain and gastroesophageal reflux. *Dig Dis Sci.* 1997;**42**(10):2138–2145.

9. Pandak WM, Arezo S, Everett S, *et al.* Short course of omeprazole: a better first diagnostic approach to noncardiac chest pain than endoscopy, manometry, or 24-hour esophageal pH monitoring. *J Clin Gastroenterol.* 2002;**35**(4):307–314.

10. Cremonini F, Wise J, Moayyedi P, *et al.* Diagnostic and therapeutic use of proton pump inhibitors in non-cardiac chest pain: a metaanalysis. *Am J Gastroenterol.* 2005;**100**(6):1226–1232.

11. Mathias SD, Colwell HH, Miller DP, *et al*. Health-related quality-of-life and quality-days incrementally gained in symptomatic nonerosive GERD patients treated with lansoprazole or ranitidine. *Dig Dis Sci.* 2001;**46** (11):2416–2423.

12. Richter JE, Kahrilas PJ, Johanson J, *et al*. Efficacy and safety of esomeprazole compared with omeprazole in GERD patients with erosive esophagitis: a randomized controlled trial. *Am J Gastroenterol.* 2001;**96**(3):656–665.

13. Gillessen A, Schoffel L, Naumburger A. [Financial restrictions in health care systems could affect treatment quality of GERD-patients.] *Z Gastroenterol.* 2006;**44**(5):379–385.

14. Scholten T, Gatz G, Hole U. Once-daily pantoprazole 40 mg and esomeprazole 40 mg have equivalent overall efficacy in relieving GERD-related symptoms. *Aliment Pharmacol Ther.* 2003;**18**(6):587–594.

15. Monnikes H, Pfaffenberger B, Gatz G, *et al*. Novel measurement of rapid treatment success with ReQuest: first and sustained symptom relief as outcome parameters in patients with endoscopy-negative GERD receiving 20 mg pantoprazole or 20 mg esomeprazole. *Digestion.* 2005;**71** (3):152–158.

16. Klok RM, Postma MJ, van Hout BA, *et al*. Meta-analysis: comparing the efficacy of proton pump inhibitors in short-term use. *Aliment Pharmacol Ther.* 2003;**17**(10):1237–1245.

17. Tsou VM, Baker R, Book L, *et al*. Multicenter, randomized, double-blind study comparing 20 and 40 mg of pantoprazole for symptom relief in adolescents (12 to 16 years of age) with gastroesophageal reflux disease (GERD). *Clin Pediatr (Philadelphia).* 2006;**45**(8):741–749.

18. Bacak BS, Patel M, Tweed E, *et al*. What is the best way to manage GERD symptoms in the elderly? *J Fam Pract.* 2006;**55**(3):251–254, 258.

19. Faybush EM, Fass R. Gastroesophageal reflux disease in noncardiac chest pain. *Gastroenterol Clin North Am.* 2004;**33**(1):41–54.

20. Rhee PL. Treatment of noncardiac chest pain. *J Gastroenterol Hepatol.* 2005;**20**(Suppl):S18–S19.

21. Scholten T, Dekkers CP, Schutze K, *et al*. On-demand therapy with pantoprazole 20 mg as effective long-term management of reflux disease in patients with mild GERD: the ORION trial. *Digestion.* 2005;**72**(2–3):76–85.

22. Johnson DA, Orr WC, Crawley JA, *et al*. Effect of esomeprazole on nighttime heartburn and sleep quality in patients with GERD: a randomized, placebo-controlled trial. *Am J Gastroenterol.* 2005;**100**(9):1914–1922.

23. Qadeer MA, Phillips CO, Lopez AR, *et al*. Proton pump inhibitor therapy for suspected GERD-related chronic laryngitis: a meta-analysis of randomized controlled trials. *Am J Gastroenterol.* 2006;**101**(11):2646–2654.

24. Earnest D, Robinson M, Rodriguez-Stanley S, *et al*. Managing heartburn at the "base" of the GERD "iceberg": effervescent ranitidine 150 mg b.d. provides faster and better heartburn relief than antacids. *Aliment Pharmacol Ther.* 2000;**14**(7):911–918.

25. Bate CM, Green JR, Axon AT, *et al*. Omeprazole is more effective than cimetidine in the prevention of recurrence of GERD-associated heartburn and the occurrence of underlying oesophagitis. *Aliment Pharmacol Ther.* 1998;**12**(1):41–47.

26. Wong WM. Use of proton pump inhibitor as a diagnostic test in NCCP. *J Gastroenterol Hepatol.* 2005;**20**(Suppl):S14–S17.

27. Richter JE. Review article: the management of heartburn in pregnancy. *Aliment Pharmacol Ther.* 2005;**22**(9):749–757.

28. Castell D, Silvers D, Littlejohn T, *et al*. Cisapride 20mg b.d. for preventing symptoms of GERD induced by a provocative meal. The CIS-USA-89 Study Group. *Aliment Pharmacol Ther.* 1999;**13**(6):787–794.

29. Richter JE, Sabesin SM, Kogut DG, *et al*. Omeprazole versus ranitidine or ranitidine/metoclopramide in poorly responsive symptomatic gastroesophageal reflux disease. *Am J Gastroenterol.* 1996;**91**(9):1766–1772.

30. Tolman KG, Chandramouli J, Fang JC. Proton pump inhibitors in the treatment of gastro-oesophageal reflux disease. *Expert Opin Pharmacother* 2000;**1**(6):1171–1194.

31. Hibbs AM, Lorch SA. Metoclopramide for the treatment of gastroesophageal reflux disease in infants: a systematic review. *Pediatrics.* 2006;**118**(2):746–752.

32. Kim YS, Kim TH, Choi CS, *et al*. Effect of itopride, a new prokinetic, in patients with mild GERD: a pilot study. *World J Gastroenterol.* 2005;**11**(27):4210–4214.

33. Tutuian R, Castell DO. Review article: oesophageal spasm: diagnosis and management. *Aliment Pharmacol Ther.* 2006;**23**(10):1393–1402.

Hemorrhoids and perianal pain

BENJAMIN A. WHITE AND STEPHEN H. THOMAS

■ Agents

- Sitz baths
- Laxatives
- Nitroglycerin
- Calcium channel blockers
- Local anesthetics
- NSAIDs
- Opioids

■ Evidence

This chapter addresses perianal painful conditions encountered in the ED setting. The most common such conditions are external hemorrhoids, anal fissures, and infectious processes (i.e. perianal abscess). Since the last is treated primarily with incision and drainage (with post-discharge **stool softeners**), most of this discussion's literature addresses relief of external hemorrhoids and perianal fissures. The significant overlap in pain relief of these two conditions warrants their consideration in a single chapter. Other conditions, particularly systemic disorders such as Crohn's disease, are also mentioned in brief here; the reader is also referred to the chapter on mucositis and stomatitis (p. 254). This chapter assumes that ED providers have executed surgical therapy where appropriate (e.g. incision and clot removal for thrombosed external hemorrhoids).

Hot baths (sitz baths), in which the patient immerses the hips and buttocks in a few inches of water or saline solution, have been widely recommended for a variety of perianal pain conditions (e.g. anal fissures, perianal hematomas, post-hemorrhoidectomy pain). However, manometry on normal subjects undergoing hot-water perineal immersion finds no sitz bath-associated decrease in anal pressures either at rest or during voluntary contraction.[1]

Furthermore, RCT evidence found that for patients with acute anal fissures who were taking *psyllium fiber* **laxatives** there was no pain improvement from adding sitz baths for 10 min (once post-defecation in the morning, and once at night).[2] Patients randomized to sitz baths do have significantly higher satisfaction, however, and adverse events from sitz baths are both uncommon and mild (mostly perianal rash).[2] The findings regarding sitz bath use for anal fissures – marginal pain improvement yet significant increase in patient satisfaction – are also reported for use of sitz baths post-hemorrhoidectomy.[3]

Laxatives are the initial therapy for perianal pain from a variety of conditions. Cochrane review of seven RCTs found that the evidence, although of suboptimal quality, consistently indicated a significant and persistent pain relief advantage from use of fiber-containing (e.g. *psyllium*) **laxatives**.[4] Use of the fiber-containing **laxatives** halves the chances of continuing hemorrhoid pain.[4] Given the low side effect rate and frequent symptomatic relief, a trial of **laxatives** is appropriate for most patients with perianal pain.

In addition to sitz baths and **laxatives**, many ED patients are candidates for **astringents** such as *witch hazel* (*Hamamelis*).[5] These over-the-counter topical preparations do provide some pain relief, particularly for mild discomfort, and can be tried if they have not already been used prior to ED presentation.[6]

Given the influence of internal anal sphincter hypertonia on perianal pain, pharmacologic measures to relieve sphincter tone form the mainstay of drug therapy for most patients with perianal disorders. The general approaches most often discussed in the literature are *nitroglycerin* (*glyceryl trinitrate*) and **calcium channel blockers**. In both cases, the drugs are best administered locally (i.e. topically) to minimize systemic side effects. *Nitroglycerin*, the more traditional therapy, will be discussed first.

Topically applied *nitroglycerin* (0.2–0.5% ointment) is widely recommended for pain caused by either anal fissures or thrombosed external hemorrhoids.[7–9] The topical preparation is worth trying even in patients with advanced external hemorrhoidal disease; response may still occur and *nitroglycerin* use can occasionally obviate surgical excision.[10]

Compared with the surgical options of excision (not in the ED armamentarium) and incision, topical *nitroglycerin* prescription gives the ED provider an opportunity to institute what has been termed "reversible chemical sphincterotomy."[11] Trial evidence shows that, while not as effective as excision in long-term follow-up, topical *nitroglycerin* ointment (0.2%) provides significantly better pain relief than does incision.[12] When topical *nitroglycerin* is used for chronic anal fissure, significant pain relief occurs in about two thirds of patients; symptom relief may be achieved even if anal fissures and ulcers are not healed.[8,9,11] The existence of conflicting data must be acknowledged. An RCT in patients receiving **stool softeners** and sitz baths (see below) found no additional symptom relief from addition of topical *nitroglycerin* in either a 0.2% or 0.4% concentration.[13] The bulk of the evidence, however, suggests that administration of *nitroglycerin* can provide rapid (within 2–6 h) and significant relief of pain from anal fissures, ulcers, or external hemorrhoids.[9] Furthermore, RCT data show that topical *nitroglycerin* provides better relief than many alternative therapies. For instance, when used for treatment of chronic anal fissures, topical *nitroglycerin* provides significantly better pain relief than application of placebo (*petrolatum*), **topical anesthetic** (*lidocaine* 5%), or a compound of *hydrocortisone*, *heparin*, *framycetin sulfate*, *esculoside*, *ethoform*, and *butoform*.[14]

Although the occasionally conflicting data about *nitroglycerin*'s efficacy is responsible for some clinicians' decision to avoid the drug, side effects are a more important consideration. Even when administered topically, *nitroglycerin* use risks headache development. The cephalalgia rate varies, and it must be acknowledged that one RCT found no difference between headache rates for patients using *nitroglycerin* and those using placebo (20% in both groups).[15] However, most of the available data suggest a 10–20% incremental incidence of headache in *nitroglycerin* users. Unlike *nitroglycerin* use in acute coronary syndromes, where the risk-to-benefit ratio favors *nitroglycerin* use even at a cost of headache, patients with perianal conditions may not wish to take extra (anti-headache) analgesics and thus will not use the *nitroglycerin*.[10,13,16–18]

There are routes to control headache risk in patients in whom clinicians wish to use *nitroglycerin*. First, the literature suggests that the lower concentrations (i.e. 0.2%) of *nitroglycerin* are effective. Thus, clinicians choosing to use *nitroglycerin* should institute therapy with 0.2% ointment, twice daily.

Second, healthcare providers should be aware of the significant diversity in actual concentrations of *nitroglycerin* in ointments, which are often prepared by compounding pharmacies. A recent study of two dozen pharmacies indicated that nearly half of the *nitroglycerin* ointments failed to meet US *Pharmacopoeia* specifications for potency or content uniformity.[7] Attention to proper preparation can at least assure clinicians what concentration a patient is getting, and thus further decision-making can progress on correct assumptions about what has already been tried. Finally, a trial examining the use of an applicator that directs (into the anus) a TID dose of *nitroglycerin* (0.75 ml of 0.3% *nitroglycerin* ointment, providing 2.25 mg *nitroglycerin*) demonstrated reduced headache incidence (with no reduction in efficacy) compared with gloved-finger application of the same *nitroglycerin* dose.[18]

In at least one group, those with post-hemorrhoidectomy pain, RCT data suggest that topical *nitroglycerin* (0.2%, applied BID) provides minimal pain relief when given in the first four to six weeks after the operation.[15] Therefore, for post-hemorrhoidectomy (especially those patients who have failed *nitroglycerin* therapy), ED recommended therapy includes PO **NSAIDs** (e.g. *indomethacin*) with rescue **opioids** (e.g. *oxycodone*) only if necessary.[19] Use of topical **calcium channel blockers** is also recommended (see below).

The utility of **NSAIDs** in post-hemorrhoidectomy pain is further demonstrated by trials of perioperative administration of agents such as *ketorolac* and *diflunisal*.[20,21] A Belgian RCT found that *diclofenac* provided some post-hemorrhoidectomy pain relief, but that the **NSAID** was outperformed by *betamethasone* in terms of **opioid**-sparing effect.[22] The conclusion based upon available data and clinical experience (e.g. taking into account the unhelpful constipating effects of **opioids**) is that **NSAIDs** constitute the optimal systemic approach to perianal pain when local therapy fails. **Opioids** can then be used as rescue therapy. Any **opioid**-sparing effect accrued with **NSAIDs** is particularly important in post-hemorrhoidectomy pain, given the importance of avoiding constipation and straining (which increases risk of postoperative hemorrhage).

For patients with chronic anal fissure or painful external hemorrhoids who fail *nitroglycerin* therapy, or who have intolerable side effects to the drug, **calcium channel blockers** have been recommended as an alternative means to reduce anal tone and relieve symptoms. In fact, evidence shows this class may be preferable to *nitroglycerin* for prescription from the ED. One study found that *nifedipine* ointment relieves fissure pain at least as well as topical *nitroglycerin*, and is associated with significantly fewer side effects.[23] Another trial found that the **calcium channel blocker diltiazem** (2% topically) actually relieved anal fissure pain better than did topical *nitroglycerin* (0.2%).[24] Further evidence of the **calcium channel blockers'** superiority over *nitroglycerin* is found in a study assessing care of patients with *nitroglycerin*-refractory external hemorrhoid pain. This study's data show that BID topical *diltiazem* gel (700 mg of a 2% preparation) relieves pain and related symptoms effectively after failure of *nitroglycerin* therapy.[25] Even in the post-hemorrhoidectomy population, in whom perianal pain relief can be particularly challenging, RCT data demonstrate topical *diltiazem* (2%) is efficacious.[26] Therefore, we conclude that the **calcium channel blockers** are a reasonable choice for first-line therapy in patients with perianal pain from either hemorrhoids or anal fissures.

The **local anesthetics** are the next class of agents occasionally recommended for perianal pain. These drugs may be administered by injection or topical application, as monotherapy or in conjunction with other agents.

Other than for use as procedural anesthesia (i.e. for incision of hemorrhoids or abscesses), there is little ED role for perianal injection of **local anesthetics**. There is essentially no evidence on ED use of (non-procedural) **local anesthetic** injection therapy for perianal pain, and the data from the perioperative setting are not suggestive of utility. When injected at the close of hemorrhoidectomy, agents such as *bupivacaine* provide only a little analgesic benefit, and no significant **opioid**-sparing effect.[27,28] There is anecdotal evidence of use of injected **local anesthetics** (e.g. *bupivacaine* 0.25%) into acute (but not chronic) anal fissures, with further relief of pain achieved by incision into the sphincter. No high-level evidence can be found addressing use of this technique in the ED, but experience is consistent with some success and little risk.

There may be a role for topical application of **local anesthetics** for improving perianal pain, but most trials find that other therapies provide faster healing and better pain relief. One RCT suggested that the modest pain relief from topical application of *lidocaine* (5%) ointment can be augmented by addition of *minoxidil* (0.5%).[29] Another study found that addition of *nifedipine* (0.3%) to *lidocaine* (1.5%) significantly improved pain relief provided by topical application of the **local anesthetic**.[30] The combination of **calcium channel blocker** and **local anesthetic** is anecdotally of utility in post-hemorrhoidectomy pain, especially if the operative procedure included sphincterotomy. Case report evidence suggests utility in topical application of *eutectic mixture of local anesthetics (EMLA)* for external hemorrhoid pain.[31] However, RCT data have shown no benefit to *EMLA* application when used to reduce pain of infiltration anesthesia for hemorrhoidectomy.[32] Consequently, it seems premature to endorse *EMLA* or any other **local anesthetic** for regular use in ED therapy of perianal pain.

Some approaches for perianal pain from hemorrhoids or fissures may provide a degree of symptom relief, but ED recommendation awaits further study. A nonblinded study showed significant relief of both resting and movement pain from application of a paste comprising *heparin* and *trypsin/chymotrypsin*.[33] The ED utility of this approach is rendered unlikely by the need to compound the paste.

Another therapy with limited high-grade evidence is use of *carraghenates*. Suppository or cream formulations both seem to provide some relief, but data are insufficient to endorse ED use.[34]

Given the uncertainties surrounding absorption of topically applied agents during pregnancy, the ED provider considering follow-up for gravida with painful hemorrhoids can feel comfortable recommending consultative referral for surgical therapy, which is both safe and effective in pregnancy.[35] Complete prolapse of the anal ring of hemorrhoids may occur in late pregnancy. This condition usually resolves postpartum, so surgical therapy is not required. An **astringent** such as *witch hazel* may be used to temporize, with consideration of addition of a **calcium channel blocker** if pain relief is incomplete.

The remainder of this chapter addresses diagnoses or therapeutic approaches that are unlikely to be in the purview of ED providers. The first such entity is Crohn's disease. *Thalidomide* has been found useful in a recent trial of patients with perianal pain from Crohn's disease (or HIV), but this approach is limited by side effects.[27,36,37] Another therapy for perianal

Crohn's disease, topical *metronidazole* (10%), may provide significant relief but is also best instituted only in close conjunction with follow-up providers.[38] One difference with Crohn's disease, compared with other perianal conditions, is that anti-diarrheals may actually be indicated if severe diarrhea risks causing hemorrhoidal prolapse.

Perianal pain may also be the presenting complaint for patients with *Condylomata acuminatum*. Repeated application of topical caustics (e.g. *trichloroacetic acid, liquid nitrogen*) or other agents such as *isotretinoin* or *interferon* may relieve pain, but prescription and use of these agents (as well as the usually necessary surgical intervention) fall outside the scope of the ED provider.[39,40]

The systemic condition lichen sclerosus, usually treated with potent topical **corticosteroids**, causes perianal (and vulvar) pain that can be significantly alleviated with topical 1% *pimecrolimus* cream.[41] There is no systemic absorption of the *pimecrolimus*, and the authors conclude that lichen sclerosus can be effectively relieved without resort to potent **corticosteroids**.[41] The unfamiliarity of most ED providers with lichen sclerosus (not to mention *pimecrolimus*) means that institution of therapy for the disease should occur as part of a long-range care plan.

Proctosis fugax is a poorly understood disease in which acute perianal pain of short duration occurs in the absence of organic disease or previous perianal surgery. While there are no RCT data to guide therapy, non-controlled analysis indicates that topical *nitroglycerin* or sublingual *nifedipine* (10 mg) provide relief in about half of patients.[42]

■ Summary and recommendations

First line: fiber-containing laxative (e.g. psyllium powder 5–15 mL PO QD–TID); topical diltiazem gel (700 mg of a 2% preparation applied BID)

Reasonable: other topical calcium channel blocker (e.g. nifedipine 0.3% preparation applied BID)

Pregnancy: fiber-containing laxative (e.g. psyllium powder 5–15 mL PO QD–TID)

Pediatric: fiber-containing laxative (e.g. psyllium powder 5 mL PO QD–TID)

Special cases:

- *history of successful nitroglycerin therapy*: nitroglycerin ointment (0.2%, applied BID)
- *post-hemorrhoidectomy pain*: diltiazem gel (700 mg of a 2% preparation applied BID); NSAIDs (e.g. ibuprofen 400–600 mg PO QID) with consideration of opioid rescue (e.g. oxycodone 5–10 mg PO q4–6 h)
- *failure of local therapy*: NSAIDs (e.g. ibuprofen 400–600 mg PO QID) with opioid rescue (e.g. oxycodone 5–10 mg PO q4–6 h)
- *any case in which opioids are prescribed*: stool softeners should be prescribed (e.g. docusate 50–300 mg PO, with dose halved and divided into 1–4 daily PO administrations for children); patients should be warned that constipation-associated discomfort can offset analgesic efficacy of opioids.

References

1. Pinho M, Correa JC, Furtado A, *et al.* Do hot baths promote anal sphincter relaxation? *Dis Colon Rectum.* 1993;**36**(3):273–274.
2. Gupta P. Randomized, controlled study comparing sitz-bath and no-sitz bath treatments in patients with acute anal fissures. *ANZ J Surg.* 2006;**76**(8):718–721.
3. Gupta PJ. Effects of warm water sitz bath on symptoms in post-anal sphincterotomy in chronic anal fissure: a randomized and controlled study. *World J Surg.* 2007;**31**(7):1480–1484.
4. Alonso-Coello P, Guyatt G, Heels-Ansdell D, *et al.* Laxatives for the treatment of hemorrhoids. *Cochrane Database Syst Rev.* 2005(4):CD004649.
5. Lenhard BH. [Hemorrhoids. Differential diagnosis and therapy.] *Hautarzt.* 2004;**55**(3):240–247.
6. [Drug therapy of hemorrhoids. Proven results of therapy with a hamamelis containing hemorrhoid ointment. Results of a meeting of experts. Dresden, 30 August 1991.] *Fortschr Med Suppl.* 1991;**116**:1–11.
7. Azarnoff DL, Lee JC, Lee C, *et al.* Quality of extemporaneously compounded nitroglycerin ointment. *Dis Colon Rectum.* 2007;**50**(4):509–516.
8. Farouk R, Gunn J, Duthie GS. Changing patterns of treatment for chronic anal fissure. *Ann R Coll Surg Engl.* 1998;**80**(3):194–196.

9. Gorfine SR. Treatment of benign anal disease with topical nitroglycerin. *Dis Colon Rectum.* 1995;**38**(5):453–456; discussion 456–457.

10. van den Berg M, Stroeken HJ, Hoofwijk AG. [Favorable results of conservative treatment with isosorbide dinitrate in 25 patients with fourth-degree hemorrhoids: a pilot study.] *Ned Tijdschr Geneeskd.* 2003;**147**(20):971–973.

11. Lund JN, Scholefield JH. A randomised, prospective, double-blind, placebo-controlled trial of glyceryl trinitrate ointment in treatment of anal fissure. *Lancet.* 1997;**349**(9044):11–14.

12. Cavcic J, Turcic J, Martinac P, *et al.* Comparison of topically applied 0.2% glyceryl trinitrate ointment, incision and excision in the treatment of perianal thrombosis. *Dig Liver Dis.* 2001;**33**(4):335–340.

13. Weinstein D, Halevy A, Negri M, *et al.* [A prospective, randomized double-blind study on the treatment of anal fissures with nitroglycerin ointment.] *Harefuah.* 2004;**143**(10):713–717, 767, 766.

14. Maan MS, Mishra R, Thomas S, *et al.* Randomized, double-blind trial comparing topical nitroglycerine with xylocaine and Proctosedyl in idiopathic chronic anal fissure. *Indian J Gastroenterol.* 2004;**23**(3):91–93.

15. Elton C, Sen P, Montgomery AC. Initial study to assess the effects of topical glyceryl trinitrate for pain after haemorrhoidectomy. *Int J Surg Invest.* 2001;**2**(5):353–357.

16. Patti R, Arcara M, Padronaggio D, *et al.* [Efficacy of topical use of 0.2% glyceryl trinitrate in reducing post-haemorrhoidectomy pain and improving wound healing.] *Chir Ital.* 2005;**57**(1):77–85.

17. Tankova L, Yoncheva K, Muhtarov M, *et al.* Topical mononitrate treatment in patients with anal fissure. *Aliment Pharmacol Ther.* 2002;**16**(1):101–103.

18. Torrabadella L, Salgado G. Controlled dose delivery in topical treatment of anal fissure: pilot study of a new paradigm. *Dis Colon Rectum.* 2006;**49**(6):865–868.

19. Limb RI, Rudkin GE, Luck AJ, *et al.* The pain of haemorrhoidectomy: a prospective study. *Ambul Surg.* 2000;**8**(3):129–134.

20. Place RJ, Coloma M, White PF, *et al.* Ketorolac improves recovery after outpatient anorectal surgery. *Dis Colon Rectum.* 2000;**43**(6):804–808.

21. Jalovaara P, Kiviniemi H, Stahlberg M. Comparison of diflunisal and dextropropoxyphene napsylate in the treatment of postoperative pain. *Ann Chir Gynaecol.* 1985;**74**(5):228–232.

22. Kisli E, Baser M, Guler O, *et al.* Comparison of the analgesic effect of betamethasone and diclofenac potassium in the management of postoperative haemorrhoidectomy pain. *Acta Chir Belg.* 2005;**105**(4):388–391.

23. Ezri T, Susmallian S. Topical nifedipine vs. topical glyceryl trinitrate for treatment of chronic anal fissure. *Dis Colon Rectum.* 2003;**46**(6):805–808.

24. Shrivastava UK, Jain BK, Kumar P, *et al.* A comparison of the effects of diltiazem and glyceryl trinitrate ointment in the treatment of chronic anal fissure: a randomized clinical trial. *Surg Today.* 2007;**37**(6):482–485.

25. Jonas M, Speake W, Scholefield JH. Diltiazem heals glyceryl trinitrate-resistant chronic anal fissures: a prospective study. *Dis Colon Rectum.* 2002;**45** (8):1091–1095.

26. Silverman R, Bendick PJ, Wasvary HJ. A randomized, prospective, double-blind, placebo-controlled trial of the effect of a calcium channel blocker ointment on pain after hemorrhoidectomy. *Dis Colon Rectum.* 2005;**48** (10):1913–1916.

27. Chester JF, Stanford BJ, Gazet JC. Analgesic benefit of locally injected bupivacaine after hemorrhoidectomy. *Dis Colon Rectum.* 1990;**33** (6):487–489.

28. Vinson-Bonnet B, Coltat JC, Fingerhut A, *et al.* Local infiltration with ropivacaine improves immediate postoperative pain control after hemorrhoidal surgery. *Dis Colon Rectum.* 2002;**45**(1):104–108.

29. Muthukumarassamy R, Robinson SS, Sarath SC, *et al.* Treatment of anal fissures using a combination of minoxidil and lignocaine: a randomized, double-blind trial. *Indian J Gastroenterol.* 2005;**24**(4):158–160.

30. Perrotti P, Antropoli C, Molino D, *et al.* Conservative treatment of acute thrombosed external hemorrhoids with topical nifedipine. *Dis Colon Rectum.* 2001;**44**(3):405–400.

31. Perez P, Abengoechea JM, Marques MD. [New uses of EMLA: anesthesia for relief of pain caused by hemorrhoid thrombosis.] *Rev Esp Anestesiol Reanim.* 2001;**48**(8):397–398.

32. Roxas MF, Talip BN, Crisostomo AC. Double-blind, randomized, placebo-controlled trial to determine the efficacy of eutectic lidocaine/prilocaine (EMLA) cream for decreasing pain during local anaesthetic infiltration for out-patient haemorrhoidectomy. *Asian J Surg.* 2003;**26**(1):26–30.

33. Gupta PJ. Use of enzyme and heparin paste in acute haemorrhoids. *Rom J Gastroenterol.* 2002;**11**(3):191–195.

34. Yang XD, Wang JP, Kang JB, *et al.* [Comparison of the efficacy and safety of compound carraghenates cream and compound carraghenates suppository in the treatment of mixed hemorrhoids.] *Zhonghua Wei Chang Wai Ke Za Zhi.* 2005;**8**(3):220–222.

35. Saleeby RG, Jr., Rosen L, Stasik JJ, *et al.* Hemorrhoidectomy during pregnancy: risk or relief? *Dis Colon Rectum.* 1991;**34**(3):260–261.

36. Plamondon S, Ng SC, Kamm MA. Thalidomide in luminal and fistulizing Crohn's disease resistant to standard therapies. *Aliment Pharmacol Ther.* 1 2007;**25**(5):557–567.

37. Soler RA, Migliorati C, van Waes H, *et al.* Thalidomide treatment of mucosal ulcerations in HIV infection. *Arch Dis Child.* 1996;**74**(1):64–65.

38. Stringer EE, Nicholson TJ, Armstrong D. Efficacy of topical metronidazole (10 percent) in the treatment of anorectal Crohn's disease. *Dis Colon Rectum.* 2005;**48**(5):970–974.

39. Metcalf A. Anorectal disorders. Five common causes of pain, itching, and bleeding. *Postgrad Med.* 1995;**98**(5):81–84, 87–89, 92–94.

40. Trombetta LJ, Place RJ. Giant condyloma acuminatum of the anorectum: trends in epidemiology and management: report of a case and review of the literature. *Dis Colon Rectum.* 2001;**44**(12):1878–1886.

41. Nissi R, Eriksen H, Risteli J, *et al.* Pimecrolimus cream 1% in the treatment of lichen sclerosus. *Gynecol Obstet Invest.* 2007;**63**(3):151–154.

42. Gracia Solanas JA, Ramirez Rodriguez JM, Elia Guedea M, *et al.* Sequential treatment for proctalgia fugax. Mid-term follow-up. *Rev Esp Enferm Dig.* 2005;**97**(7):491–496.

Migraine and undifferentiated headache

SOHAN PAREKH AND ANDY JAGODA

■ Agents

- Ergots
- Antiemetics
- Triptans
- NSAIDs
- Opioids
- Steroids

■ Evidence

The ED physician frequently encounters patients with migraine headache (MH). Many patients have carried the diagnosis for years, but in some cases there may be uncertainty as to the precise type of cephalalgia present. In fact, in the ED population, about a third of patients with headache cannot be precisely differentiated.[1] Other chapters address other headache etiologies, but the ED physician should be reassured by acute care literature demonstrating that headache type differentiation is not always necessary for successful treatment. If patients have uncertain etiology, or other headache etiologies besides those covered in other chapters in this text, the acute care provider may find the "anti-migraine" therapies useful.[2] This recommendation assumes the ED physician administers disease-specific treatments where appropriate (e.g. **corticosteroids** for tumor-related swelling, **decongestants** for sinusitis).

The **ergot alkaloids**, available in myriad formulations, are among the oldest drugs used for MH. Data addressing efficacy of the oldest such agent, *ergotamine*, is mixed at best. *Ergotamine* exhibits inconsistent efficacy in numerous studies of varying methodological rigor; the overall picture from available evidence is one of doubtful efficacy (and no ED role) for *ergotamine*.[3,4]

There is a limited acute care role for the ergot derivative *dihydroergotamine* (*DHE*). Trials show that the nasal spray formulation (2 mg IN) provides MH relief that is better than placebo but inferior to that achieved with either **antiemetics** or **triptans**.[3,5–7]

Years ago, routine MH care included **antiemetic** pretreatment to prevent nausea induced by the **ergots**. Clinicians noted that MH pain was often alleviated before the "real" analgesic was administered, prompting interest in the use of **antiemetics** as stand-alone therapy.[7,8] Among the **antiemetics** RCT data show to be highly effective for MH are *metoclopramide* (10 mg IV) and *prochlorperazine* (10 mg IV).[9,10] *Prochlorperazine* is more sedating than *metoclopramide*, which may be related to the higher success seen with the former.[11,12] *Metoclopramide* remains quite useful, however, being demonstratedly more effective than the **opioid** *meperidine* (*pethidine*) in patients with undifferentiated headaches.[13]

Prochlorperazine's superiority over other **antiemetics** is also found for non-IV administration routes. However, some patients may lack IV access, and migraineurs' frequent nausea limits the utility of PO medications. Administration of 10 mg *prochlorperazine* by either IM or PR suppository provides at least partial relief of MH.[11,14–16] An additional route of administration for *prochlorperazine* is the orally disintegrating buccal tablet (3 mg dose). A small study evaluating the use of this preparation for MH showed promising results.[17] Trials involving IM and PR *metoclopramide* formulations have failed to demonstrate superiority of either approach over placebo.[11,18]

One of the advantages of the **antiemetics** is their efficacy in a broad range of benign headache syndromes. As noted in this chapter's introduction, precise differentiation between benign tension and vascular headache syndromes tends to be both difficult and unnecessary.[1,2] Previous ED investigators have reported efficacy of *metoclopramide* and *prochlorperazine* in a variety of headache syndromes (including undifferentiated cephalalgia).[13,15,16]

The phenothiazine *chlorpromazine*, one of the earliest agents assessed for headache treatment, has been rendered obsolete by the emergence of other options for ED treatment of MH. *Chlorpromazine* (12.5 mg IV) is efficacious, but its administration is associated with a high incidence of untoward side effects (e.g. hypotension, deep sedation, extrapyramidal reactions).[19,20]

Serotonin 5-HT1$_{B/D}$ agonists, collectively known as the **triptans**, are specifically targeted toward MH pathophysiology. Dozens of studies have addressed varying formulations and administration routes of the **triptans**. *Sumatriptan* is the best-studied agent for MH, although a burgeoning literature (including large multicenter trials) demonstrates *zolmitriptan*'s safety and efficacy.[21,22]

Placebo-controlled trials have found *sumatriptan* to be effective via SC, PO, IN, and PR routes.[23–29] Subcutaneous *sumatriptan* (6 mg), while more effective than the PO route, is associated with a higher incidence of adverse effects.[30,31] Perhaps *sumatriptan*'s best administration route is via the naris (10 or 30 mg IN); this formulation causes few side effects and achieves efficacy comparable to that of the PO preparation.[26,27] Preliminary evidence suggests PR administration of *sumatriptan* (12.5 or 25 mg) is also efficacious and has few side effects.[29]

In addition to *sumatriptan*, many other **triptans** offer similar MH relief and side effect profiles.[32,33] There is a substantial body of evidence supporting use of *zolmitriptan* as a first-line agent. Administered by a variety of routes, *zolmitriptan* achieves MH relief as fast as 10–15 min after IN administration (of 5 mg).[34] Administration of an easily used orally dissolving tablet (of 2.5 or 5 mg) allows *zolmitriptan* to achieve MH pain relief in less than 30 minutes.[35,36] *Zolmitriptan* (2.5 mg PO) is also effective in menstruation-associated MH.[37]

Although the underlying literature is noted to be methodologically mixed, both *sumatriptan* and *zolmitriptan* are recommended by various authorities on pediatric MH.[38–40] One evidence review concluded that the data are strongest for *sumatriptan* administered by the IN route; there is insufficient data to conclusively recommend a 5 mg or 20 mg IN dose in children.[41]

Some of the other **triptans** that are efficacious in MH include *almotriptan*, *eletriptan*, *frovatriptan*, *naratriptan*, and *rizatriptan*. These agents appear relatively equal in their relief of MH and associated symptoms such as nausea and phono- and photophobia.[33]

Like the **antiemetics**, the **triptans** are useful in myriad benign headache syndromes. Clinical trial evidence from the ED demonstrates *sumatriptan*'s equal efficacy in migraine, probable migraine, and tension-type headaches.[42]

The utility of the **triptans** in cluster headache is outlined in a separate chapter of this text.

Vasospasm-mediated serious adverse effects such as stroke and myocardial infarction have been reported with **triptan** use.[43,44] The risk of these serious adverse effects can be reduced to acceptably low levels by limiting use of **triptans** to patients lacking history of, or significant risk factors for, vascular disease.[45]

Combination therapy with PO *sumatriptan* (85 mg) and the **NSAID** *naproxen* (500 mg) results in significantly better pain relief than monotherapy with either agent.[31]

Controlled trials demonstrate efficacy of multiple **NSAIDs** for MH pain. Among those drugs performing better than placebo are *aspirin*, *ibuprofen*, *tolfenamic acid*, *diclofenac*, and *naproxen*.[46–53] *Ketorolac* offers the advantage of parenteral administration. Although no placebo-controlled data are available, this injectable **NSAID** appears to be effective either IV or IM.[53,54]

Patients presenting to ED with MH usually require a more potent analgesic than *acetaminophen* (*paracetanol*). There are RCT data demonstrating utility of *acetaminophen*.[55] The primary use will be for occasional cases in which patients have not tried pre-ED analgesia. Investigators report some MH pain relief from combination therapy with *acetaminophen* and a mild **opioid**, although **opioids** such as *codeine* may exacerbate MH-associated nausea.[56]

Despite their non-specific mechanism of action, **opioids** are frequently used for MH. Evidence supporting use of this class is limited, and rigorous placebo-controlled trials are lacking. Data addressing use of *meperidine* consistently find this **opioid** to be no better than (and often inferior to) alternative non-opioid drugs.[13,57] Intranasal administration of *butorphanol* achieves better MH relief than placebo, but the agonist–antagonist can cause problematic side effects such as nausea and dysphoria.[58]

While there is no good evidence to prove benefit of **opioids** for MH (or other headache syndromes), it is hard to conceive of providing ED care without having access to this class, at least for rescue therapy. Many chronic headache sufferers report allergies or non-effectiveness of non-opioid regimens. Additionally, many primary care physicians send patients to the ED for treatment with **opioids**. It is often difficult or impossible to separate the drug seeker from the true migraineur. So ultimately, clinical judgment must guide the ED provider's decision as to when and how to use **opioids** in the treatment of this difficult condition. Although previously mentioned data suggest **opioids** are often ineffective for MH, preliminary evidence from one small RCT points to potential utility for an IV formulation of the mixed-mechanism agent *tramadol* (administered 100 mg IV, in 100 mL saline, over 30 minutes). Nearly three quarters of patients receiving *tramadol* had significant pain relief, with about a third achieving complete analgesia after the single 100 mg IV dose.[59]

Corticosteroid therapy has been suggested to be of potential utility in patients with intractable MH. There is some evidence to suggest that *dexamethasone* (8 mg IV) may be useful for resistant MH, but currently available data do not support a recommendation for routine ED use.[60]

Medication overuse headaches are encountered in the ED with increasing frequency. While overuse of non-specific analgesics tends to cause tension-type headache pain, **triptan** overuse is usually manifest as recurrent MH.[61] For these patients, discontinuation of pharmacotherapy is the best approach.

Prophylactic medications that may have ED utility in the earliest stages of migraine include the **beta-blockers** (e.g. *metoprolol*, *propranolol*) and the **calcium channel blockers** (e.g. *flunarizine*).[33,38] A variety of other agents, including **antidepressants** (e.g. *amitriptyline*) **antiepileptics** (e.g. *topiramate*), **vitamins** (e.g. *niacin*) and even *botulinum toxin*, have been assessed for MH but have no acute care indication.[62,63]

■ Summary and recommendations

First line: prochlorperazine (10 mg IV)

Reasonable:

- metoclopramide (10 mg IV)
- sumatriptan (6 mg SC) or other triptan (e.g. zolmitriptan 2.5 mg PO or 5 mg IN)
- combination therapy: oral sumatriptan (25 mg PO) *plus* naproxen 500 mg

Pregnancy: metoclopramide (10 mg IV)

Pediatric:

- ibuprofen (10 mg/kg PO)
- acetaminophen (10–15 mg/kg PO)
- intranasal sumatriptan (5 mg IN if < 25 kg, 10 mg if 25–50 kg, 20 mg if > 50 kg)

Special cases:

- *undifferentiated cephalalgia*: antiemetic
- *wish to avoid drowsiness*: triptan (e.g. sumatriptan 6 mg SC)
- *vascular disease presence or significant risk factors*: avoid triptans
- *nuisance adverse effects from SC sumatriptan*: sumatriptan IN (20 mg IN)
- *menstruation-associated migraine*: triptan (e.g. sumatriptan 6 mg SC)

References

1. Friedman BW, Hochberg ML, Esses D, *et al.* Applying the International Classification of Headache Disorders to the emergency department: an assessment of reproducibility and the frequency with which a unique diagnosis can be assigned to every acute headache presentation. *Ann Emerg Med.* 2007;**49**:409–419, e401–409.

2. Thomas S, Stone C. Emergency department treatment of migraine, tension, and mixed-type headache. *J Emerg Med.* 1994;**12**:657–664.

3. Dihydroergotamine Nasal Spray Multicenter Investigators. Efficacy, safety, and tolerability of dihydroergotamine nasal spray as monotherapy in the treatment of acute migraine. *Headache.* 1995;**35**:177–184.

4. Dahlof C. Placebo-controlled clinical trials with ergotamine in the acute treatment of migraine. *Cephalalgia.* 1993;**13**:166–171.

5. Gallagher RM. Acute treatment of migraine with dihydroergotamine nasal spray. Dihydroergotamine Working Group. *Arch Neurol.* 1996;**53**:1285–1291.

6. Touchon J, Bertin L, Pilgrim AJ, *et al.* A comparison of subcutaneous sumatriptan and dihydroergotamine nasal spray in the acute treatment of migraine. *Neurology.* 1996;**47**:361–365.

7. Colman I, Brown MD, Innes GD, *et al.* Parenteral dihydroergotamine for acute migraine headache: a systematic review of the literature. *Ann Emerg Med.* 2005;**45**:393–401.

8. Lane R, Ross R. Intravenous chlorpromazine: preliminary results in acute migraine. *Headache.* 1985;**25**:302–304.

9. Ellis G, Delaney J, DeHart D, *et al.* The efficacy of metoclopramide in the treatment of migraine headache. *Ann Emerg Med.* 1993;**22**:191–195.

10. Tek D, McClellan D, Olshaker J, *et al.* A prospective, double-blind study of metoclopramide hydrochloride for the control of migraine in the emergency department. *Ann Emerg Med.* 1990;**19**:1083–1087.

11. Jones J, Pack S, Chun E. Intramuscular prochlorperazine versus metoclopramide as single-agent therapy for the treatment of acute migraine headache. *Am J Emerg Med.* 1996;**14**:262–264.

12. Coppola M, Yealy D, Leibold R. Randomized, placebo-controlled evaluation of prochlorperazine versus metoclopramide for emergency department treatment of migraine headache. *Ann Emerg Med.* 1995;**26**:541–546.

13. Cicek M, Karcioglu O, Parlak I, *et al.* Prospective, randomised, double blind, controlled comparison of metoclopramide and pethidine in the emergency treatment of acute primary vascular and tension type headache episodes. *Emerg Med J.* 2004;**21**:323–326.

14. Jones E, Gonzalez E, Boggs J, *et al.* Safety and efficacy of rectal prochlorperazine for the treatment of migraine in the emergency department. *Ann Emerg Med.* 2004;**24**:237–241.

15. Thomas S, Stone C, Ray V, *et al.* Intravenous vs. rectal prochlorperazine for the treatment of benign vascular or tension headache. *Ann Emerg Med.* 1994;**23**:923–927.

16. Jones J, Sklar D, Dougherty J, *et al.* Randomized double-blind trial of intravenous prochlorperazine for the treatment of acute headache. *JAMA.* 1989;**261**:1174–1176.

17. Sharma S. Efficacy and tolerability of prochlorperazine buccal tablets in treatment of acute migraine. *Headache.* 2002;**42**:896–902.

18. Tfelt-Hansen P, Olesen J, Aebelholt-Krabbe A, *et al.* A double-blind study of metoclopramide in the treatment of migraine attacks. *J Neurol Neurosurg Psychiatry.* 1980;**43**:369–371.

19. Bell R, Montoya D, Shuaib A, *et al.* A comparative trial of three agents in the treatment of acute migraine headache. *Ann Emerg Med.* 1990;**19**:1079–1082.

20. Cameron J, Lane P, Speechley M. Intravenous chlorpromazine vs intravenous metoclopramide in acute migraine headache. *Acad Emerg Med.* 1995;**2**:597–602.

21. Diener HC, Evers S. Effectiveness and satisfaction with zolmitriptan 5 mg nasal spray for treatment of migraine in real-life practice: results of a postmarketing surveillance study. *Clin Drug Invest.* 2007;**27**:59–66.

22. Gawel M, Aschoff J, May A, *et al*. Treatment satisfaction with zolmitriptan nasal spray for migraine in a real life setting: results from phase two of the REALIZE study. *J Headache Pain*. 2005;**6**:405–411.

23. Akpunonu BE, Mutgi AB, Federman DJ, *et al*. Subcutaneous sumatriptan for treatment of acute migraine in patients admitted to the emergency department: a multicenter study. *Ann Emerg Med*. 1995;**25**:464–469.

24. Cutler N, Mushet GR, Davis R, *et al*. Oral sumatriptan for the acute treatment of migraine: evaluation of three dosage strengths. *Neurology*. 1995;**45**(Suppl 7):S5–S9.

25. Sargent J, Kirchner JR, Davis R, *et al*. Oral sumatriptan is effective and well tolerated for the acute treatment of migraine: results of a multicenter study. *Neurology*. 1995;**45**(Suppl 7):S10–S14.

26. Ryan R, Elkind A, Baker CC, *et al*. Sumatriptan nasal spray for the acute treatment of migraine. Results of two clinical studies. *Neurology*. 1997;**49**:1225–1230.

27. Salonen R, Ashford E, Dahlof C, *et al*. Intranasal sumatriptan for the acute treatment of migraine. International Intranasal Sumatriptan Study Group. *J Neurol*. 1994;**241**:463–469.

28. Bertin L, Brion N, Farkkila M, *et al*. A dose-defining study of sumatriptan suppositories in the acute treatment of migraine. *Int J Clin Pract*. 1999;**53**:593–598.

29. Tepper SJ, Cochran A, Hobbs S, *et al*. Sumatriptan suppositories for the acute treatment of migraine. S2B351 Study Group. *Int J Clin Pract*. 1998;**52**:31–35.

30. Carpay HA, Matthijsse P, Steinbuch M, *et al*. Oral and subcutaneous sumatriptan in the acute treatment of migraine: an open randomized cross-over study. *Cephalalgia*. 1997;**17**:591–595.

31. Gruffydd-Jones K, Hood CA, Price DB. A within-patient comparison of subcutaneous and oral sumatriptan in the acute treatment of migraine in general practice. *Cephalalgia*. 1997;**17**:31–36.

32. Ferrari MD, Roon KI, Lipton RB, *et al*. Oral triptans (serotonin 5-HT(1B/1D) agonists) in acute migraine treatment: a meta-analysis of 53 trials. *Lancet*. 2001;**358**:1668–1675.

33. Diener H. Pharmacological approaches to migraine. *J Neural Transm Suppl*. 2003;**64**:35–63.

34. Dodick D, Brandes J, Elkind A, *et al*. Speed of onset, efficacy and tolerability of zolmitriptan nasal spray in the acute treatment of migraine: a randomised, double-blind, placebo-controlled study. *CNS Drugs*. 2005;**19**:125–136.

35. Loder E, Freitag FG, Adelman J, *et al.* Pain-free rates with zolmitriptan 2.5 mg ODT in the acute treatment of migraine: results of a large double-blind placebo-controlled trial. *Curr Med Res Opin.* 2005;**21**:381–389.

36. Spierings EL, Rapoport AM, Dodick DW, *et al.* Acute treatment of migraine with zolmitriptan 5 mg orally disintegrating tablet. *CNS Drugs.* 2004;**18**:1133–1141.

37. Tuchman M, Hee A, Emeribe U, *et al.* Efficacy and tolerability of zolmitriptan oral tablet in the acute treatment of menstrual migraine. *CNS Drugs.* 2006;**20**:1019–1026.

38. Lewis DW, Winner P. The pharmacological treatment options for pediatric migraine: an evidence-based appraisal. *NeuroRx.* 2006;**3**:181–191.

39. Rothner AD, Wasiewski W, Winner P, *et al.* Zolmitriptan oral tablet in migraine treatment: high placebo responses in adolescents. *Headache.* 2006;**46**:101–109.

40. Linder SL, Dowson AJ. Zolmitriptan provides effective migraine relief in adolescents. *Int J Clin Pract.* 2000;**54**:466–469.

41. Lewis D, Ashwal S, Hershey A, *et al.* Practice parameter: pharmacological treatment of migraine headache in children and adolescents: report of the American Academy of Neurology Quality Standards Subcommittee and the Practice Committee of the Child Neurology Society. *Neurology.* 2004;**63**:2215–2224.

42. Miner JR, Smith SW, Moore J, *et al.* Sumatriptan for the treatment of undifferentiated primary headaches in the ED. *Am J Emerg Med.* 2007;**25**:60–64.

43. Jayamaha JE, Street MK. Fatal cerebellar infarction in a migraine sufferer whilst receiving sumatriptan. *Intensive Care Med.* 1995;**21**:82–83.

44. O'Connor P, Gladstone P. Oral sumatriptan-associated transmural myocardial infarction. *Neurology.* 1995;**45**:2274–2276.

45. Hall GC, Brown MM, Mo J, *et al.* Triptans in migraine: the risks of stroke, cardiovascular disease, and death in practice. *Neurology.* 24 2004;**62**:563–568.

46. Lipton RB, Goldstein J, Baggish JS, *et al.* Aspirin is efficacious for the treatment of acute migraine. *Headache.* 2005;**45**:283–292.

47. Lipton RB, Stewart WF, Ryan RE, Jr., *et al.* Efficacy and safety of acetaminophen, aspirin, and caffeine in alleviating migraine headache pain: three double-blind, randomized, placebo-controlled trials. *Arch Neurol.* 1998;**55**:210–217.

48. Kellstein DE, Lipton RB, Geetha R, *et al.* Evaluation of a novel solubilized formulation of ibuprofen in the treatment of migraine headache: a randomized,

double-blind, placebo-controlled, dose-ranging study. *Cephalalgia*. 2000;**20**:233–243.

49. Kloster R, Nestvold K, Vilming ST. A double-blind study of ibuprofen versus placebo in the treatment of acute migraine attacks. *Cephalalgia*. 1992;**12**:169–171; discussion 128.

50. Myllyla VV, Havanka H, Herrala L, *et al*. Tolfenamic acid rapid release versus sumatriptan in the acute treatment of migraine: comparable effect in a double-blind, randomized, controlled, parallel-group study. *Headache*. 1998;**38**:201–207.

51. Diener HC, Montagna P, Gacs G, *et al*. Efficacy and tolerability of diclofenac potassium sachets in migraine: a randomized, double-blind, cross-over study in comparison with diclofenac potassium tablets and placebo. *Cephalalgia*. 2006;**26**:537–547.

52. Andersson PG, Hinge HH, Johansen O, *et al*. Double-blind study of naproxen vs placebo in the treatment of acute migraine attacks. *Cephalalgia*. 1989;**9**:29–32.

53. Shrestha M, Singh R, Moreden J, *et al*. Ketorolac vs chlorpromazine in the treatment of acute migraine without aura. A prospective, randomized, double-blind trial. *Arch Intern Med*. 1996;**156**:1725–1728.

54. Seim MB, March JA, Dunn KA. Intravenous ketorolac vs intravenous pro-chlorperazine for the treatment of migraine headaches. *Acad Emerg Med*. 1998;**5**:573–576.

55. Lipton RB, Baggish JS, Stewart WF, *et al*. Efficacy and safety of acetaminophen in the treatment of migraine: results of a randomized, double-blind, placebo-controlled, population-based study. *Arch Intern Med*. 2000;**160**:3486–3492.

56. Boureau F, Joubert JM, Lasserre V, *et al*. Double-blind comparison of an acetaminophen 400 mg–codeine 25 mg combination versus aspirin 1000 mg and placebo in acute migraine attack. *Cephalalgia*. 1994;**14**:156–161.

57. Colman I, Rothney A, Wright SC, *et al*. Use of narcotic analgesics in the emergency department treatment of migraine headache. *Neurology*. 2004;**62**:1695–1700.

58. Hoffert MJ, Couch JR, Diamond S, *et al*. Transnasal butorphanol in the treatment of acute migraine. *Headache*. 1995;**35**:65–69.

59. Alemdar M, Pekdemir M, Selekler HM. Single-dose intravenous tramadol for acute migraine pain in adults: a single-blind, prospective, randomized, placebo-controlled clinical trial. *Clin Ther*. 2007;**29**:1441–1447.

60. Gallagher RM. Emergency treatment of intractable migraine. *Headache*. 1986;**26**:74–75.

61. Rabe K, Katsarava Z. [Medication-overuse headache.] *MMW Fortschr Med.* 2006;**148**:37–38.

62. Evers S, Frese A. Recent advances in the treatment of headaches. *Curr Opin Anaesthesiol.* 2005;**18**:563–568.

63. Prousky J, Seely D. The treatment of migraines and tension-type headaches with intravenous and oral niacin (nicotinic acid): systematic review of the literature. *Nutr J.* 2005;**4**:3.

Mucositis and stomatitis

KELLY YOUNG

■ Agents

- Opioids
- Topical anesthetics
- NSAIDs
- Sucralfate
- Amlexanox
- Corticosteroids

■ Evidence

Available evidence for treating pain caused by mucositis (inflammation of the digestive tract's lining) and stomatitis (mucositis involving the mouth) can be categorized into two general categories, depending on whether or not the stomatitis is related to cancer therapy (either chemo- or radiation therapy). This chapter is thus divided into two sections. The initial portion of the discussion addresses cancer treatment-associated stomatitis (CTAM). The chapter concludes with an overview of the evidence, lesser in quality and quantity, addressing non-CTAM stomatitis (e.g. from aphthous ulcers or viral agents).

For the purposes of this chapter, the term mucositis will be used with the understanding that the major focus of discussed evidence is on oral disease (i.e. stomatitis). As is the case with many disease states, the line between treating pain and treating the disease's pathophysiology can be indistinct. This chapter deals mostly with topical approaches and systemic analgesics, with the understanding that disease-specific systemic therapy (e.g. *acyclovir* [aciclovir] for herpetic gingivostomatitis) may be warranted in some cases.

CANCER TREATMENT-ASSOCIATED MUCOSITIS

For CTAM, which can be a substantial (treatment-limiting) complication in oncology, prophylactic therapy is often used; these approaches are not discussed here. For CTAM that does develop, pain can be severe and **opioids** are the therapeutic mainstay. In fact, CTAM pain often necessitates IV *morphine* and even hospitalization and institution of a PCA regimen.[1] Cochrane review found that the **opioid** PCA regimen, while providing no better overall pain relief than standard-regimen IV **opioids**, was associated with lower medication dosages per hour and a shorter pain duration.[2] It is likely that in many hospitals, ED utilization of PCA will be limited by a variety of factors (e.g. relatively short duration of ED stay, physician and nursing familiarity with PCA, availability of PCA pumps). However, for those settings with access to (and expertise in) PCA use, the earlier institution of this analgesia modality is desirable.

Methodologically rigorous comparisons of *morphine*, *hydromorphone*, and *sufentanil* PCA for mucositis find each of the therapies generally efficacious, but *morphine* exhibits advantages in safety and side effects.[1] *Hydromorphone* is the next most desirable **opioid** for PCA-administered mucositis pain; *sufentanil*'s disadvantage (as demonstrated in adults) is a greater susceptibility to tolerance.[1,3,4] As is the case in other conditions in which PCA may be useful in the ED, initial pain reduction should be achieved with IV bolus **opioid** therapy before instituting a PCA regimen.

While the IV route is preferred for severe pain, other methods of **opioid** delivery have been studied for CTAM. Transdermal *fentanyl* in doses of up to 50 μg/h is ineffective for CTAM.[5] Results have been better with the oral topical route for **opioids**. *Morphine* mouthwash is demonstrated safe and effective in multiple trials.[6–8] Oral rinsing with 15 mL *morphine* (2.1000) reduces patients' pain scores by an average of 80%; pain relief occurs within 30 min and lasts nearly 4 h.[8] Serum levels of *morphine* after the mouth rinse are negligible, and neither systemic drug effects nor toxicity are seen in extant studies.[7]

Besides *morphine*, other topical approaches for CTAM have been tried, but they tend to fall short of the **opioids** in safety, efficacy, or both. The **NSAIDs** may have some promise, and *doxepin* may have utility in refractory cases, but trials of other approaches have been disappointing.

The **NSAIDs** that have been investigated for topical application in CTAM include various preparations of *indomethacin* and *benzydamine*. More evidence is needed for definitive recommendations, but small uncontrolled studies of topical *indomethacin* formulations (one a gel, the other a 0.25% spray) have reported that its application reduced both pain and need for **opioids** in CTAM.[9,10] The *indomethacin* spray is well tolerated and has few or no significant side effects, although the potential for systemic absorption (and accompanying toxicity) must be acknowledged.[10] *Benzydamine*, available in some countries as a mouthwash, may have some prophylactic utility for CTAM mucositis but a 2007 Cochrane review found no role for the agent in acute care pain relief.[2,11]

One trial of an oral rinse with *doxepin* (5 mg/mL) showed effective CTAM relief as soon as 15 minutes after dosing.[12] At least for refractory CTAM pain, *doxepin* rinse seems to have a role for acute care prescription. Pain relief persists for at least 3–4 h after the mouthwash, and the average patient's pain decreases by 70%.[12] The capsule form of *doxepin* is not as effective, being shown to be substantially inferior to PO **opioids**.[13]

Preliminary reports suggest CTAM utility for topical rinse with *ketamine*.[14] No methodologically rigorous trial data exist but *ketamine*, like *doxepin*, may be a reasonable choice for refractory CTAM pain.

Local anesthetics such as *tetracaine* or *lidocaine* (in a viscous formulation) are often recommended for CTAM, but their utility is not definitively demonstrated.[15–18] A preliminary (phase II) trial suggests topical *tetracaine* gel reduces the pain of radiation-related CTAM in about 80% of patients.[19] Further studies may demonstrate utility of the **local anesthetics**. This class does exhibit some systemic absorption after topical oral therapy, but toxicity is unexpected given the minimal blood concentrations. One trial has shown that rinsing for 1 min (followed by expectoration) with 5 mL of a 2% *lidocaine* solution results in subtherapeutic blood levels of the drug.[20]

The **local anesthetics** have also been applied topically as part of multidrug compounds. One such compound is administered as a mucosal adhesive water-soluble film, containing *tetracaine, ofloxacine, miconazole, guaiazulene,* and *triacetin*. The preparation is effective at relieving CTAM, but the evidence is insufficient to warrant a recommendation for ED use of the preparation.[21]

Perhaps the best known multidrug compound incorporating **local anesthetics** is "*magic mouthwash*," which comprises equal parts viscous *lidocaine*, *diphenydramine*, and *magnesium/aluminum hydroxide*. *Magic mouthwash* is often recommended for CTAM.[22] However, data reveal that *magic mouthwash* is no better than simpler mixtures, and substantially inferior to *morphine* rinses. An RCT in CTAM found *magic mouthwash* no more effective than mouth rinses with either *chlorhexidine* or *salt plus soda* (½ teaspoon of table salt and 2 teaspoons of baking soda in four cups of water).[23] Another CTAM trial, comparing *morphine* rinse with *magic mouthwash*, found the latter substantially inferior in pain relief, with nearly half of patients receiving the *magic mouthwash* complaining of local side effects.[6] Cochrane review concluded that there is no benefit to *magic mouthwash* in CTAM.[2]

Though a previously cited trial found *chlorhexidine* rinses were as effective as *magic mouthwash*, results from CTAM trials focusing on *chlorhexidine* are disappointing. The **topical antimicrobial**, in the form of a mouth rinse or antibiotic oral lozenge, is generally ineffective in the treatment of CTAM.[2,17,18,23]

Sucralfate is no more effective than placebo or *salt plus soda* mouthwash in reducing the pain of CTAM.[2,24-26]

MUCOSITIS NOT ASSOCIATED WITH CANCER TREATMENT

Most of the data dealing with non-CTAM mucositis addresses aphthous ulcer (AU) treatment; assumptions about viral stomatitis therapy generally represent extrapolation from AU trials. While **opioids** are acknowledged to be superior for the severe pain of CTAM, agents with lesser potency (e.g. **NSAIDs**) may be effective for the milder pain of viral stomatitis or AU.[22] Approaches that are not effective for CTAM may, in fact, have some utility for other, non-oncologic etiologies of mucositis.

Topical *sucralfate* is an example of an approach that is not successful in CTAM but which is found useful in AU. A crossover RCT found *sucralfate* to be more effective than either *antacids* or placebo in the treatment of AU.[27] Supporting evidence for *sucralfate*'s effectiveness in non-CTAM mucositis is found in a RCT in patients with Behçet's disease, which demonstrated effective pain control with *sucralfate* suspension.[28]

For some treatments found not useful for CTAM, there is simply insufficient evidence to support use in AU or viral stomatitis. *Magic mouthwash* (see above) is often recommended for non-CTAM mucositis such as viral stomatitis.[22] However, results for this preparation in CTAM are disappointing, and there are no data to support claims of efficacy for non-CTAM stomatitis.

The anti-inflammatory, anti-allergic agent *amlexanox* in a 5% topical paste (applied as a 100 mg dose QID) is effective for reducing the pain (and the time to healing) of recurrent AU.[29-31] Application during the prodromal stage of AU formation reduces pain by as much as 85%.[30] *Amlexanox* comes in a variety of forms (e.g. mucoadhesive patch), all of which offer similar pain relief advantage over control.[31] Pooled analysis of data from four trials indicate that *amlexanox* consistently accelerates time to pain resolution, with effects seen after as little as one day of therapy.[32]

Trial evidence, as well as expert reviews, suggest efficacy of topical **corticosteroids** for AU treatment.[33] Preliminary data suggest that the paste form of *clobetasol* is more effective than an oral ointment or swallowed form of the drug.[34] Although **corticosteroids** have no effect on AU recurrence, topically applied *clobetasol* and *beclomethasone* are well tolerated and effective at pain reduction.[34,35] Other topical **corticosteroids** (e.g. *triamcinolone acetonide*, 0.1%) are likely equally effective.

■ Summary and recommendations

CANCER THERAPY-ASSOCIATED MUCOSITIS

First line:

- morphine oral rinse (2:1000 concentration), every 2-4 h
- opioid (e.g. morphine initial dose 4-6 mg IV, then titrate), with PCA if available

Reasonable: indomethacin 0.25% spray applied q4-6 h

Pregnancy: morphine oral rinse (2:1000 concentration) or IV (initial dose 4-6 mg IV, then titrate)

Pediatric: morphine oral rinse (2:1000 concentration) or IV (initial dose 0.05-0.1 mg/kg IV, then titrate)

Special cases:

- *refractory CTAM*: doxepin (5 mg/mL oral rinse q4–6 h)

MUCOSITIS NOT ASSOCIATED WITH CANCER

First line:

- amlexanox (5% topical paste, applied in 100 mg dose QID)
- steroid (e.g. clobetasol propionate 0.05% applied 1:1 with dental paste BID)

Reasonable: sucralfate oral rinse (5–10 mL suspension, equal to 500–1000 mg, with 2–3 min rinse QID)

Pregnancy: sucralfate oral rinse (5–10 mL suspension, equal to 500–1000 mg, with 2–3 min rinse QID)

Pediatric:

- sucralfate oral rinse (5 mL suspension, equal to 500 mg, with 2–3 min rinse QID)
- steroid (e.g. clobetasol propionate 0.05% applied 1:1 with dental paste BID)

References

1. Coda BA, O'Sullivan B, Donaldson G, *et al*. Comparative efficacy of patient-controlled administration of morphine, hydromorphone, or sufentanil for the treatment of oral mucositis pain following bone marrow transplantation. *Pain*. 1997;**72**(3):333–346.
2. Clarkson JE, Worthington HV, Eden OB. Interventions for treating oral mucositis for patients with cancer receiving treatment. *Cochrane Database Syst Rev*. 2007(2):CD001973.
3. Collins JJ, Geake J, Grier HE, *et al*. Patient-controlled analgesia for mucositis pain in children: a three-period crossover study comparing morphine and hydromorphone. *J Pediatr*. 1996;**129**(5):722–728.
4. Dunbar PJ, Chapman CR, Buckley FP, *et al*. Clinical analgesic equivalence for morphine and hydromorphone with prolonged PCA. *Pain*. 1996;**68**(2–3):265–270.

5. Demarosi F, Lodi G, Soligo D, *et al.* Transdermal fentanyl in HSCT patients: an open trial using transdermal fentanyl for the treatment of oral mucositis pain. *Bone Marrow Transplant.* 2004;**33**(12):1247–1251.

6. Cerchietti LC, Navigante AH, Bonomi MR, *et al.* Effect of topical morphine for mucositis-associated pain following concomitant chemoradiotherapy for head and neck carcinoma. *Cancer.* 15 2002;**95**(10):2230–2236.

7. Cerchietti LC, Navigante AH, Korte MW, *et al.* Potential utility of the peripheral analgesic properties of morphine in stomatitis-related pain: a pilot study. *Pain.* 2003;**105**(1–2):265–273.

8. Cerchietti L. Morphine mouthwashes for painful mucositis. *Support Care Cancer.* 2007;**15**(1):115–116; author reply 117.

9. Momo K, Shiratsuchi T, Taguchi H, *et al.* Preparation and clinical application of indomethacin gel for medical treatment of stomatitis. *Yakugaku Zasshi.* 2005;**125**(5):433–440.

10. Nakamura T, Aoyama T, Yanagihara Y, *et al.* [The effects of indomethacin spray on the pain of stomatitis in the patients for hematopoietic stem cell transplantation.] *Yakugaku Zasshi.* 2003;**123**(12):1023–1029.

11. Epstein JB, Silverman S, Jr., Paggiarino DA, *et al.* Benzydamine HCl for prophylaxis of radiation-induced oral mucositis: results from a multicenter, randomized, double-blind, placebo-controlled clinical trial. *Cancer.* 2001;**92**(4):875–885.

12. Epstein JB, Epstein JD, Epstein MS, *et al.* Oral doxepin rinse: the analgesic effect and duration of pain reduction in patients with oral mucositis due to cancer therapy. *Anesth Analg.* 2006;**103**(2):465–470; table of contents.

13. Ehrnrooth E, Grau C, Zachariae R, *et al.* Randomized trial of opioids versus tricyclic antidepressants for radiation-induced mucositis pain in head and neck cancer. *Acta Oncol.* 2001;**40**(6):745–750.

14. Slatkin NE, Rhiner M. Topical ketamine in the treatment of mucositis pain. *Pain Med.* 2003;**4**(3):298–303.

15. Epstein JB, Klasser GD. Emerging approaches for prophylaxis and management of oropharyngeal mucositis in cancer therapy. *Expert Opin Emerg Drugs.* 2006;**11**(2):353–373.

16. McGuire DB, Correa ME, Johnson J, *et al.* The role of basic oral care and good clinical practice principles in the management of oral mucositis. *Support Care Cancer.* 2006;**14**(6):541–547.

17. Rubenstein EB, Peterson DE, Schubert M, *et al.* Clinical practice guidelines for the prevention and treatment of cancer therapy-induced oral and gastrointestinal mucositis. *Cancer.* 2004;**100**(9 Suppl):2026–2046.

18. Barasch A, Elad S, Altman A, *et al.* Antimicrobials, mucosal coating agents, anesthetics, analgesics, and nutritional supplements for alimentary tract mucositis. *Support Care Cancer.* 2006;**14**(6):528–532.

19. Alterio D, Jereczek-Fossa BA, Zuccotti GF, *et al.* Tetracaine oral gel in patients treated with radiotherapy for head-and-neck cancer: final results of a phase II study. *Int J Radiat Oncol Biol Phys.* 2006;**64**(2):392–395.

20. Elad S, Cohen G, Zylber-Katz E, *et al.* Systemic absorption of lidocaine after topical application for the treatment of oral mucositis in bone marrow transplantation patients. *J Oral Pathol Med.* 1999;**28**(4):170–172.

21. Oguchi M, Shikama N, Sasaki S, *et al.* Mucosa-adhesive water-soluble polymer film for treatment of acute radiation-induced oral mucositis. *Int J Radiat Oncol Biol Phys.* 1998;**40**(5):1033–1037.

22. Zempsky WT, Schechter NL. Office-based pain management. The 15-minute consultation. *Pediatr Clin North Am.* 2000;**47**(3):601–615.

23. Dodd MJ, Dibble SL, Miaskowski C, *et al.* Randomized clinical trial of the effectiveness of 3 commonly used mouthwashes to treat chemotherapy-induced mucositis. *Oral Surg Oral Med Oral Pathol Oral Radiol Endod.* 2000;**90**(1):39–47.

24. Chiara S, Nobile MT, Vincenti M, *et al.* Sucralfate in the treatment of chemotherapy-induced stomatitis: a double-blind, placebo-controlled pilot study. *Anticancer Res.* 2001;**21**(5):3707–3710.

25. Dodd MJ, Miaskowski C, Greenspan D, *et al.* Radiation-induced mucositis: a randomized clinical trial of micronized sucralfate versus salt and soda mouthwashes. *Cancer Invest.* 2003;**21**(1):21–33.

26. Shenep JL, Kalwinsky DK, Hutson PR, *et al.* Efficacy of oral sucralfate suspension in prevention and treatment of chemotherapy-induced mucositis. *J Pediatr.* 1988;**113**(4):758–763.

27. Rattan J, Schneider M, Arber N, *et al.* Sucralfate suspension as a treatment of recurrent aphthous stomatitis. *J Intern Med.* 1994;**236**(3):341–343.

28. Alpsoy E, Er H, Durusoy C, *et al.* The use of sucralfate suspension in the treatment of oral and genital ulceration of Behçet disease: a randomized, placebo-controlled, double-blind study. *Arch Dermatol.* 1999;**135**(5):529–532.

29. Khandwala A, van Inwegen RG, Charney MR, *et al.* 5% amlexanox oral paste, a new treatment for recurrent minor aphthous ulcers: II. Pharmacokinetics and demonstration of clinical safety. *Oral Surg Oral Med Oral Pathol Oral Radiol Endod.* 1997;**83**(2):231–238.

30. Murray B, McGuinness N, Biagioni P, *et al.* A comparative study of the efficacy of Aphtheal in the management of recurrent minor aphthous ulceration. *J Oral Pathol Med.* 2005;**34**(7):413–419.

31. Liu J, Zeng X, Chen Q, *et al.* An evaluation on the efficacy and safety of amlexanox oral adhesive tablets in the treatment of recurrent minor aphthous ulceration in a Chinese cohort: a randomized, double-blind, vehicle-controlled, unparallel multicenter clinical trial. *Oral Surg Oral Med Oral Pathol Oral Radiol Endod.* 2006;**102**(4):475–481.

32. Bell J. Amlexanox for the treatment of recurrent aphthous ulcers. *Clin Drug Invest.* 2005;**25**(9):555–566.

33. Barrons RW. Treatment strategies for recurrent oral aphthous ulcers. *Am J Health Syst Pharm.* 2001;**58**(1):41–50; quiz 51–53.

34. Lo Muzio L, della Valle A, Mignogna MD, *et al.* The treatment of oral aphthous ulceration or erosive lichen planus with topical clobetasol propionate in three preparations: a clinical and pilot study on 54 patients. *J Oral Pathol Med.* 2001;**30**(10):611–617.

35. Thompson AC, Nolan A, Lamey PJ. Minor aphthous oral ulceration: a double-blind cross-over study of beclomethasone dipropionate aerosol spray. *Scott Med J.* 1989;**34**(5):531–532.

Neck and back pain – mechanical strain

MICHAEL TURTURRO

■ Agents

- NSAIDs
- Opioids
- Skeletal muscle relaxants
- Benzodiazepines
- Corticosteroids
- Local anesthetics

■ Evidence

Because of different therapeutic approaches, this text separates mechanical strain spinal pain (MSSP) from neck and back pain of other etiologies (e.g. spondylosis, radiculopathy). There may be some overlap in presentation, so referral to other chapters of this text addressing neck and back pain may be useful.

The **NSAIDs** are the mainstay of therapy for nonradiating mechanical back pain, and also – by extrapolation of evidence from back pain studies – for neck strain.[1-4] Cochrane review of the relevant evidence (from over 50 trials) addressing MSSP pain relief concluded that **NSAIDs** are probably more effective than placebo; there is conflicting evidence as to whether **NSAIDs** are consistently better than other MSSP treatment alternatives.[4]

There are good data supporting a contention that there are no differences in the analgesic efficacies of the different **NSAIDs** for MSSP.[4] In most cases, because of its wide availability and low cost, *ibuprofen* (600 mg PO QID or 800 mg PO TID) is a reasonable first-line therapy.

Opioids are the preferred treatment for MSSP in patients who have not responded to, or who cannot take, **NSAIDs**. Although RCTs have not specifically evaluated **opioid** therapy for MSSP, support for their use can be extrapolated from their effectiveness in managing the closely related syndrome of refractory back pain.[5]

Muscle relaxants are often prescribed for sprains and strains of the neck and back. Although agents in this class have sedative properties, they provide no direct skeletal muscle relaxation at the doses commonly used for MSSP.[6] In fact, the sedative effects of skeletal muscle relaxants are probably responsible for their efficacy (compared with placebo) as monotherapy for improving MSSP pain.[7,8] Clinicians who use **muscle relaxants** to treat MSSP should be aware that the likely mediator of symptom relief is not muscular at all, but rather the drugs' sedative actions.

Despite anecdotal suggestions of efficacy, and prevalent use in everyday acute care practice, the dual-therapy approach combining **muscle relaxants** and **NSAIDs** lacks robust evidentiary support. If widely held beliefs in this regimen's utility are indeed accurate, efficacy could be a placebo effect or a salutary combination of sedation with analgesia. There are no RCT data finding benefit of dual therapy over single-agent use of either **NSAIDs** or **muscle relaxants**.[9,10]

Commonly used **muscle relaxants** include *cyclobenzaprine* (5–10 mg PO TID), *orphenadrine* (100 mg PO BID), *metaxolone* (800 mg PO TID–QID), *methocarbamol* (1000 mg PO QID), *carisoprodol* (350 mg PO TID–QID), and *chlorzoxazone* (250–500 mg PO TID–QID). While there are no data comparing effectiveness of **muscle relaxants** for MSSP, these agents differ with respect to chemical class, pharmacology, and relative propensity to cause certain adverse effects.[11] For example, *cyclobenzaprine* and *orphenadrine* are associated with anticholinergic side effects; *chlorzoxazone* (rarely) causes hepatic toxicity, and *carisoprodol* has abuse potential.[12,13] As one of the more commonly prescribed skeletal muscle relaxants, *cyclobenzaprine* has the advantage of familiarity and is probably as good as any other **muscle relaxant;** its sedative effects can be minimized by using a lower dose (5 mg PO TID).[3]

Potential for side effects (e.g. sedation) and lack of evidence of improved pain relief over that attained with **NSAID** monotherapy relegates **muscle relaxants** to second-line use. These agents are recommended only for patients in whom they have been effective in the past, or in those who fail or who are not candidates for **NSAID** or **opioid** therapy. Because of the risk of excessive sedation, **muscle relaxants** should not be routinely used in combination with **opioids**.

Benzodiazepines have skeletal muscle-relaxing properties, and so this class (most notably *diazepam*) is occasionally prescribed for MSSP. As is the case with the **muscle relaxants**, the benefit of **benzodiazepines** for neck and back strain is largely attributable to sedative properties. There are few studies – none methodologically rigorous   supporting claims that muscle relaxation is the mechanism by which *diazepam* mediates pain relief.[14] It is likely that, at doses commonly prescribed for outpatient treatment, *diazepam* produces little or no clinically significant decrease in muscle spasm. Clinicians who use **benzodiazepines** for MSSP should be aware that, as is the case with other **muscle relaxants**, symptom relief is likely a result of the agents' sedative properties.

The manufacturer's prescribing information for *cyclobenzaprine* (see US prescribing information available with the drug) references three unpublished studies that demonstrate that agent's superiority over *diazepam* in improving patients' muscle spasm, local pain and tenderness, limitation of motion, and ability to perform activities of daily living. However, literature search fails to identify any head-to-head trials in the published literature. Whether or not *cyclobenzaprine* is more effective than *diazepam*, the limited data demonstrating **benzodiazepine** efficacy in MSSP relegate this class to second-line use. *Diazepam* should be considered in patients who fail other therapy, or in those who have responded well to **benzodiazepines** in the past.

There is no evidence supporting routine use of systemic **corticosteroids** in the acute management of MSSP.[15]

Trigger point injection with **local anesthetics** is occasionally effective for some patients with neck or back pain, but injection therapy for MSSP has been insufficiently studied to recommend its routine use. If a patient with MSSP has a particular trigger point stimulating the pain, injection therapy may be worthwhile.[16] Facet joint injections of **local anesthetics** and **corticosteroids** are occasionally beneficial, but this procedure is outside the scope of routine EM practice.

■ Summary and recommendations

First line: NSAIDs (e.g. ibuprofen 600–800 mg PO TID)

Reasonable:
- oral opioids (e.g. oxycodone 5–10 mg q4–6 h, with or without acetaminophen)
- cyclobenzaprine 5 mg PO TID *or* methocarbamol 1000 mg PO QID

Pregnancy: acetaminophen (650–1000 mg PO QID), oral opioids (e.g. oxycodone 5–10 mg PO q4–6 h), cyclobenzaprine (5 mg PO TID)

Pediatric: NSAIDs (e.g. ibuprofen 10 mg/kg PO QID)

Special cases:
- *NSAIDs and opioids not indicated, or benzodiazepines previously efficacious*: benzodiazepines (e.g. diazepam 5 mg PO QID)
- *discrete trigger points identified on examination*: injection with local anesthetics (e.g. lidocaine)
- *refractory symptoms, opioids are to be avoided*: combination therapy with NSAID (e.g. ibuprofen 600–800 mg PO TID) and a skeletal muscle relaxant (e.g. cyclobenzaprine 5 mg PO TID)

References

1. Bigos S, Bowyer O, Braen G. *Clinical Practice Guideline No. 14: Acute Low Back Problems in Adults*. [AHCPR Publication 95-0642.] Rockville, MD: Agency for Health Care Policy and Research, 1994.
2. Beebe FA, Barkin RL, Barkin S. A clinical and pharmacologic review of skeletal muscle relaxants for musculoskeletal conditions. *Am J Ther*. 2005;**12**(2): 151–171.
3. van Tulder MW, Koes BW, Bouter LM. Conservative treatment of acute and chronic nonspecific low back pain. A systematic review of randomized controlled trials of the most common interventions. *Spine*. 1997;**22**(18):2128–2156.
4. van Tulder MW, Scholten RJ, Koes BW, *et al*. Nonsteroidal anti-inflammatory drugs for low back pain: a systematic review within the framework of the Cochrane Collaboration Back Review Group. *Spine*. 2000;**25**(19):2501–2513.

5. Jamison RN, Raymond SA, Slawsby EA, *et al.* Opioid therapy for chronic noncancer back pain. A randomized prospective study. *Spine.* 1998;**23**(23):2591–2600.

6. Waldman HJ. Centrally acting skeletal muscle relaxants and associated drugs. *J Pain Symptom Manage.* 1994;**9**(7):434–441.

7. Borenstein DG, Korn S. Efficacy of a low-dose regimen of cyclobenzaprine hydrochloride in acute skeletal muscle spasm: results of two placebo-controlled trials. *Clin Ther.* 2003;**25**(4):1056–1073.

8. van Tulder MW, Touray T, Furlan AD, *et al.* Muscle relaxants for non-specific low back pain. *Cochrane Database Syst Rev.* 2003(2):CD004252.

9. Childers MK, Borenstein D, Brown RL, *et al.* Low-dose cyclobenzaprine versus combination therapy with ibuprofen for acute neck or back pain with muscle spasm: a randomized trial. *Curr Med Res Opin.* 2005;**21**(9):1485–1493.

10. Turturro MA, Frater CR, D'Amico FJ. Cyclobenzaprine with ibuprofen versus ibuprofen alone in acute myofascial strain: a randomized, double-blind clinical trial. *Ann Emerg Med.* 2003;**41**(6):818–826.

11. Chou R, Peterson K, Helfand M. Comparative efficacy and safety of skeletal muscle relaxants for spasticity and musculoskeletal conditions: a systematic review. *J Pain Symptom Manage.* 2004;**28**(2):140–175.

12. Powers BJ, Cattau EL, Jr., Zimmerman HJ. Chlorzoxazone hepatotoxic reactions. An analysis of 21 identified or presumed cases. *Arch Intern Med.* 1986;**146**(6):1183–1186.

13. Bailey DN, Briggs JR. Carisoprodol: an unrecognized drug of abuse. *Am J Clin Pathol.* 2002;**117**(3):396–400.

14. Srivastava M, Walsh D. Diazepam as an adjuvant analgesic to morphine for pain due to skeletal muscle spasm. *Support Care Cancer.* 2003;**11**(1):66–69.

15. Finckh A, Zufferey P, Schurch MA, *et al.* Short-term efficacy of intravenous pulse glucocorticoids in acute discogenic sciatica. A randomized controlled trial. *Spine.* 2006;**31**(4):377–381.

16. Alvarez DJ, Rockwell PG. Trigger points: diagnosis and management. *Am Fam Physician.* 2002;**65**(4):653–660.

Neck and back pain – radicular syndromes

ADAM LEVINE AND STEPHEN H. THOMAS

■ Agents

- NSAIDs
- Opioids
- Steroids

■ Evidence

True radiculopathy is usually caused by intervertebral disk compression and subsequent irritation of a spinal nerve root. The etiologic differences between radiating spine pain (RSP) and other causes of neck and back pain translate into differences in therapeutic approach. This chapter focuses on pharmacologic treatment modalities for RSP. Drug treatment remains the mainstay of RSP analgesia, since studies of most nonpharmacologic approaches find them ineffective or impractical for ED use.[1,2]

The **NSAID**s have been studied extensively for pain relief in undifferentiated low-back pain, but there are fewer data addressing their use in RSP. Several early studies, each with methodological limitations, failed to show consistent benefit (over placebo) for use of **NSAIDs** (e.g. *indomethacin*, *phenylbutazone*, *ketoprofen*) in acute RSP based in the lower back.[3–8] Two larger trials have reported conflicting results with regard to *piroxicam*'s efficacy.[9,10] A multicenter RCT found IM *dipyrone* outperformed both *diclofenac* PO and placebo in reducing RSP pain at 1, 6, and 48 h, but *dipyrone* cannot be recommended owing to its hematologic side effects (which resulted in its removal from the US market).[11–13]

Two recent multicenter RCTs (comprising over 1000 patients) were designed with more methodological rigor than earlier studies.[14] The first of these RCTs compared oral *meloxicam* (a **COX-2 selective NSAID**), at doses of 7.5 mg and 15 mg PO QD, with placebo; the second compared the same doses of *meloxicam* with *diclofenac* (50 mg PO TID). There was similar pain improvement (at 6 h, three days, and one week) with *diclofenac* and either *meloxicam* dosage, with both drugs outperforming placebo.

Although there are studies of use of **muscle relaxants** (e.g. **benzodiazepines**) for undifferentiated neck and back pain, no placebo-controlled trials have examined their use in acute RSP. Furthermore, since RSP is not caused by muscle spasm, there is little reason to suspect that **muscle relaxants** should be of much therapeutic benefit in these patients.

Patients with refractory RSP often require **opioid** therapy, but available evidence does not support specific recommendations. Some studies of undifferentiated neck or back pain have included subjects with RSP, but no trials have focused on **opioid** use in this population. The available data do provide guidance as to which approaches are less likely to be useful. Studies suggest no incremental benefit, compared with **NSAIDs**, for PO low-potency **opioids** (e.g. *codeine*) or agonist–antagonist agents (e.g. *meptazinol, ethoheptazine*).[15–18] We believe the main role for low-potency **opioids** in RSP is for use in patients who fail, or do not tolerate, other therapies such as **NSAIDs**.

Corticosteroids have been used for the treatment of acute RSP since the 1960s. Their use is rational, since RSP pain is caused by nerve root compression and inflammation. Nonetheless, recent evidence has questioned (though not ruled out) a role for **corticosteroids** in acute RSP.

The injection of **corticosteroids** into the epidural space is a commonly used approach. A 2005 review of 11 RCTs assessing epidural **corticosteroid** injection for acute (low back-centered) RSP concluded that, while data show a few weeks' benefit, pain tends to recur by the second post-treatment month.[19] A subsequent trial confirmed these findings, reporting significant improvement in pain scores (compared with placebo) at three weeks, but no difference by 6–52 weeks.[20] In addition to its limitation of relatively short analgesia duration, epidural **corticosteroid** injection requires resources and expertise (e.g. fluoroscopic guidance) rarely available in the acute care setting.[20]

Corticosteroids have also been administered IV for RSP, with results similar to those found for local injection: initial relief followed by pain recurrence. An RCT illustrates that the IV route for **corticosteroids** is associated with shorter analgesia duration than that achieved with epidural injection. A single dose of **methylprednisolone** (500 mg IV) significantly reduces pain scores in RSP, but the effect is small in magnitude and limited in duration (48 h at most).[21]

■ Summary and recommendations

First line: NSAIDs (e.g. meloxicam 7.5–15 mg PO QD, diclofenac 50 mg PO TID)

Reasonable: opioids (e.g. oxycodone 5–10 mg PO q4–6 h, with or without acetaminophen)

Pregnancy: acetaminophen 650–1000 mg PO QID; opioids (e.g. oxycodone 5–10 mg PO q4–6 h)

Pediatric: NSAIDs (e.g. ibuprofen 10 mg/kg PO QID)

Special case:
■ *mild pain, patient not candidate for NSAIDs*: low-potency opioid (e.g. hydrocodone 2.5–5.0 mg PO q4–6 h)

References

1. Hagen KB, Jamtvedt G, Hilde G, *et al*. The updated Cochrane Review of bed rest for low back pain and sciatica. *Spine*. 2005;**30**(5):542–546.
2. Koes B, van Tulder M. Acute low back pain. *Am Fam Physician*. 2006;**74**(5):803–805.
3. Braun H, Huberty R. [Therapy of lumbar sciatica. A comparative clinical study of a corticoid-free monosubstance and a corticoid-containing combination drug.] *Med Welt*. 1982;**33**(13):490–491.
4. Goldie I. A clinical trial with indomethacin (indomee^R) in low back pain and sciatica. *Acta Orthop Scand*. 1968;**39**(1):117–128.
5. Grevsten S, Johansson H. Phenylbutazone in treatment of acute lumbago-sciatica. *Z Rheumatol*. 1975;**34**(11–12):444–447.
6. Jacobs JH, Grayson MF. Trial of an anti-inflammatory agent (indomethacin) in low back pain with and without radicular involvement. *BMJ*. 1968;**3**(5611):158–160.

7. Radin EL, Bryan RS. Phenylbutazone for prolapsed discs? *Lancet.* 1968;**ii** (7570):736.

8. Weber H, Aasand G. The effect of phenylbutazone on patients with acute lumbago–sciatica. A double blind trial. *J Oslo City Hosp.* 1980;**30** (5): 69–72.

9. Aoki T, Kuroki Y, Kageyama T, *et al.* Multicentre double-blind comparison of piroxicam and indomethacin in the treatment of lumbar diseases. *Eur J Rheumatol Inflamm.* 1983;**6**(3):247–252.

10. Weber H, Holme I, Amlie E. The natural course of acute sciatica with nerve root symptoms in a double-blind placebo-controlled trial evaluating the effect of piroxicam. *Spine.* 1993;**18**(11):1433–1438.

11. Ribera A, Monasterio J, Acebedo G, *et al.* Dipyrone-induced immune haemolytic anaemia. *Vox Sang.* 1981;**41**(1):32–35.

12. Shinar E, Hershko C. Causes of agranulocytosis in a hospital population: identification of dipyrone as an important causative agent. *Isr J Med Sci.* 1983;**19**(3):225–229.

13. Babej-Dolle R, Freytag S, Eckmeyer J, *et al.* Parenteral dipyrone versus diclofenac and placebo in patients with acute lumbago or sciatic pain: randomized observer-blind multicenter study. *Int J Clin Pharmacol Ther.* 1994;**32**(4):204–209.

14. Dreiser RL, Le Parc JM, Velicitat P, *et al.* Oral meloxicam is effective in acute sciatica: two randomised, double-blind trials versus placebo or diclofenac. *Inflamm Res.* 2001;**50**(Suppl 1):S17–S23.

15. Brown FL, Jr., Bodison S, Dixon J, *et al.* Comparison of diflunisal and acetaminophen with codeine in the treatment of initial or recurrent acute low back strain. *Clin Ther.* 1986;**9**(Suppl C):52–58.

16. Innes GD, Croskerry P, Worthington J, *et al.* Ketorolac versus acetaminophen-codeine in the emergency department treatment of acute low back pain. *J Emerg Med.* 1998;**16**(4):549–556.

17. Sweetman BJ, Baig A, Parsons DL. Mefenamic acid, chlormezanone–paracetamol, ethoheptazine–aspirin–meprobamate: a comparative study in acute low back pain. *Br J Clin Pract.* 1987;**41**(2):619–624.

18. Videman T, Heikkila J, Partanen T. Double-blind parallel study of meptazinol versus diflunisal in the treatment of lumbago. *Curr Med Res Opin.* 1984;**9** (4):246–252.

19. McLain RF, Kapural L, Mekhail NA. Epidural steroid therapy for back and leg pain: mechanisms of action and efficacy. *Spine J.* 2005;**5**(2):191–201.

20. Arden NK, Price C, Reading I, *et al*. A multicentre randomized controlled trial of epidural corticosteroid injections for sciatica: the WEST study. *Rheumatology (Oxford)*. 2005;**44**(11):1399–1406.

21. Finckh A, Zufferey P, Schurch MA, *et al*. Short-term efficacy of intravenous pulse glucocorticoids in acute discogenic sciatica. A randomized controlled trial. *Spine*. 2006;**31**(4):377–381.

Neck and back pain – spinal spondylitic syndromes

MICHAEL WALTA AND STEPHEN H. THOMAS

■ Agents

- NSAIDs
- Opioids
- Tricyclic antidepressants
- Antiepileptics
- Corticosteroids

■ Evidence

In this chapter, neck and back pain from spinal stenosis, intervertebral disk disease, or arthritis is grouped into the category of spinal spondylitic syndromes (SSS). Acute care provider familiarity with treating SSS pain is important. Only half of medically managed patients achieve adequate outpatient analgesia, and there is little evidence to support surgical intervention for the sole purpose of obtaining pain relief.[1-4] Injection therapy (into the facet joint, epidural space, or locally) has little supporting evidence for use in SSS.[5]

Despite scant evidence support for their use in SSS, **NSAIDs** are frequently used to treat pain from these disorders. Recommendation for **NSAID** use in SSS, after *acetaminophen* (*paracetamol*) has failed, is based upon a presumed inflammatory component to the pain.[6,7] Since Cochrane review provides inconclusive evidence of **NSAIDs'** overall efficacy in spinal pain syndromes, and since patients with SSS tend to be relatively older and more susceptible to **NSAID** side effects, **NSAIDs** should be used with caution in SSS.[8] However, **NSAIDs'** common use with anecdotal success for some patients with SSS means that the acute care clinician should keep this class in mind for occasional use. **COX-2 selective NSAIDs** (the risks of which are addressed in the chapter on Arthritis) have not been studied in SSS. These agents appear to have little role in acute care management of SSS.

Few data address efficacy of **opioids** for SSS. A trial in patients with spinal osteoarthritis showed significant pain reduction compared with placebo from either regular formulation *oxycodone* (30–60 mg/day) plus *acetaminophen* (1–2 g/day), or sustained-release *oxycodone* (30–60 mg/day).[9] No adverse effects were reported, although it is well known that approximately 80% of patients experience constipation, nausea, or somnolence with chronic **opioid** use.[10] Though caution must be exercised in the elderly, **opioid** use for moderate-to-severe SSS pain is endorsed by the American Geriatric Society's clinical practice guidelines.[11]

As is the case with **opioids**, there are few studies that directly address the use of **muscle relaxants** and the chemically related **tricyclic antidepressants** for SSS. *Cyclobenzaprine* (30–60 mg/day) is known to be somewhat effective in mixed populations of patients with acute back and neck pain; these populations include patients with SSS pain but the absence of subgroup analysis limits generalization of efficacy results.[12,13] The age and comorbidity characteristics of patients with SSS dictate a need for added caution with regard to *cyclobenzaprine*'s anticholinergic effects (e.g. delirium, fall risk).[14] Other **tricyclic antidepressants**, including low-dose *amitriptyline* (25–50 mg/day) and *nortriptyline* (50–150 mg/day), are commonly used with reasonable efficacy in patient populations that include subgroups with SSS symptoms.[6,15,16]

There is preliminary evidence supporting some role for *gabapentin* (300–2400 mg/day) in cervical SSS pain. A small case series suggests borderline improvement in pain scores.[17] Endorsement of *gabapentin* use for SSS pain is based primarily upon its presumed benefit in related pain syndromes such as diabetic neuropathy (as discussed in other chapters).[18]

Corticosteroids, potentially of use in cervical radicular pain with inflammatory component, have not been studied in SSS pain.[6]

The **omega-3 fatty acids** *eicosapentaenoic acid* and *decosahexaenoic acid*, which have known anti-inflammatory properties, have been used for SSS pain of discogenic nature. Limited evidence reveals only borderline increases in self-reported pain scores over a one month period, and these agents have no role in the acute care setting.[19]

■ Summary and recommendations

First line: acetaminophen (initial dose 650–1000 mg PO QID), opioids (e.g. oxycodone 5–10 mg PO q4–6 h)

Reasonable: short course of NSAIDs (e.g. ibuprofen 600–800 mg PO TID)

Pregnancy: acetaminophen (initial dose 650–1000 mg PO QID), opioids (e.g. oxycodone 5–10 mg PO q4–6 h)

Pediatric: acetaminophen (10–15 mg/kg PO QID), opioids (e.g. hydrocodone 2.5 mg PO q4–6 h for age > 5 years)

Special case:
■ *if other agents fail and side effect risk favorable*: cyclobenzaprine (5 mg PO TID) or tricyclic antidepressants (e.g. nortriptyline 50–150 mg PO qHS)

References

1. Gore J, Corrao J, Goldberg R, *et al*. Feasibility and safety of emergency inter-hospital transport of patients during early hours of acute myocardial infarction. *Arch Intern Med*. 1989;**149**(2):353–355.
2. Rao R. Neck pain, cervical radiculopathy, and cervical myelopathy: pathophysiology, natural history, and clinical evaluation. *Instr Course Lect*. 2003;**52**:479–488.
3. Kadanka Z, Mares M, Bednanik J, *et al*. Approaches to spondylotic cervical myelopathy: conservative versus surgical results in a 3-year follow-up study. *Spine*. 2002;**27**(20):2205–2210; discussion 2210–2211.
4. Sampath P, Bendebba M, Davis JD, *et al*. Outcome of patients treated for cervical myelopathy. A prospective, multicenter study with independent clinical review. *Spine*. 2000;**25**(6):670–676.
5. Nelemans PJ, de Bie RA, de Vet HC, *et al*. Injection therapy for subacute and chronic benign low back pain. *Cochrane Database Syst Rev*. 2000(2):CD001824.
6. Mazanec D, Reddy A. Medical management of cervical spondylosis. *Neurosurgery*. 2007;**60**(1 Suppl 1):S43–S50.
7. Clyman BB. Osteoarthritis: new roles for drug therapy and surgery. Interview by Peter Pompei. *Geriatrics*. 1996;**51**(9):32–36.

8. van Tulder MW, Scholten RJ, Koes BW, *et al.* Nonsteroidal anti-inflammatory drugs for low back pain: a systematic review within the framework of the Cochrane Collaboration Back Review Group. *Spine.* 2000;**25**(19):2501–2513.

9. Caldwell JR, Hale ME, Boyd RE, *et al.* Treatment of osteoarthritis pain with controlled release oxycodone or fixed combination oxycodone plus acetaminophen added to nonsteroidal antiinflammatory drugs: a double blind, randomized, multicenter, placebo controlled trial. *J Rheumatol.* 1999;**26**(4):862–869.

10. Kalso E, Edwards JE, Moore RA, *et al.* Opioids in chronic non-cancer pain: systematic review of efficacy and safety. *Pain.* 2004;**112**(3):372–380.

11. American Geriatrics Society Panel on Persistent Pain in Older Persons. The management of persistent pain in older persons. *J Am Geriatr Soc.* 2002;**50**(6 Suppl):S205–S224.

12. Borenstein DG, Korn S. Efficacy of a low-dose regimen of cyclobenzaprine hydrochloride in acute skeletal muscle spasm: results of two placebo-controlled trials. *Clin Ther.* 2003;**25**(4):1056–1073.

13. Childers MK, Borenstein D, Brown RL, *et al.* Low-dose cyclobenzaprine versus combination therapy with ibuprofen for acute neck or back pain with muscle spasm: a randomized trial. *Curr Med Res Opin.* 2005;**21**(9):1485–1493.

14. Browning R, Jackson JL, O'Malley PG. Cyclobenzaprine and back pain: a meta-analysis. *Arch Intern Med.* 2001;**161**(13):1613–1620.

15. Atkinson JH, Slater MA, Williams RA, *et al.* A placebo-controlled randomized clinical trial of nortriptyline for chronic low back pain. *Pain.* 1998;**76**(3):287–296.

16. Pheasant H, Bursk A, Goldfarb J, *et al.* Amitriptyline and chronic low-back pain. A randomized double-blind crossover study. *Spine.* 1983; **8**(5):552–557.

17. Sist TC, Filadora VA, 2nd, Miner M, *et al.* Experience with gabapentin for neuropathic pain in the head and neck: report of ten cases. *Reg Anesth.* 1997;**22**(5):473–478.

18. Morello CM, Leckband SG, Stoner CP, *et al.* Randomized double-blind study comparing the efficacy of gabapentin with amitriptyline on diabetic peripheral neuropathy pain. *Arch Intern Med.* 1999;**159**(16): 1931–1937.

19. Maroon JC, Bost JW. Omega-3 fatty acids (fish oil) as an anti-inflammatory: an alternative to nonsteroidal anti-inflammatory drugs for discogenic pain. *Surg Neurol.* 2006;**65**(4):326–331.

Neuropathy – complex regional pain syndrome

DAVID CLINE

■ Agents

- Bisphosphonates
- Calcitonin
- Gabapentin
- Corticosteroids

■ Evidence

This chapter covers both types (1 and 2) of complex regional pain syndrome (CRPS). Although the discussion follows the common practice of discussing CRPS type 1 (reflex sympathetic dystrophy, RSD) in the context of neuropathy, it should be noted that RSD is not technically neuropathic since there is no nerve lesion. CRPS type 2, also known as causalgia, is a true neuropathy.

Of all of the types of neuropathic pain, CRPS (either type) is the most resistant to pharmacotherapy. Even traditionally endorsed approaches such as sympathetic blockade are found poorly efficacious in Cochrane review.[1] In fact, RCT evidence does not conclusively confirm utility for *any* agent for CRPS.[2,3]

For CRPS type 2, two trials of IV infusion of **bisphosphonates** find that pain may be reduced by *alendronate* (7.5 mg IV daily) or *clodronate* (300 mg IV daily).[4,5]

Evidence addressing IN *calcitonin* use for CRPS is inconsistent but suggests a possible role for this approach in some patients. The hormone can also be administered IV, SC, or IM; some protocols for neuropathic pain involve administering 200 IU IV over 20 min, followed by a second infusion if pain relief is incomplete. For CRPS type 1, meta-analysis of 21 RCTs, acknowledging limitations in available data, concluded that IN *calcitonin* (administered in a dose of 200 IU) is the only therapy warranting endorsement.[6] For CRPS type 2, administration of 400 IU *calcitonin* IN was found unhelpful by one group.[7] However, another study found that, in patients receiving physical therapy, addition of 300 IU IN *calcitonin* significantly alleviated CRPS type 2 pain.[8]

The **anticonvulsant gabapentin**, effective in a broad range of neuropathic pain syndromes, is of little utility in CRPS.[9]

There is limited evidence for use of systemic **corticosteroids** for CRPS type 2. One small trial, assessing PO *prednisone* (10 mg TID), found some benefit compared with placebo.[10]

■ Summary and recommendations

First line: calcitonin (200 IU IV, SC, or IM QD)

Reasonable: alendronate (7.5 mg IV QD) or clodronate (300 mg IV QD), if
   follow-up is arranged (optimally with pain specialist)

Pregnancy:
■ calcitonin and bisphosphonates are both Pregnancy Category C; therapy
   with these agents should not be instituted by acute care providers
■ acetaminophen (650–1000 mg PO QID) and opioids (e.g. hydrocodone
   5–10 mg PO q4–6 h) may be used as temporizing therapy

Pediatric: safe/effective use of calcitonin or bisphosphonates has not been
   established in children; although there are few applicable studies,
   prednisone (0.14 mg/kg PO QD) may be the best therapeutic option for
   CRPS type 2

Special case:
■ *CRPS type 2, failure of bisphosphonates and calcitonin*: prednisone (10 mg
   PO TID)

References

1. Cepeda MS, Carr DB, Lau J. Local anesthetic sympathetic blockade for complex regional pain syndrome. *Cochrane Database Syst Rev*. 2005(4):CD004598.
2. Bennicky S, Tajti J, Timea Varga E, *et al*. Evidence-based pharmacological treatment of neuropathic pain syndromes. *J Neural Transm*. 2005;**112**(6):735–749.

3. Finnerup NB, Otto M, McQuay HJ, *et al*. Algorithm for neuropathic pain treatment: an evidence based proposal. *Pain*. 2005;**118**(3):289–305.

4. Adami S, Fossaluzza V, Gatti D, *et al*. Bisphosphonate therapy of reflex sympathetic dystrophy syndrome. *Ann Rheum Dis*. 1997;**56**(3):201–204.

5. Varenna M, Zucchi F, Ghiringhelli D, *et al*. Intravenous clodronate in the treatment of reflex sympathetic dystrophy syndrome. A randomized, double blind, placebo controlled study. *J Rheumatol*. 2000;**27**(6):1477–1483.

6. Perez RS, Kwakkel G, Zuurmond WW, *et al*. Treatment of reflex sympathetic dystrophy (CRPS type 1): a research synthesis of 21 randomized clinical trials. *J Pain Symptom Manage*. 2001;**21**(6):511–526.

7. Bickerstaff DR, Kanis JA. The use of nasal calcitonin in the treatment of posttraumatic algodystrophy. *Br J Rheumatol*. 1991;**30**(4):291–294.

8. Gobelet C, Waldburger M, Meier JL. The effect of adding calcitonin to physical treatment on reflex sympathetic dystrophy. *Pain*. 1992;**48**(2):171–175.

9. Serpell MG. Gabapentin in neuropathic pain syndromes: a randomised, double-blind, placebo-controlled trial. *Pain*. 2002;**99**(3):557–566.

10. Christensen K, Jensen EM, Noer I. The reflex dystrophy syndrome response to treatment with systemic corticosteroids. *Acta Chir Scand*. 1982;**148**(8):653–655.

Neuropathy – diabetic

DAVID CLINE

■ Agents

- Opioids
- Tricyclic antidepressants
- SSRIs
- Selective serotonin–norepinephrine reuptake inhibitors
- Anticonvulsants
- Local anesthetics

■ Evidence

Treatment decisions regarding diabetic neuropathy (DN) can be based upon useful evidence. Many agents have been assessed for therapy of DN pain, and many have some role in relief of symptoms. The breadth of therapeutic options is fortunate, given the often-refractory nature of the pain. The difficulty of controlling DN is ameliorated by the availability of several non-pharmacologic approaches (e.g. transcutaneous electrical nerve stimulator [TENS] units) that can improve pain relief provided by drug therapy.[1,2]

Although their side effects may relegate them to second-line use, the **opioids** do help in DN. Data from RCTs have demonstrated the utility of controlled-release *oxycodone* (starting dose 10 mg PO BID, with up-titration to a maximum of 60 mg daily).[3]

The **opioid** *tramadol*, which has additional (monoamine-related) mechanisms of analgesia, has particular utility in DN. Data from RCTs show that one in four patients achieves significant pain relief; analgesic benefit lasts for months.[4] Up-titration may be necessary. One RCT found that the average daily dose of *tramadol* required for significant relief of DN was 210 mg.[5]

As noted in other chapters of this text, the **tricyclic antidepressants (TCAs)** are among the most consistently effective therapy for neuropathic pain. Systematic review of studies including patients with DN (among others) confirms the utility of once-daily HS doses of **TCAs** such as *amitriptyline* (75 mg) or *imipramine* (titrated up to 150 mg).[6,7]

Multiple RCTs have demonstrated the efficacy of the **serotonin-norepinephrine reuptake inhibitor** (**SNRI**) *duloxetine* in the treatment of DN.[8-11] The initial dose of *duloxetine* for DN is 60 mg QD; if the initial QD dose is well tolerated but insufficient at controlling pain, 60 mg may be taken BID (some authorities use a single HS dose of 120 mg). In elderly patients, or those with renal impairment, or any patient for whom tolerability may be a concern, a starting dose of 20 mg QD may be slowly advanced to 40–60 mg daily (administered in either one or two doses). The **SNRI** *venlafexine* is also effective for DN, with a dose in the range 75–225 mg QD. With the **SNRIs**, pain relief may occur as early as one to two weeks after institution of therapy, though some patients may not see a full effect for up to six weeks. A withdrawal syndrome can occur if the **SNRIs** are abruptly discontinued.

Anticonvulsants are a valuable therapeutic option in DN. *Gabapentin*'s utility is demonstrated consistently in multiple RCTs; significant pain relief is found in approximately one in four patients.[12-14] The PO dosing of *gabapentin* for DN follows an advancing regimen: 300 mg HS on day one, followed by 300 mg BID on day two, then 300 mg TID on day three. The drug can then be titrated up to 1800 mg/day over two weeks.

Pregabalin (in a daily dose of 300–600 mg, administered in two or three divided doses) is effective for DN as well; approximately five patients must be treated for pain relief to be achieved in one.[15-17] When used in neuropathic pain, *pregabalin* achieves pain reduction by the end of therapy's first week, maximal analgesia is reached within four weeks.[18]

Topical application of **local anesthetics** may be useful in patients with focal DN pain. Patch application of *lidocaine* (5% preparation, applied for up to 4 h alternating with 12 h off), is known to be effective in DN; about one in four patients will respond.[19,20]

Intravenously injected **local anesthetics** have been reported potentially useful in DN. For example, bolus doses of *lidocaine* (a 5 mg/kg dose) are reported to achieve DN pain relief for up to three weeks post-injection.[21] However, *lidocaine* injection's overall risk-to-benefit ratio is not as favorable as those of other therapies, so there is little role for bolus *lidocaine* in ED treatment of DN.

■ Summary and recommendations

First line:

- duloxetine (60 mg PO QD)
- gabapentin (300 mg PO HS on day one, followed by 300 mg BID on day two, then 300 mg TID; up-titration to 1800 mg/day maximum)

Reasonable:

- tramadol (50 mg PO q6–8 h)
- pregabalin (150 mg PO BID)
- lidocaine patch (5% preparation, on for 2–4 h and off for 12 h)

Pregnancy:

- acetaminophen (650–1000 mg PO QID) plus opioid (e.g. hydrocodone 5–10 mg PO q4–6 h)
- topical lidocaine
- there are insufficient data to recommend most of the anticonvulsants or antidepressants for neuropathic pain use in pregnancy; acute care clinicians should consult with appropriate specialists before prescribing these agents for neuropathic pain.

Pediatric:

- gabapentin (5 mg/kg PO TID)
- lidocaine patch (5% preparation, on for 2–4 h and off for 12 h)

Special case:

- *if pain interferes with sleep:* antidepressants (e.g. duloxetine 60 mg PO QD)

References

1. Hamza MA, White PF, Craig WF, *et al*. Percutaneous electrical nerve stimulation: a novel analgesic therapy for diabetic neuropathic pain. *Diabetes Care*. 2000;**23**(3):365–370.

2. Alvaro M, Kumar D, Julka IS. Transcutaneous electrostimulation: emerging treatment for diabetic neuropathic pain. *Diabetes Technol Ther*. 1999;**1**(1):77–80.

3. Gimbel JS, Richards P, Portenoy RK. Controlled-release oxycodone for pain in diabetic neuropathy: a randomized controlled trial. *Neurology.* 2003;**60** (6):927–934.

4. Harati Y, Gooch C, Swenson M, *et al.* Maintenance of the long-term effectiveness of tramadol in treatment of the pain of diabetic neuropathy. *J Diabetes Complications.* 2000;**14**(2):65–70.

5. Harati Y, Gooch C, Swenson M, *et al.* Double-blind randomized trial of tramadol for the treatment of the pain of diabetic neuropathy. *Neurology.* 1998;**50**(6):1842–1846.

6. Beniczky S, Tajti J, Timea Varga E, *et al.* Evidence-based pharmacological treatment of neuropathic pain syndromes. *J Neural Transm.* 2005;**112** (6):735–749.

7. Finnerup NB, Otto M, McQuay HJ, *et al.* Algorithm for neuropathic pain treatment: an evidence based proposal. *Pain.* 2005;**118**(3):289–305.

8. Arnold LM, Lu Y, Crofford LJ, *et al.* A double-blind, multicenter trial comparing duloxetine with placebo in the treatment of fibromyalgia patients with or without major depressive disorder. *Arthritis Rheum.* 2004;**50**(9):2974–2984.

9. Goldstein DJ, Lu Y, Detke MJ, *et al.* Duloxetine vs. placebo in patients with painful diabetic neuropathy. *Pain.* 2005;**116**(1–2):109–118.

10. Raskin J, Pritchett YL, Wang F, *et al.* A double-blind, randomized multicenter trial comparing duloxetine with placebo in the management of diabetic peripheral neuropathic pain. *Pain Med.* 2005;**6**(5):346–356.

11. Wernicke JF, Pritchett YL, D'Souza DN, *et al.* A randomized controlled trial of duloxetine in diabetic peripheral neuropathic pain. *Neurology.* 2006;**67** (8):1411–1420.

12. Backonja M, Beydoun A, Edwards KR, *et al.* Gabapentin for the symptomatic treatment of painful neuropathy in patients with diabetes mellitus: a randomized controlled trial. *JAMA.* 1998;**280**(21): 1831–1836.

13. Backonja M, Glanzman RL. Gabapentin dosing for neuropathic pain: evidence from randomized, placebo-controlled clinical trials. *Clin Ther.* 2003;**25**(1):81–104.

14. Bone M, Critchley P, Buggy DJ. Gabapentin in postamputation phantom limb pain: a randomized, double-blind, placebo-controlled, cross-over study. *Reg Anesth Pain Med.* 2002;**27**(5):481–486.

15. Rosenstock J, Tuchman M, LaMoreaux L, *et al.* Pregabalin for the treatment of painful diabetic peripheral neuropathy: a double-blind, placebo-controlled trial. *Pain.* 2004;**110**(3):628–638.

16. Lesser H, Sharma U, LaMoreaux L, *et al.* Pregabalin relieves symptoms of painful diabetic neuropathy: a randomized controlled trial. *Neurology.* 2004;**63**(11):2104–2110.

17. Richter RW, Portenoy R, Sharma U, *et al.* Relief of painful diabetic peripheral neuropathy with pregabalin: a randomized, placebo-controlled trial. *J Pain.* 2005;**6**(4):253–260.

18. Freynhagen R, Busche P, Konrad C, *et al.* [Effectiveness and time to onset of pregabalin in patients with neuropathic pain.] *Schmerz.* 2006;**20**(4):285–288, 290–282.

19. Barbano RL, Herrmann DN, Hart-Gouleau S, *et al.* Effectiveness, tolerability, and impact on quality of life of the 5% lidocaine patch in diabetic polyneuropathy. *Arch Neurol.* 2004;**61**(6):914–918.

20. Meier T, Wasner G, Faust M, *et al.* Efficacy of lidocaine patch 5% in the treatment of focal peripheral neuropathic pain syndromes: a randomized, double-blind, placebo-controlled study. *Pain.* 2003;**106**(1–2):151–158.

21. Kastrup J, Petersen P, Dejgard A, *et al.* Intravenous lidocaine infusion: a new treatment of chronic painful diabetic neuropathy? *Pain.* 1987;**28**(1):69–75.

Neuropathy – HIV related

DAVID CLINE AND STEPHEN H. THOMAS

■ Agents

- Antidepressants
- Anticonvulsants
- Acetyl-L-carnitine
- Cannibis
- Memantine
- Intravenous immunoglobulin
- Capsaicin
- Lidocaine
- Thalidomide

■ Evidence

Neuropathy is common in patients infected with HIV. Unfortunately, HIV-related neuropathy (HIVNP) is resistant to many of the drugs that are generally helpful in neuropathic conditions. Cochrane review has found, for instance, that **antidepressants** are ineffective for treating HIVNP.[1]

Data are mixed with respect to use of the **anticonvulsant** *lamotrigine* (titrated to 600 mg PO daily) in HIVNP. It appears that *lamotrigine* reduces HIVNP, but only in patients who are also receiving neurotoxic antiretroviral drugs (didanosine, zalcitabine, or stavudine).[2] Cochrane review of the literature addressing *lamotrigine* in HIVNP concluded that there is insufficient evidence to support recommendation for its routine use.[3]

Available evidence on the utility of *gabapentin* for HIVNP is conflicting. A large trial of various types of neuropathy demonstrated relief with *gabapentin* in the overall study population but failed to reveal utility of the drug in subgroup analysis of patients with HIVNP.[4] Conversely, a small RCT ($n = 29$) focusing on HIVNP reported effective pain relief with *gabapentin* (2400 to

3600 mg/day); a high (80%) somnolence rate was also seen.[5] Evidence from other trials also supports utility of *gabapentin* for HIVNP.[6]

Neurotoxic neuropathic pain (i.e. that from antiviral agents) is improved by treatment with the neurotrophic support drug *acetyl-L-carnitine* (500 mg IM BID).[4–6]

An RCT assessing use of *cannabis* cigarettes found this approach – not realistic for the acute care setting – reduced pain compared with placebo.[7] Anonymous questionnaires suggest that *cannabis* reduces HIVNP in up to 90% of respondents.[8]

Multicenter RCT evidence demonstrated lack of utility of the N-methyl-D-aspartate (NMDA) antagonist *memantine* for HIVNP.[9]

Although *intravenous immunoglobulin* (*IVIG*) is often used for treating HIVNP, critical reviews of available data reveal insufficient evidence to support a recommendation for its acute care administration for this indication.[10,11]

Topical therapy with *capsaicin* is recommended for HIVNP by some editorialists and expert reviews.[12,13] However, Cochrane review of the available evidence concluded that there are no data supporting use of *capsaicin* for HIVNP.[14,15]

Data from RCT also demonstrated failure of topical *lidocaine* (5% gel) in treatment of HIVNP.[16]

The antineoplastic agent *thalidomide* has been used for HIVNP, but its known toxicity outweighs any evidence-supported benefit for its use in this condition.[17]

■ Summary and recommendations

First line: gabapentin (300 mg PO HS on day 1; 300 mg PO BID on day 2; 300 mg PO TID thereafter with up-titration as needed, to 1800 mg/day maximum)

Reasonable: if HIVNP is from toxic antiviral drugs, acetyl-L-carnitine (500 mg IM BID)

Pregnancy: weighing risks and benefits of gabapentin, lamotrigine, and acetyl-L-carnitine therapy during pregnancy may result in a decision to delay institution of optimal therapy until after delivery; acetaminophen and (in some cases) opioids may be used as temporizing measures

Special case:

■ *if patient taking neurotoxic antiviral drugs and* N-*acetyl-*L-*carnitine fails*: lamotrigine (600 mg PO QD)

References

1. Saarto T, Wiffen PJ. Antidepressants for neuropathic pain. *Cochrane Database Syst Rev*. 2005(3):CD005454.

2. Simpson DM, McArthur JC, Olney R, *et al*. Lamotrigine for HIV associated painful sensory neuropathies: a placebo-controlled trial. *Neurology*. 2003;**60**(9):1508–1514.

3. Wiffen PJ, Rees J. Lamotrigine for acute and chronic pain. *Cochrane Database Syst Rev*. 2007(2):CD006044.

4. Serpell MG. Gabapentin in neuropathic pain syndromes: a randomised, double-blind, placebo-controlled trial. *Pain*. 2002;**99**(3):557–566.

5. Hahn K, Arendt G, Braun JS, *et al*. A placebo-controlled trial of gabapentin for painful HIV-associated sensory neuropathies. *J Neurol*. 2004;**251**(10):1260–1266.

6. La Spina I, Porazzi D, Maggiolo F, *et al*. Gabapentin in painful HIV-related neuropathy: a report of 19 patients, preliminary observations. *Eur J Neurol*. 2001;**8**(1):71–75.

7. Abrams DI, Jay CA, Shade SB, *et al*. Cannabis in painful HIV-associated sensory neuropathy: a randomized placebo-controlled trial. *Neurology*. 2007;**68**(7):515–521.

8. Woolridge E, Barton S, Samuel J, *et al*. Cannabis use in HIV for pain and other medical symptoms. *J Pain Symptom Manage*. 2005;**29**(4):358–367.

9. Schifitto G, Yiannoutsos CT, Simpson DM, *et al*. A placebo-controlled study of memantine for the treatment of human immunodeficiency virus-associated sensory neuropathy. *J Neurovirol*. 2006;**12**(4):328–331.

10. Gorshtein A, Levy Y. Intravenous immunoglobulin in therapy of peripheral neuropathy. *Clin Rev Allergy Immunol*. 2005;**29**(3):271–279.

11. Darabi K, Abdel-Wahab O, Dzik WH. Current usage of intravenous immune globulin and the rationale behind it: the Massachusetts General Hospital data and a review of the literature. *Transfusion*. 2006; **46**(5):741–753.

12. Letendre S, Ellis RJ. Neurologic complications of HIV disease and their treatments. *Top HIV Med.* 2006;**14**(1):21–26.

13. Neuropathy treatment shows promise. *AIDS Patient Care STDs.* 2004;**18**(6):370.

14. Liu JP, Manheimer E, Yang M. Herbal medicines for treating HIV infection and AIDS. *Cochrane Database Syst Rev.* 2005(3):CD003937.

15. Paice JA, Ferrans CE, Lashley FR, *et al.* Topical capsaicin in the management of HIV-associated peripheral neuropathy. *J Pain Symptom Manage.* 2000;**19**(1):45–52.

16. Estanislao L, Carter K, McArthur J, *et al.* A randomized controlled trial of 5% lidocaine gel for HIV-associated distal symmetric polyneuropathy. *J Acquir Immune Defic Syndr.* 2004;**37**(5):1584–1586.

17. Matthews SJ, McCoy C. Thalidomide: a review of approved and investigational uses. *Clin Ther.* 2003;**25**(2):342–395.

Neuropathy – overview

SHARON E. MACE

■ Agents

- Acetaminophen
- NSAIDs
- Antidepressants
- Anticonvulsants
- Local anesthetics
- Corticosteroids

■ Evidence

The diagnosis of neuropathic pain (NP) encompasses a broad array of conditions. Many of these conditions are considered in individual chapters in this text; the diagnosis-specific chapters should be consulted for pertinent recommendations. Some principles of the pharmacologic approach to NP are applicable to multiple causes of neuropathy. This chapter covers some of these overarching topics.

For the acute care provider, the goals of NP therapy are to decrease persistent pain and to suppress breakthrough pain. The challenge lies in selecting a regimen that provides effective symptom relief while not causing unacceptable drug-related risks or side effects. The prescriber's task is complicated by the fact that the typical failure of single-analgesic therapy for NP means that multiple drugs will be required. The optimal approach usually includes combining two or more drugs that exert effects via different mechanisms. One recommended strategy for NP treatment is to begin therapy simultaneously with two drugs: an analgesic (e.g. mild **opioid**) and an adjuvant (e.g. an **antidepressant**). If the multidrug approach is used, the patient is instructed to gradually taper the **opioid** as pain relief is achieved.

OVER-THE-COUNTER ANALGESICS

Although there are no large randomized, double-blind studies of NP treatment with common non-opioid analgesics (i.e. **NSAIDs**, *acetaminophen* [*paracetamol*]), there are logical arguments for these drugs having a beneficial effect in neuropathy. *Acetaminophen* is known to block peripheral pain impulse generation; it also inhibits CNS prostaglandin synthesis. **NSAIDs'** inhibition of prostaglandin synthesis results in both peripheral and central analgesia.[1] Particularly relevant to the NP situation, in which long-term therapy may be indicated, is the fact that **NSAIDs** and *acetaminophen* can have a synergistic effect with – and thus having a sparing effect upon – the **opioids**.[2]

Topical over-the-counter drugs have the potential advantage of avoiding the complications and side effects of systemically administered agents. The topical approach is probably most useful when the peripheral nervous system is the predominate pain locus. Although the prescription agent *lidocaine* (see below) is useful for NP, the evidence supporting nonprescription topical agents is mixed or absent. *Capsaicin*, extracted from hot chili peppers, may be the most promising of the group. Its putative aid in musculoskeletal and postsurgical NP, as well as its possible utility in arthritis (see the chapter on arthritis) is based on *capsaicin*'s depletion of peripheral substance P levels (substance P activates dorsal horn nociceptive ganglia). Against any salutary effect of *capsaicin* must be weighed the nontrivial pain caused by the drug's application. All things considered, it seems premature for the acute care provider to recommend *capsaicin* (or any of the other nonprescription topical agents) at this time.

OPIOIDS

Traditional teaching holds that NP is "**opioid** resistant" and that **opioids** are more appropriately prescribed for nocioceptive (as opposed to neuropathic) pain.[3] Recent studies dispel this postulate, since several placebo-controlled trials have demonstrated **opioids'** utility in many types of NP, including some neuropathy etiologies (e.g. multiple sclerosis, spinal cord injury) in which other agents usually fail.[4–8]

Opioid doses in NP may be relatively higher than customary for non-NP indications, and in fact varying types of NP (as outlined in specific chapters) may warrant different **opioid** dosages.[4,5,7] While there is probably not too much difference between the various **opioids** in terms of efficacy for NP, efficacy and side effects in individual patients tend to vary between different agents. Some longer-acting **opioids** not traditionally used in the ED may be useful in NP. For instance, the long-acting agent *levorphanol* (in either low dose of 2.7 mg QD, or at a high daily dose of 8.9 mg) has been found effective in a wide variety of NP disorders.[8]

The clinical model upon which NP treatment with **opioids** is based is the use of this class for cancer pain. Some components of the cancer pain treatment approach are worth reiterating. First, sustained-release **opioids** are administered on a scheduled (rather than an as-needed) basis. This approach minimizes drug-related complications, since such problems are often a function of high peak **opioid** levels.[2] Second, the same **opioid** that is prescribed in sustained-release form should be prescribed in a shorter-acting form for relief of breakthrough pain. A recommended starting dose for rescue drug therapy is approximately 10–15% of the total daily **opioid** dose, administered every 3–4 h as needed.

If the patient can tolerate oral medications, the PO route for **opioids** is preferred since these formulations are easily administered, cost effective, and may be available in several preparations (e.g. liquid as well as pill form). In patients unable to tolerate oral medications, there are other choices (e.g. sublingual, transdermal).

Although it has mu receptor activity, and is associated with some abuse potential, *tramadol* is not a pure **opioid**. It is likely that *tramadol*'s inhibition of monoamine reuptake contributes to its uility in NP. For generalized polyneuropathy, and for specific NP indications as outlined in other chapters, *tramadol* (up to 200 mg PO BID for polyneuropathy) can be quite useful.[9]

ANTIDEPRESSANTS

Antidepressants are of substantial clinical utility in NP. The main subgroups used are the **tricyclic** drugs (**TCAs**), the **SSRIs**, and the **serotonin–norepinephrine reuptake inhibitors** (**SNRIs**).

The **TCAs,** the "first generation" of drugs used to treat depression, include such agents as *amitryptyline*, *imipramine*, *nortriptyline*, and *doxepin*. Their mechanism of action involves inhibition of the reuptake of serotonin and norepinephrine; increased synaptic levels of these monoamines augments pain inhibitory pathways. Well-designed trials have shown the **TCAs** to be effective in the treatment of NP associated with many different conditions. Some of the many types of NP for which **TCAs** are clinically useful are post-mastectomy and post-stroke pain, as well as non-diabetic polyneuropathy.[10-12] The **TCAs** are relatively less effective in spinal cord injury and HIV-related neuropathy.

Although they are useful in NP, **TCAs** do incur risk of side effects.[11] Patients (such as the elderly) at particular risk for adverse drug effects should be started at low doses and gradually titrated upward to a therapeutic range. Fortunately, **TCA** dosages required for effective NP treatment may be lower than those used for depression. Specific recommendations for NP therapy with **TCAs** are found in other chapters. In general, for NP management, the usual oral daily (HS) doses of the **TCAs** are 50–150 mg for *amitriptyline* or *nortriptyline*, and 100 mg for *imipramine*.

The **SSRIs** are the "second generation" of antidepressants. Examples of this drug class include *fluoxetine*, *paroxetine*, *sertraline*, and *citalopram*. As their name implies, the **SSRIs** inhibit the reuptake of serotonin only. The limitation of SSRI activity to serotonin, compared with the broader mono-amine augmentation provided by the **TCAs**, is probably responsible for the superiority of the **SSRIs** class in NP. The interclass difference becomes clear when one assesses the number of patients needed to treat in order to achieve at least 50% pain relief: Placebo-controlled trials comparing **TCAs** and **SSRIs** produced a figure of approximately 1.4 for the **TCAs** and a figure ranging as high as 7 for the SSRIs.[11,12]

The **SNRIs** (e.g. *venlafaxine*, *duloxetine*) are the newest ("third-generation") class of **antidepressants**. Like the **TCAs**, these drugs inhibit the reuptake of both norepinephrine and serotonin; their broader monoamine reuptake inhibition explains their **TCA**-like efficacy (and improved performance over **SSRIs**) in the treatment of NP.[13-15] Although the early evidence for the analgesic utility of the **SNRIs** is for patients with diabetic neuropathy, there are also multicenter trial data supporting use of this class for other diagnoses (e.g. fibromyalgia).[14,16] The doses of **SNRIs**, like those of **TCAs**, should be reduced in high-risk populations (e.g. advanced age, renal disease). Pain relief may start in one or two weeks, but over a month may elapse before the full effect.

ANTICONVULSANTS

In a manner similar to that which occurred with the **antidepressants**, NP treatment with **anticonvulsants** began with early-generation agents and evolved to include newer drugs. The **anticonvulsants** exert their effects by three mechanisms: modulation of the voltage-gated sodium and calcium channels, enhancement of the inhibitory effects of GABA, and inhibition of excitatory glutaminergic transmission. The **anticonvulsants** are also membrane-stabilizing medications.

Used for trigeminal neuralgia since the 1970s, *carbamazepine* was one of the first drugs employed in NP. Notable for its structural similarities to the **TCAs**, *carbamazine* remains a drug of choice for acute pain that is lancinating or tic-like. Clinical research and scientific approval processes being less rigorous four decades ago than today, some of the studies supporting *carbamazepine* use in NP are small. A Cochrane review of *carbamazepine*'s use in neuropathic conditions, evaluating 12 trials, found the number needed to treat in order to achieve at least 50% pain relief of 1.8 for trigeminal neuralgia and minimal high-quality evidentiary support for other diagnoses for which the drug is often used (e.g. glossopharyngeal neuralgia, diabetic neuropathy, multiple sclerosis).[17] As a general guide, dosing of *carbamazepine* for NP starts at 100 mg PO BID, with titration up to a maximum of 1200 mg daily.

Other first-generation **anticonvulsants** occasionally used in NP are *phenytoin* and *valproic acid*. A randomized controlled crossover trial demonstrated *phenytoin*'s effectiveness in relieving NP, although *carbamazepine* remained superior to either *phenytoin* or *valproic acid* for trigeminal neuralgia.[18] In fact, there are no large-scale trials demonstrating *valproic acid*'s utility for NP.[19] Overall, the first-generation **anticonvulsants** are less effective for NP than other choices (e.g. newer **anticonvulsants**, **TCAs**, **SNRIs**).

Gabapentin and *pregabalin* are the main newer-generation **anticonvulsants** with utility in NP. These agents work by inhibiting calcium channels and the release of neurotransmitters (e.g. substance P).

Gabapentin's effectiveness in a variety of types of NP is shown in multiple RCTs.[20–22] High potential for broad clinical application of *gabapentin* for NP is indicated by numerous human and animal NP studies delineating the drug's utility (and its superiority over other **anticonvulsants**). The usual dose of *gabapentin* for NP is 600–1200 mg PO TID; for patients with resistant NP, optimal pain relief is achieved with a combination approach of an **opioid** and *gabapentin*.[23]

Pregabalin is similar to *gabapentin* in both mechanism of action and breadth of potential application in NP.[24–26] *Pregabalin* is reported to be useful in some types of NP (e.g. after spinal cord injury) that are historically refractory to pharmacotherapy.[26] The daily dose of *pregabalin* for NP starts at 150 mg PO (typical dosage range is 50–100 mg PO TID).

When used for NP, *gabapentin* and *pregabalin* are expected to decrease pain scores by at least 50% after one week of therapy; some effect is seen even earlier.[24]

The pain relief efficacy of the newer-generation **anticonvulsants** is complemented by the fact that, compared with many therapeutic alternatives in NP, *gabapentin* and *pregabalin* are safer. The newer agents have lesser toxicity and fewer side effects. Drug interactions are less of a risk, and ongoing hepatic or hematologic monitoring is unnecessary. Both *gabapentin* and *pregabalin* undergo renal metabolism, necessitating dosage adjustment in patients with renal failure. *Pregabalin* does offer a few advantages over *gabapentin*. It has faster onset, and starting doses are more likely to be clinically effective. *Pregabalin* can also be rapidly titrated upward in patients needing more pain relief. Neither drug should be stopped abruptly, but instead should be tapered over at least one week to prevent withdrawal symptoms.

There is also evidence addressing use of another new-generation **anticonvulsant**, *lamotrigine*, for NP. A 2007 Cochrane review of available data found no role for *lamotrigine* for the general patient population with NP, or for any NP subgroups.[27]

LOCAL ANESTHETICS

By stabilizing sodium channels, **local anesthetics** block spontaneous ectopic impulses in the axons of peripheral first-order neurons. They may also have **opioid**-like effects, and may alter N-methyl-D-aspartate (NMDA) receptor activity. This class of drugs may be most effective in a partially injured nerve with excess sodium channnels. Clinically, patients with allodynia are potential candidates for **local anesthetic** use, since allodynia implies presence of functional, yet damaged, peripheral nocioceptors. If there are no remaining peripheral nocioceptors (i.e. complete deafferentation), **local anesthetics** will not work. The concentrations at which **local anesthetics** suppress nociceptive impulses are lower than those in which they suppress normal sensorimotor impulses. Cochrane review found that oral or parenteral **local anesthetics** exhibit both safety and efficacy in non-ED treatment of the the general NP population.[28]

Of the **local anesthetics**, *lidocaine* is the most studied. Other agents (e.g. *tocainide*) have occasionally been discussed for NP therapy, but the lack of supporting evidence and potential risk of side effects relegate these agents to use outside the acute care setting. The most cited use of topical *lidocaine* in NP is for post-herpetic neuralgia.[29] However, the topical *lidocaine* approach has also been the found effective in other NP conditions. A trial in mixed-etiology focal painful polyneuropathy found that *lidocaine's* number needed to treat to achieve 50% pain relief was 4.4 (95% confidence interval, 2.5–17.5).[30] Advantages of the *lidocaine* patch are its size and shape flexibility and the physical protection that allodynic skin receives from the covering patch.

Although mild local skin reactions may occur after topical application of local anesthetics, systemic absorption of *lidocaine* is minimal when the drug is used in topical form for NP. Intravenous *lidocaine* (5 mg/kg) is sometimes used for NP, but the data are insufficient to warrant a recommendation for ED use of this approach.[31]

Local anesthetics may also be useful in NP when administered in the form of regional nerve blocks. The regional block approach has some appeal for acute care, especially for those nerve blocks commonly provided in the ED.

However, there is little evidence supporting first-line use of nerve blocks for the ED treatment of NP. Similar reservations preclude recommendation for ED providers to apply transcutaneous electrical nerve stimulation (TENS).

CORTICOSTEROIDS

Since inflammatory mediators sensitize nociception, the anti-inflammatory **corticosteroids** have been used for NP. **Corticosteroids** also decrease local edema, thus reducing pressure on peripheral nerves. As *dexamethasone* has relative few mineralocorticoid effects, it is preferred by many who use **corticosteroids** in NP.

Despite widespread use and theoretical benefits, controlled trials of **corticosteroids** in NP are lacking. There is a trial that demonstrated effectiveness of oral *prednisone* for one type of NP (chronic regional pain syndrome).[32] With this possible exception, there is insufficient evidence to support any recommendation for ED initiation of **corticosteroids** for NP.

MISCELLANEOUS AGENTS

The **alpha-2-adrenergic agents** (e.g. *clonidine*) decrease nociceptive input into the CNS by activating α_2-adrenoceptors in the spinal cord and brainstem. They also decrease sympathetic tone, which makes them potentially valuable in patients with complex regional pain syndrome. Animal models and preliminary work suggest *clonidine* may have a therapeutic role in NP (e.g. as an **opioid**-sparing agent), but there is insufficient evidence to support a recommendation for ED prescription of **alpha-2-adrenergic agents** for NP.[33,34]

Other approaches to NP that may have current or future utility include agents with agonism at NMDA or gamma-aminobutyric acid (GABA) receptors. Despite occasional clinical utility for some of these drugs (e.g. *baclofen* for spasticity), there is no evidence supporting ED prescription of these agents for NP.

Cannabinoids include agents such as *delta*-trans-*tetrahydrocannabinol* (*THC*). These drugs may have analgesic effects (including synergism with

opioids), with sites of action in the periphery, spinal cord, and brain. At least one RCT suggests that **cannabinoids** have a greater analgesic effect than placebo.[35] However, in addition to a paucity of evidence, limitations to this class include CNS depression and the concern over potential abuse.

Proinflammatory interleukins (e.g. tumor necrosis factor-alpha) have a role in inflammatory NP. It is premature to recommend agents intended to counter these effects, but there is preliminary animal data to support a possible future NP role for drugs like *thalidomide* (which inhibits tumor necrosis factor-alpha production).[36-38]

■ Summary and recommendations

See other chapters for diagnosis-specific recommendations for various NP etiologies.

First line: mild opioid (e.g. hydrocodone 5–10 mg PO q4–6 h) plus SNRI (e.g. venlafaxine 75 mg PO QD)

Reasonable: opioid plus pregabalin (starting dose 50 mg PO TID)

Pregnancy:

■ acetaminophen (650–1000 mg PO QID) and opioid (e.g. hydrocodone 5–10 mg PO q4–6 h)
■ there is insufficient data to recommend most of the anticonvulsants or antidepressants for NP use in pregnancy; acute care clinicians should consult with appropriate specialists before prescribing these agents for NP

Pediatric: mild analgesic (NSAID or acetaminophen) with addition of pregabalin (50 mg PO TID) if necessary (for patients aged at least 12 years)

Special case:

■ *if pain interferes with sleep:* antidepressants (e.g. nortriptyline 50 mg PO HS) are recommended as adjuvant therapy

References

1. Samad TA, Moore KA, Sapirstein A, *et al.* Interleukin-1beta-mediated induction of Cox-2 in the CNS contributes to inflammatory pain hypersensitivity. *Nature.* 2001;**410**(6827):471–475.

2. Miaskowski C, Cleary J, Burney R. *Cancer Pain Management Guideline Panel. Guideline for the Management of Cancer Pain in Adults and Children*, 5th edn. Glenview, IL: American Pain Society, 2005.

3. Arner S, Meyerson BA. Lack of analgesic effect of opioids on neuropathic and idiopathic forms of pain. *Pain.* 1988;**33**(1):11–23.

4. Gimbel JS, Richards P, Portenoy RK. Controlled-release oxycodone for pain in diabetic neuropathy: a randomized controlled trial. *Neurology.* 2003;**60**(6):927–934.

5. Watson CP, Babul N. Efficacy of oxycodone in neuropathic pain: a randomized trial in postherpetic neuralgia. *Neurology.* 1998;**50**(6): 1837–1841.

6. Raja SN, Haythornthwaite JA, Pappagallo M, *et al.* Opioids versus antidepressants in postherpetic neuralgia: a randomized, placebo-controlled trial. *Neurology.* 2002;**59**(7):1015–1021.

7. Huse E, Larbig W, Flor H, *et al.* The effect of opioids on phantom limb pain and cortical reorganization. *Pain.* 2001;**90**(1–2):47–55.

8. Rowbotham MC, Twilling L, Davies PS, *et al.* Oral opioid therapy for chronic peripheral and central neuropathic pain. *N Engl J Med.* 2003;**348**(13):1223–1232.

9. Sindrup SH, Andersen G, Madsen C, *et al.* Tramadol relieves pain and allodynia in polyneuropathy: a randomised, double-blind, controlled trial. *Pain.* 1999;**83**(1):85–90.

10. Watson CP, Vernich L, Chipman M, *et al.* Nortriptyline versus amitriptyline in postherpetic neuralgia: a randomized trial. *Neurology.* 1998;**51**(4):1166–1171.

11. Sindrup SH, Jensen TS. Efficacy of pharmacological treatments of neuropathic pain: an update and effect related to mechanism of drug action. *Pain.* 1999;**83**(3):389–400.

12. Max M. Thirteen consecutive well-designed randomized trials show that antidepressants reduce pain in diabetic neuropathy and postherpetic neuralgia. *Pain Forum.* 1995;**4**:248–253.

13. Sindrup SH, Bach FW, Madsen C, *et al.* Venlafaxine versus imipramine in painful polyneuropathy: a randomized, controlled trial. *Neurology.* 2003;**60**(8):1284–1289.

14. Arnold LM, Lu Y, Crofford LJ, *et al.* A double-blind, multicenter trial comparing duloxetine with placebo in the treatment of fibromyalgia patients with or without major depressive disorder. *Arthritis Rheum.* 2004;**50**(9):2974–2984.

15. Raskin J, Pritchett YL, Wang F, *et al.* A double-blind, randomized multicenter trial comparing duloxetine with placebo in the management of diabetic peripheral neuropathic pain. *Pain Med.* 2005;**6**(5):346–356.

16. Goldstein DJ, Lu Y, Detke MJ, *et al.* Duloxetine vs. placebo in patients with painful diabetic neuropathy. *Pain.* 2005;**116**(1–2):109–118.

17. Wiffen PJ, McQuay HJ, Moore RA. Carbamazepine for acute and chronic pain. *Cochrane Database Syst Rev.* 2005(3):CD005451.

18. McCleane GJ. Intravenous infusion of phenytoin relieves neuropathic pain: a randomized, double blinded, placebo-controlled, crossover study. *Anesth Analg.* 1999;**89**(4):985–988.

19. Guieu R, Mesdjian E, Rochat H, *et al.* Central analgesic effect of valproate in patients with epilepsy. *Seizure.* 1993;**2**(2):147–150.

20. Backonja M, Glanzman RL. Gabapentin dosing for neuropathic pain: evidence from randomized, placebo-controlled clinical trials. *Clin Ther.* 2003;**25**(1):81–104.

21. Rowbotham M, Harden N, Stacey B, *et al.* Gabapentin for the treatment of postherpetic neuralgia: a randomized controlled trial. *JAMA.* 1998;**280**(21):1837–1842.

22. Hahn K, Arendt G, Braun JS, *et al.* A placebo-controlled trial of gabapentin for painful HIV associated sensory neuropathies. *J Neurol.* 2004;**251**(10):1260–1266.

23. Gilron I, Bailey JM, Tu D, *et al.* Morphine, gabapentin, or their combination for neuropathic pain. *N Engl J Med.* 2005;**352**(13):1324–1334.

24. Freynhagen R, Strojek K, Griesing T, *et al.* Efficacy of pregabalin in neuropathic pain evaluated in a 12-week, randomised, double-blind, multicentre, placebo-controlled trial of flexible- and fixed-dose regimens. *Pain.* 2005;**115**(3):254–263.

25. Dworkin RH, Corbin AE, Young JP, Jr., *et al.* Pregabalin for the treatment of postherpetic neuralgia: a randomized, placebo-controlled trial. *Neurology.* 2003;**60**(8):1274–1283.

26. Siddall PJ, Cousins MJ, Otte A, *et al.* Pregabalin in central neuropathic pain associated with spinal cord injury: a placebo-controlled trial. *Neurology.* 2006;**67**(10):1792–1800.

27. Wiffen PJ, Rees J. Lamotrigine for acute and chronic pain. *Cochrane Database Syst Rev.* 2007(2):CD006044.

28. Challapalli V, Tremont-Lukats IW, McNicol ED, *et al.* Systemic administration of local anesthetic agents to relieve neuropathic pain. *Cochrane Database Syst Rev.* 2005(4):CD003345.

29. Galer BS, Rowbotham MC, Perander J, *et al.* Topical lidocaine patch relieves postherpetic neuralgia more effectively than a vehicle topical patch: results of an enriched enrollment study. *Pain.* 1999;**80**(3):533–538.

30. Meier T, Wasner G, Faust M, *et al.* Efficacy of lidocaine patch 5% in the treatment of focal peripheral neuropathic pain syndromes: a randomized, double-blind, placebo-controlled study. *Pain.* 2003;**106**(1–2):151–158.

31. Tremont-Lukats IW, Hutson PR, Backonja MM. A randomized, double-masked, placebo-controlled pilot trial of extended IV lidocaine infusion for relief of ongoing neuropathic pain. *Clin J Pain.* 2006;**22**(3):266–271.

32. Christensen K, Jensen EM, Noer I. The reflex dystrophy syndrome response to treatment with systemic corticosteroids. *Acta Chir Scand.* 1982;**148**(8):653–655.

33. Khasar SG, Green PG, Chou B, *et al.* Peripheral nociceptive effects of alpha 2-adrenergic receptor agonists in the rat. *Neuroscience.* 1995;**66**(2):427–432.

34. Goudas L, Carr D, Filos K. The spinal clonidine–opioid analgesic interaction: from laboratory animals to the postoperative ward. A review of preclinical and clinical evidence. *Analgesia.* 1998;**3**:277–290.

35. Karst M, Salim K, Burstein S, *et al.* Analgesic effect of the synthetic cannabinoid CT-3 on chronic neuropathic pain: a randomized controlled trial. *JAMA.* 2003;**290**(13):1757–1762.

36. George A, Marziniak M, Schafers M, *et al.* Thalidomide treatment in chronic constrictive neuropathy decreases endoneurial tumor necrosis factor-alpha, increases interleukin-10 and has long-term effects on spinal cord dorsal horn met enkephalin. *Pain.* 2000;**88**(3):267–275.

37. Sommer C, Marziniak M, Myers RR. The effect of thalidomide treatment on vascular pathology and hyperalgesia caused by chronic constriction injury of rat nerve. *Pain.* 1998;**74**(1):83–91.

38. Ribeiro RA, Vale ML, Ferreira SH, *et al.* Analgesic effect of thalidomide on inflammatory pain. *Eur J Pharmacol.* 2000;**391**(1–2):97–103.

Neuropathy – phantom limb pain

DAVID CLINE

■ Agents

- Opioids
- Calcitonin
- Antidepressants
- Anticonvulsants

■ Evidence

Acute care providers need to be familiar with phantom limb pain (PLP) as the complaint occurs in up to 80% of patients after amputation and it is important to institute early and effective intervention: prompt treatment minimizes the chances of chronic pain development.[1] Unfortunately, despite the high prevalence of PLP, there is no consensus on an effective and reliable analgesic approach. Experts contend that the inconsistent results with peripheral analgesics should prompt a refocus of pain relief research efforts, with emphasis on approaches that reverse (or prevent the formation of) central memory processes.[2] Interesting trials are demonstrating utility of novel approaches such as biofeedback and "mirror therapy."[3–5] This chapter centers on drug therapy.

Opioids are commonly recommended for acute treatment of PLP.[1] Oral **opioids**, usually in combination with another agent (e.g. *calcitonin*), form the mainstay of PLP therapy.[1] Particularly in refractory cases, PLP may require high doses of **opioids** such as *morphine*; the range of daily oral *morphine* needed is reported to be 70–300 mg.[6,7] Case series data also supports the use of long-acting **opioids** such as *methadone* (2–5 mg PO BID or TID) for PLP.[8]

Randomized double-blind crossover trial data, as well as case reports, have found that PLP is successfully treated with *calcitonin* (the anti-nociceptive activity of which is related in part to elevation of beta-endorphins).[9–11] Expert reviews conclude that infusion of salmon *calcitonin* (one or two IV doses of

200 IU) is a treatment of choice for acute PLP flares.[1,12] As with other agents with which ED providers may not be familiar, quick reference for safety purposes (e.g. withholding of *calcitonin* in hypocalcemic patients) is necessary. For patients with hypersensitivity to fish (in whom the nasal salmon preparation is contraindicated), a human *calcitonin* preparation may be used.

The **benzodiazepines**, which potentiate the spinal neuronal inhibitory effects of gamma-aminobutyric acid (GABA), may ameliorate pain from acute PLP flares. Case reports suggest that both *clonazepam* and *midazolam* are effective.[13,14] The familiarity of ED providers with safe use of *midazolam* makes this an attractive choice. Slow infusion of up to 3–5 mg (over 10–20 min, with meticulous ventilatory monitoring), is supported by the available case series data.[14,15]

Midazolam is not the only procedural sedation drug with potential utility for PLP. Multiple case series reports support *ketamine* use for acute PLP flares.[16,17]

In contradistinction to their utility in other forms of neuropathic pain, **antidepressants** have only a limited role for acute PLP; they may be useful as an aid to chronic management.[1] The exception may be the **heterocyclic antidepressant** *mirtazapine*, for which there is open-label case series evidence suggesting reduction in PLP via central mechanisms.[18]

The **anticonvulsants** have been investigated for PLP, with mixed results. *Carbamazepine* is postulated to be of utility, but supporting evidence for its use in PLP is anecdotal.[19] There is stronger evidence for *gabapentin* prescription in PLP. Case series evidence suggests utility for *gabapentin*, and a clinical trial calculated that about one in four patients will achieve significant pain relief with *gabapentin*.[20,21] Another RCT suggested limited *gabapentin* efficacy. In this RCT, although over half of participants had a meaningful pain decrease during the *gabapentin* phase (compared with 20% in the placebo phase), no predefined efficacy endpoints were met.[22]

The oral dosing of *gabapentin* for NP follows an advancing regimen: 300 mg HS on day one, followed by 300 mg BID on day two, then 300 mg TID on day three. The drug can then be titrated up to 1800 mg/day over two weeks.

Another **anticonvulsant**, *topiramate*, is found useful in individual time-series analyses. Three out of four amputee participants receiving *topiramate* had statistically significant decreases in pain (peak effects occurred at 800 mg daily).[23]

The *N*-methyl-D-aspartate (NMDA) antagonist *memantine* attenuates phantom pain memory formation, but its utility seems to be limited to early post-amputation prevention rather than in acute (ED) therapy. Trials find little or no efficacy when the drug is used to treat acute PLP flares.[24-26]

■ Summary and recommendations

First line: salmon calcitonin (one or two IV doses of 200 IU, administered as a 20 min infusion) with as-needed opioids

Reasonable: gabapentin (300 mg PO HS on day one, followed by 300 mg PO BID on day two, then 300 mg PO TID)

Pregnancy:
- the majority of the drugs discussed above are Pregnancy Category C or D; weighing risks and benefits of PLP therapy during pregnancy may result in a decision to delay institution of optimal therapy until after delivery
- opioid monotherapy may be used during pregnancy
- calcitonin (which may be used with appropriate consultation in pregnancy) suppresses lactation and should not be used in breastfeeding patients

Pediatrics: salmon calcitonin (one or two IV doses of 200 IU, administered as a 20 min infusion) with as-needed opioids

Special case:
- *closely monitored setting*: slow IV administration of midazolam (2–5 mg) or ketamine (1 mg/kg)
- *PLP refractory to other therapies*: topiramate (starting dose 25 mg PO QD or BID, with planned up-titration on follow-up)

References

1. Baron R, Wasner G, Lindner V. Optimal treatment of phantom limb pain in the elderly. *Drugs Aging*. 1998;**12**(5):361–376.

2. Flor H. Phantom-limb pain: characteristics, causes, and treatment. *Lancet Neurol.* 2002;**1**(3):182–189.

3. Harden RN, Houle TT, Green S, *et al.* Biofeedback in the treatment of phantom limb pain: a time-series analysis. *Appl Psychophysiol Biofeedback.* 2005;**30**(1):83–93.

4. MacLachlan M, McDonald D, Waloch J. Mirror treatment of lower limb phantom pain: a case study. *Disabil Rehabil.* 2004;**26**(14–15): 901–904.

5. Brodie EE, Whyte A, Niven CA. Analgesia through the looking-glass? A randomized controlled trial investigating the effect of viewing a "virtual" limb upon phantom limb pain, sensation and movement. *Eur J Pain.* 2007;**11**(4):428–436.

6. Mishra S, Bhatnagar S, Singhal AK. High-dose morphine for intractable phantom limb pain. *Clin J Pain.* 2007;**23**(1):99–101.

7. Huse E, Larbig W, Flor H, *et al.* The effect of opioids on phantom limb pain and cortical reorganization. *Pain.* 2001;**90**(1–2):47–55.

8. Bergmans L, Snijdelaar DG, Katz J, *et al.* Methadone for phantom limb pain. *Clin J Pain.* 2002;**18**(3):203–205.

9. Shapiro S, Kundhal P, Barua M, *et al.* Calcitonin treatment for phantom limb pain. *Can J Psychiatry.* 2004;**49**(7):499.

10. Jaeger H, Maier C. Calcitonin in phantom limb pain: a double-blind study. *Pain.* 1992;**48**(1):21–27.

11. Fiddler DS, Hindman BJ. Intravenous calcitonin alleviates spinal anesthesia-induced phantom limb pain. *Anesthesiology.* 1991;**74**(1):187–189.

12. Wall GC, Heyneman CA. Calcitonin in phantom limb pain. *Ann Pharmacother.* 1999;**33**(4):499–501.

13. Bartusch SL, Sanders BJ, D'Alessio JG, *et al.* Clonazepam for the treatment of lancinating phantom limb pain. *Clin J Pain.* 1996;**12**(1):59–62.

14. Vichitrananda C, Pausawasdi S. Midazolam for the treatment of phantom limb pain exacerbation: preliminary reports. *J Med Assoc Thai.* 2001;**84**(2):299–302.

15. Tessler MJ, Kleiman SJ. Spinal anaesthesia for patients with previous lower limb amputations. *Anaesthesia.* 1994;**49**(5):439–441.

16. Stannard CF, Porter GE. Ketamine hydrochloride in the treatment of phantom limb pain. *Pain.* 1993;**54**(2):227–230.

17. Knox DJ, McLeod BJ, Goucke CR. Acute phantom limb pain controlled by ketamine. *Anaesth Intensive Care.* 1995;**23**(5):620–622.

18. Kuiken TA, Schechtman L, Harden RN. Phantom limb pain treatment with mirtazapine: a case series. *Pain Pract.* 2005;**5**(4):356–360.

19. Patterson JF. Carbamazepine in the treatment of phantom limb pain. *South Med J.* 1988;**81**(9):1100–1102.

20. Bone M, Critchley P, Buggy DJ. Gabapentin in postamputation phantom limb pain: a randomized, double-blind, placebo-controlled, cross-over study. *Reg Anesth Pain Med.* 2002;**27**(5):481–486.

21. Rusy LM, Troshynski TJ, Weisman SJ. Gabapentin in phantom limb pain management in children and young adults: report of seven cases. *J Pain Symptom Manage.* 2001;**21**(1):78–82.

22. Smith DG, Ehde DM, Hanley MA, *et al*. Efficacy of gabapentin in treating chronic phantom limb and residual limb pain. *J Rehabil Res Dev.* 2005;**42**(5):645–654.

23. Harden RN, Houle TT, Remble TA, *et al*. Topiramate for phantom limb pain: a time-series analysis. *Pain Med.* 2005;**6**(5):375–378.

24. Schley M, Topfner S, Wiech K, *et al*. Continuous brachial plexus blockade in combination with the NMDA receptor antagonist memantine prevents phantom pain in acute traumatic upper limb amputees. *Eur J Pain.* 2007;**11**(3):299–308.

25. Wiech K, Kiefer RT, Topfner S, *et al*. A placebo-controlled randomized cross-over trial of the N-methyl-D-aspartic acid receptor antagonist, memantine, in patients with chronic phantom limb pain. *Anesth Analg.* 2004;**98**(2):408–413; table of contents.

26. Maier C, Dertwinkel R, Mansourian N, *et al*. Efficacy of the NMDA-receptor antagonist memantine in patients with chronic phantom limb pain: results of a randomized double blinded, placebo-controlled trial. *Pain.* 2003;**103**(3):277–283.

Ocular inflammation

STEPHEN H. THOMAS

■ Agents

- NSAIDs
- Corticosteroids
- Antihistamines
- Decongestants
- Mast cell stabilizers
- Local anesthetics
- Cycloplegics
- Opioids

■ Evidence

This chapter addresses ocular inflammatory conditions such as conjunctivitis (allergic and infectious) and keratitis. Related information on topical anesthetics is found in the chapter on corneal abrasion. This chapter does not address systemic therapy for disease-specific causes of ocular pain (e.g. *cyclosporine* [*ciclosporin*] for ocular pemphigoid).[1] This discussion also does not include general care measures (e.g. irrigation for chemical exposures), which may contribute to, or completely achieve, pain relief.[2,3]

General guidelines for treating ocular inflammation of both infectious and noninfectious origin emphasize the utility of topical **NSAIDs**, which avoid the complications (e.g. local immunocompromise) of the traditional topical alternative, **corticosteroids**.[4,5] Furthermore, the effective application of these topical agents can reduce or eliminate the need for potent systemic therapy such as **opioids**.

For nearly all types of ocular inflammatory pain, ranging from traumatic inflammation to edema to allergic conjunctivitis, the topical **NSAIDs** have proven useful.[6–8] *Ketorolac* (0.5%) and *indomethacin* (0.1%) are the most-studied agents, with significant efficacy compared with placebo.[9–14] Other topical **NSAIDs** useful for corneal abrasion, and by extension likely of use for general ocular inflammation, include *diclofenac* (0.1%), *flurbiprofen* (0.03%), and *piroxicam* (0.5%).[15-19] The only noted adverse effect in studies of topical **NSAIDs** is transient (minor) stinging.

An RCT illustrating **NSAIDs'** utility in mechanical irritation addressed use of *indomethacin* (0.1%) in painfully inflamed pterygia or pinguecula. Topical *indomethacin* (0.1%) was significantly less painful than, and provided equally good pain relief to, the topical **corticosteroid** *dexamethasone phosphate* (0.1%); both agents were administered six times daily for three days, then QID for 11 days.[20]

Topical **NSAIDs** also provide effective pain relief for allergic conjunctivitis. Although there is probably little difference between various **NSAIDs**, *indomethacin* (0.1% QID) performs at least as well as, and may be associated with earlier symptom relief than, *ketorolac* (0.5% QID).[7]

The topical **NSAIDs** relieve pain in infectious conjunctivitis. In hemorrhagic (presumably coxsackieviral) conjunctivitis treated with antibiotic drops, the addition of *piroxicam* (0.5%, 1 drop QID) is associated with significant improvement in pain as well as a variety of other endpoints.[21]

As is the case with corneal abrasion, there are no studies on the use of oral or parenteral **NSAIDs** in ocular inflammation. However, there is intuitive basis for some benefit to their use, given the utility of topically administered **NSAIDs**. There are few studies specifically addressing use of the topical ophthalmic **NSAIDs** in children, but the available evidence suggests that this class is safe in children.[22]

When **corticosteroids** are to be applied topically for infectious conjunctivitis, RCT evidence supports the use of *dexamethasone*. A trial comparing combination therapy with BID-applied topical antibiotic (*tobramycin*, 0.3%) and either *dexamethasone* (0.1%) or *loteprednol* (0.5%) found better pain and symptom reduction with *dexamethasone*.[23] **Corticosteroids** applied topically are also useful in exposures from land- and marine-based stinging exposures such as from bees or coral.[24,25] Topical **corticosteroids** are anecdotally useful adjuncts for ultraviolet keratitis, as they hasten the relief of swelling and also tend to provide some relief from the burning pain and photophobia that accompany this.[26]

Other RCT data have demonstrated that painful symptoms of adenoviral conjunctivitis are significantly reduced with topical **antihistamine/decongestant** drops; symptom duration is also reduced, from eight to five days.[27] Typical combination drops include *naphazoline hydrochloride* (0.025%) and *pheniramine* (0.3%); the combination therapy is administered in a dose of 1–2 drops QID.

For seasonal allergic conjunctivitis, RCT data comparing two topical **antihistamines** demonstrated superiority (at assessment at both 5 and 21 days) of BID *ketotifen fumarate* (0.025%) ophthalmic solution over *olopatadine hydrochloride* (0.1%) ophthalmic solution.[28] Large-scale RCT evidence has demonstrated efficacy, as well as safety, of *ketotifen* (0.025%) in adults and children.[29] A relatively nonsedating **antihistamine**, *mizolastine* (10 mg PO QD), is demonstrated by RCT data to provide significant relief (compared with placebo) for allergic rhinoconjunctivitis; the additional symptom relief for rhinitis is an additional advantage to this agent.[30]

In an RCT assessing QID topical therapy for allergic conjunctivitis, the antimetabolite *mitomycin C* (0.2 mg/10 mL) was more effective than the topical **antihistamine** *azelastine* (0.02%) for both symptom relief and resolution of signs; the use of topical *mitomycin C* in such low doses does not cause any significant adverse effect.[31]

The **mast cell stabilizer** *lodoxamide* appears to be somewhat useful, but only if given very early in, or even as prophylaxis against, allergic conjunctivitis.[32] Another **mast cell stabilizer**, *nedocromil sodium* (2%), is also effective in reducing burning (and other symptoms) of allergic conjunctivitis.[33] Because of their primary utility as preventive agents, the **mast cell stabilizers** are not first-line choices for ED therapy of allergic conjunctivitis, unless there are reasons to avoid other agents (and even then, only if patients present very early in the disease course).

For keratoconjunctivitis photoelectrica (ultraviolet light injury such as from welding), consensus guidelines acknowledge the limited available evidence but endorse limited (i.e. in the ED) use of topically applied **local anesthetics** such as *proparacaine* (0.5%).[34] Their application in the ED provides 15–20 min of anesthesia, which facilitates physical examination, and the **local anesthetics** have been reported useful for ocular pain indications as unusual as conjunctivitis occurring after eye exposure to spider venom.[35] As long as they are used in moderation, the **local anesthetics** have broad utility in relieving ocular pain, but prolonged use risks significant corneal epithelial complications and these agents should not be prescribed for outpatient use by the ED physician.[36]

The historical role of **cycloplegics** in ocular conditions is based on their reduction of ciliary spasm-associated pain. Agents such as *cyclopentolate* (1.0%, 1 drop TID) are used in a variety of ocular inflammatory conditions, having been reported useful adjuncts for conditions ranging from keratoconjunctivitis-related ulcers to fungal iritis and plant sap-related conjunctivitis.[37–39] The **cycloplegics** are particularly useful in traumatic or other etiologies of iritis.[40] While some systemic absorption may be prevented by instructing patients to occlude the lacrimal drainage system with the index finger while instilling drops, the potential for unwanted systemic anticholinergic and neurotoxic effects must be remembered.[41] Some RCT data have demonstrated that sufficient cycloplegic effect is obtainable with a single drop rather than two or three drops and that the single-drop dosage reduces side effects.[42] Also contraindicated is the use of **cycloplegics** in patients with potential for angle-closure glaucoma.

Opioids have not been directly assessed as analgesics for ocular inflammation, but (as is the case with corneal abrasion), agents such as *oxycodone* may be useful for refractory ocular pain.[18] Especially since **local anesthetics** are not prescribed on an outpatient basis, and because relief from other topical approaches may be incomplete, systemic **opioids** may be needed for the initial day or two post-ED care.

Eye patching, not recommended for corneal abrasion treatment (see the chapter on corneal abrasion), is also not recommended for other forms of ocular inflammation, but with severe photophobia and light-induced ciliary constriction pain, light patching may be useful for 12–24 h.

■ Summary and recommendations

First line: topical NSAID (e.g. indomethacin 0.1% 1 drop QID, ketorolac 0.5% 1 drop QID)

Reasonable: oral NSAID (e.g. ibuprofen 400–600 mg PO QID)

Pregnancy: acetaminophen (1000 mg PO QID) with as-needed opioid (e.g. hydrocodone 5–10 mg PO q4–6 h)

Pediatric:

■ acetaminophen (15 mg/kg PO QID) or NSAID (e.g. ibuprofen 10 mg/kg PO QID)

■ topical NSAID (e.g. ketorolac 0.5% 1 drop QID)

Special cases:

■ *pain control for short-term (ED) evaluation:* proparacaine 0.5% 1–2 drops q15–20 min, repeated 2–3 times

■ *pain from sting or envenomation*: dexamethasone 0.1% 1–2 drops BID

■ *allergic conjunctivitis*: 1–2 drops QID of combination preparation of topical antihistamine (e.g. pheniramine 0.3%) and decongestant (e.g. naphazoline hydrochloride 0.025%)

■ *allergic conjunctivitis with rhinitis*: corticosteroid (e.g. prednisone 1 mg/kg PO QD)

■ *iritis or ciliary spasm-associated pain*: to other regimen, add cycloplegic (e.g. cyclopentolate 1.0% 1 drop TID)

■ *severe pain unrelieved by topical outpatient regimen*: oral opioids (e.g. 5–10 mg oxycodone PO q4–6 h)

References

1. Alonso A, Bignone ML, Brunzini M, *et al.* Ocular autoimmune pemphigoid and cyclosporin A. *Allergol Immunopathol (Madrid)*. 2006;**34**(3): 113–115.
2. Bradberry SM, Proudfoot AT, Vale JA. Glyphosate poisoning. *Toxicol Rev.* 2004;**23**(3):159–167.
3. Eisenkraft A, Robenshtok E, Luria S, *et al.* [Medical aspects of the lacrimator CS.] *Harefuah.* 2003;**142**(6):464–468, 484, 483.
4. Colin J. The role of NSAIDs in the management of postoperative ophthalmic inflammation. *Drugs.* 2007;**67**(9):1291–1308.
5. Chan CM, Theng JT, Li L, *et al.* Microsporidial keratoconjunctivitis in healthy individuals: a case series. *Ophthalmology.* 2003;**110**(7):1420–1425.
6. Nichols J, Snyder RW. Topical nonsteroidal anti-inflammatory agents in ophthalmology. *Curr Opin Ophthalmol.* 1998;**9**(4):40–44.

7. Tauber J, Raizman MB, Ostrov CS, *et al*. A multicenter comparison of the ocular efficacy and safety of diclofenac 0.1% solution with that of ketorolac 0.5% solution in patients with acute seasonal allergic conjunctivitis. *J Ocul Pharmacol Ther*. 1998;**14**(2):137–145.

8. Koay P. The emerging roles of topical non-steroidal anti-inflammatory agents in ophthalmology. *Br J Ophthalmol*. 1996;**80**(5):480–485.

9. Donnenfeld ED, Selkin BA, Perry HD, *et al*. Controlled evaluation of a bandage contact lens and a topical nonsteroidal anti-inflammatory drug in treating traumatic corneal abrasions. *Ophthalmology*. 1995;**102**(6): 979–984.

10. Goyal R, Shankar J, Fone DL, *et al*. Randomised controlled trial of ketorolac in the management of corneal abrasions. *Acta Ophthalmol Scand*. 2001;**79**(2):177–179.

11. Kaiser PK. A comparison of pressure patching versus no patching for corneal abrasions due to trauma or foreign body removal. Corneal Abrasion Patching Study Group. *Ophthalmology*. 1995;**102**(12):1936–1942.

12. Alberti MM, Bouat CG, Allaire CM, *et al*. Combined indomethacin/gentamicin eyedrops to reduce pain after traumatic corneal abrasion. *Eur J Ophthalmol*. 2001;**11**(3):233–239.

13. Patrone G, Sacca SC, Macri A, *et al*. Evaluation of the analgesic effect of 0.1% indomethacin solution on corneal abrasions. *Ophthalmologica*. 1999;**213**(6):350–354.

14. Solomon A, Halpert M, Frucht-Perry J. Comparison of topical indomethacin and eye patching for minor corneal trauma. *Ann Ophthalm*. 2000;**32**:316–319.

15. Brahma AK, Shah S, Hillier VF, *et al*. Topical analgesia for superficial corneal injuries. *J Accid Emerg Med*. 1996;**13**(3):186–188.

16. Jayamanne DG, Fitt AW, Dayan M, *et al*. The effectiveness of topical diclofenac in relieving discomfort following traumatic corneal abrasions. *Eye*. 1997;**11**(Pt 1):79–83.

17. Le Sage N, Verreault R, Rochette L. Efficacy of eye patching for traumatic corneal abrasions: a controlled clinical trial. *Ann Emerg Med*. 2001;**38**(2):129–134.

18. Szucs PA, Nashed AH, Allegra JR, *et al*. Safety and efficacy of diclofenac ophthalmic solution in the treatment of corneal abrasions. *Ann Emerg Med*. 2000;**35**(2):131–137.

19. Vigasio F, Giroletti G. Piroxicam 0.5% topico e corpi estranei corneali. *Minerva Oftalmol*. 1986;**28**(1):59–62.

20. Frucht-Pery J, Siganos CS, Solomon A, *et al.* Topical indomethacin solution versus dexamethasone solution for treatment of inflamed pterygium and pinguecula: a prospective randomized clinical study. *Am J Ophthalmol.* 1999;**127**(2):148–152.

21. Kosrirukvongs P. Topical piroxicam and conjunctivitis. *J Med Assoc Thai.* 1997;**80**(5):287–292.

22. Chung I, Buhr V. Topical ophthalmic drugs and the pediatric patient. *Optometry.* 2000;**71**(8):511–518.

23. Rhee SS, Mah FS. Comparison of tobramycin 0.3%/dexamethasone 0.1% and tobramycin 0.3%/loteprednol 0.5% in the management of blepharo-kerato-conjunctivitis. *Adv Ther.* 2007;**24**(1):60–67.

24. Keamy J, Umlas J, Lee Y. Red coral keratitis. *Cornea.* 2000;**19**(6): 859–860.

25. Grub M, Mielke J, Schlote T. [Bee sting of the cornea: a case report.] *Klin Monatsbl Augenheilkd.* 2001;**218**(11):747–750.

26. Komericki P, Fellner P, El-Shabrawi Y, *et al.* Keratopathy after ultraviolet B phototherapy. *Wien Klin Wochenschr.* 2005;**117**(7–8):300–302.

27. Majeed A, Naeem Z, Khan DA, *et al.* Epidemic adenoviral conjunctivitis report of an outbreak in a military garrison and recommendations for its management and prevention. *J Pak Med Assoc.* 2005;**55**(7):273–275.

28. Ganz M, Koll E, Gausche J, *et al.* Ketotifen fumarate and olopatadine hydrochloride in the treatment of allergic conjunctivitis: a real-world comparison of efficacy and ocular comfort. *Adv Ther.* 2003; **20**(2):79–91.

29. Abelson MB, Chapin MJ, Kapik BM, *et al.* Ocular tolerability and safety of ketotifen fumarate ophthalmic solution. *Adv Ther.* 2002;**19**(4): 161–169.

30. Bachert C, Brostoff J, Scadding GK, *et al.* Mizolastine therapy also has an effect on nasal blockade in perennial allergic rhinoconjunctivitis. RIPERAN Study Group. *Allergy.* 1998;**53**(10):969–975.

31. Sodhi PK, Pandey RM, Ratan SK. Efficacy and safety of topical azelastine compared with topical mitomycin C in patients with allergic conjunctivitis. *Cornea.* 2003;**22**(3):210–213.

32. Dekaris I, Gabric N, Lazic R, *et al.* [Evaluation of the efficacy and safety of lodoxamide in patients with allergic eye diseases.] *Acta Med Croatica.* 2002;**56** (3):93–98.

33. Tauber J. Nedocromil sodium ophthalmic solution 2% twice daily in patients with allergic conjunctivitis. *Adv Ther.* 2002;**19**(2):73–84.

34. van der Weele GM, Rietveld RP, Wiersma T, *et al.* [Summary of the practice guideline "The red eye" (first revision) of the Dutch College

of General Practitioners (NHG).] *Ned Tijdschr Geneeskd.* 2007;**151**(22): 1232-1237.

35. Isbister GK. Acute conjunctival inflammation following contact with squashed spider contents. *Am J Ophthalmol.* 2003;**136**(3):563-564.

36. Pharmakakis NM, Katsimpris JM, Melachrinou MP, *et al.* Corneal complications following abuse of topical anesthetics. *Eur J Ophthalmol.* 2002;**12** (5):373-378.

37. Gedik S, Akova YA, Gur S. Secondary bacterial keratitis associated with shield ulcer caused by vernal conjunctivitis. *Cornea.* 2006;**25**(8): 974-976.

38. Hwang JM, Pian D. Iritis presumed as secondary to disseminated coccidioidomycosis. *Optometry.* 2006;**77**(11):547-553.

39. Eke T, Al-Husainy S, Raynor MK. The spectrum of ocular inflammation caused by euphorbia plant sap. *Arch Ophthalmol.* 2000;**118**(1):13-16.

40. He D, Blomquist PH, Ellis E, 3rd. Association between ocular injuries and internal orbital fractures. *J Oral Maxillofac Surg.* 2007;**65**(4):713-720.

41. Jimenez-Jimenez FJ, Alonso-Navarro H, Fernandez-Diaz A, *et al.* [Neurotoxic effects induced by the topical administration of cycloplegics. A case report and review of the literature.] *Rev Neurol.* 2006;**43**(10):603-609.

42. Bagheri A, Givrad S, Yazdani S, *et al.* Optimal dosage of cyclopentolate 1% for complete cycloplegia: a randomized clinical trial. *Eur J Ophthalmol.* 2007;**17** (3):294-300.

Odontalgia

MICHAEL T. SCHULTZ AND MICHAEL S. RUNYON

■ Agents

- NSAIDs
- Opioids
- Acetaminophen
- Local anesthetics
- Eugenol
- Vitamin C

■ Evidence

Patients with odontogenic pain (OP) represent a broad spectrum of both disease etiology and severity. From the infant with teething to the older patient with denture-related OP, cases of tooth-related discomfort require an individualized approach, tailored to the patient and the diagnosis. This chapter does not attempt to assess all of the symptomatic therapies for all of the potential causes of OP. Instead, the goal is to overview the most important systemic, parenteral, and topical analgesic choices available to the acute care provider trying to relieve OP. The use and applicability of the three pharmacologic approaches for OP is sufficiently variable that the chapter is divided into three subsections: systemic, local injection, and topical therapy. Regardless of the analgesic modality selected, ED relief of OP is usually provided with the understanding that acute care is intended only as a bridge to appropriate dental follow-up.

SYSTEMIC ANALGESICS

NSAIDs are among the most widely used and well-studied drug classes used in management of acute and chronic OP, or odontalgia.[1] Data demonstrate superiority of **NSAIDs** over most other approaches for OP. For post-extraction pain, trial evidence has found either *ibuprofen* (400 mg PO) or *ketorolac* (10 mg PO) provides relief superior to that achieved with *acetaminophen* (*paracetamol*; 600 mg PO) alone or in combination with *codeine* (60 mg PO).[2] Another study found that *ketorolac* (10 mg PO) monotherapy was significantly more efficacious than treatment with *acetaminophen* (625 mg) plus *codeine* (15 mg PO).[3] Other trials in OP have demonstrated the equivalence or superiority of *ibuprofen* (400 mg PO) to *acetaminophen* (600 mg), *aspirin* (650 mg PO), *codeine* (up to 60 mg PO), and even combination therapy comprising *codeine* (60 mg PO) and either *aspirin* or *ibuprofen*.[4,5] Given the efficacy of the 400 mg PO of *ibuprofen*, and the increased incidence of adverse effects associated with higher doses, we recommend 400 mg of this NSAID as the initial approach for OP.

The literature fails to identify any significant differences in efficacy between the various **NSAID** classes for OP. There are, however, several **NSAIDs** (e.g. *naproxen*, *etodolac*, *piroxicam*) that are attractive for OP use given their extended dosing intervals.

Among the **NSAIDs** demonstrated to provide better pain relief than placebo is parenteral *ketorolac*.[6] While *ketorolac*'s general acute care efficacy may not differ from that achieved with other **NSAIDs**, assessments of the agent's parenteral use in acute care suggest it is highly effective in OP.[7] This agent's IV or IM administration may be useful when patients, owing to oral pain or other reason, cannot take PO therapy. The full effect of *ketorolac* analgesia, which can take as long as an hour even after IV administration, can be accelerated and even augmented by administering the **NSAID** directly into the periapical space.[8–10] The periapical injection of *ketorolac* is promising for application in acute care, but its recommendation for ED use must await further safety and efficacy data.

Trials suggest that there is no reason to employ the **COX-2 selective NSAIDs**. Compared with these agents, nonselective **NSAIDs** such as *ibuprofen* provide superior pain relief while incurring no extra short-term side effects. Consequently, we agree with dental expert reviews that find no reason to use the **COX-2 selective NSAIDs** in lieu of agents such as *ibuprofen*.[11,12]

Although the action mechanism is unknown, it is clear that addition of *caffeine* improves *ibuprofen*'s analgesic efficacy in OP. The combination of

100 mg *caffeine* and 200 mg *ibuprofen* achieves significantly greater OP relief than **NSAID** monotherapy.[13] Adding *caffeine* to *ibuprofen* improves analgesic potency (by 2.4–2.8 times), speeds onset of analgesia, and prolongs pain relief.[13]

Although a previously cited trial found that addition of mild **opioids** (e.g. *codeine*) to **NSAIDs** did not reliably improve OP relief, there is conflicting evidence on the subject.[4,14] The minimum dose of **opioid** needed to improve analgesia, while minimizing side effects, remains unknown. Both clinical studies and ED experience bear out some utility of potent **opioids** (e.g. *oxycodone*) for OP.[15–17] The use of these agents is recommended for those patients for whom other approaches (e.g. **NSAIDs**) have failed or are contraindicated.[1,18,19] Routine addition of **opioids** to **NSAIDs** is not warranted, given the overall risk-to-benefit ratio of dual therapy over treatment with **NSAIDs** alone.

The mixed-mechanism drug *tramadol* provides pain relief that is partially mediated by **opioid** receptors. As a single-agent approach to OP, *tramadol* seems to offer little advantage and we do not recommend it for monotherapy.[20] However, combination therapy with *tramadol* and a mild non-opioid analgesic represents an attractive therapeutic option for OP. Dual therapy with *tramadol* and either *flurbiprofen* or *acetaminophen* provides superior pain relief to monotherapy with any of these drugs.[21] The combination approach also allows a reduction in *tramadol* dose. A trial assessing combination therapy with *tramadol* (75 mg PO) plus *acetaminophen* (650 mg PO) found the dual regimen far superior to monotherapy with a larger dose of *tramadol* (100 mg PO).[20]

The OP of alveolar osteitis is usually treated with topical therapy (see below). In one study, mega-dose *vitamin C* (4000 mg/day) was found to provide complete resolution of alveolar osteitis symptoms within four days. The study's authors, who found that a majority of patients have complete relief within 48 h, postulate that the *vitamin C* works by facilitating granulation tissue formation.[22]

LOCAL INJECTION THERAPY

The supraperiosteal infiltration of **local anesthetics** (e.g. *lidocaine, bupivacaine*) usually provides suitable anesthesia when OP is emanating from a single maxillary tooth. Infiltration is only necessary on the buccal side; lingual injection increases discomfort without improving pain relief.[23] The relative thickness of the mandibular bone, compared with the maxillary bone, provides more of a barrier to diffusion of the injected agent (i.e. to the apical nerve). Therefore, an inferior alveolar nerve block is recommended for anesthesia of ipsilateral mandibular tooth-related OP. Both accessory innervation and operator technique contribute to a failure rate of at least 20% for inferior alveolar nerve blocks.[24]

Although discussion of the procedural approach to providing regional anesthesia is outside this text's scope, some notes about medication selection are in order. First, neither the selected **local anesthetic** nor its volume and concentration appear to impact the rate of anesthetic success.[25,26] Second, as long as some vasoconstricting *epinephrine* is coadministered, the concentration (1:50 000, 1:80 000, 1:100 000) does not appear critical.[27] Finally, *bupivacaine*'s extended duration of action, while advantageous in some respects, is associated with buccal trauma risks related to prolonged anesthesia. For safety reasons, we do not believe bilateral inferior alveolar nerve blocks should be provided.

Injection of **local anesthetics** is a legitimate, well-studied mechanism for providing relief of OP. This route may not be the approach of first choice in every patient. However, it is sufficiently efficacious for most causes of dental pain that it can be ethically recommended by the ED physician who is concerned about potential (inappropriate) drug-seeking behavior on the part of the patient with OP.

While there is insufficient evidence to recommend their routine use by the acute care provider, locally injected **opioids** may in the future prove useful for some cases of OP. One trial found that administration of low-dose (0.4 to 1.2 mg) *morphine* into the intraligamentary space provided relief in chronic, but not in acute, OP.[28]

Since there is no indication for routine addition of **antibiotics** for all patients with OP, it is not surprising that *penicillin* therapy usually has no impact on pain unless there is obvious infection. Trial evidence from OP series shows that *penicillin* neither alleviates pain nor reduces the amount of other analgesics required.[29,30]

TOPICAL THERAPY

Topical preparations are frequently, if only partially, efficacious for OP. For some OP etiologies (e.g. pericoronitis, infant teething), topical monotherapy will often suffice. For other conditions (e.g. severe pain from alveolar osteitis pain), topical drug application can be important adjunctive therapy. Remember the contraindication of topical therapies in the setting of tooth fractures (risk of sterile abscess development).

Alveolar osteitis is one cause of OP in which topical therapy is the approach of choice. In alveolar osteitis, or "dry socket," a focal osteomyelitis occurs after premature lysis of a post-extraction clot. Abundant literature addresses perioperative prevention, but there is a paucity of high-level evidence assessing acute treatment. One approach incorporates socket irrigation (with 0.9% saline) followed by packing with a dry socket paste. The paste constituents vary, but *benzocaine* and *eugunol* (i.e. *clove oil extract*) are recommended. The *eugunol* has an anesthetic effect on alveolar bone and seems more effective than *chlorhexidine* mouthwashes or *lidocaine* ointment.[31]

In addition to its potential use in alveolar osteitis, *benzocaine* (available in a variety of gel and paste concentrations ranging up to 20%) is efficacious in other causes of OP. In fact, so long as *benzocaine* is used for a limited time period (less than a week), its application no more than four times daily has a favorable risk-to-benefit ratio for myriad causes of OP. For example, application of *benzocaine* for carious disease relieves pain in over 80% of patients (compared with 16% for placebo).[32] Topical *benzocaine* (applied no more than four times daily) is also useful in infant teething; a few drops of the liquid preparation are usually recommended for this indication. Pain related to dental appliances can be treated by applying *benzocaine* paste to the (dried) appliance before its placement in the oral cavity.

Another topical agent, *choline salicylate*, has been used for nearly a half-century for its analgesia and anti-inflammatory effects.[33] The lack of more up-to-date evidence, the theoretical risk of complications, and the availability of other effective approaches mean that there is no role for ED use of *choline salicylate* at this time.

■ Summary and recommendations

First line: NSAID (e.g. ibuprofen 400–600 mg PO q6–8 h)

Reasonable:

■ mild opioid (e.g. hydrocodone 2.5–5 mg PO QID) with acetaminophen (325–650 mg PO QID)
■ topical benzocaine 10–20% (depending on etiology)

Pregnancy: acetaminophen (325–650 mg PO QID) with or without opioid (e.g. hydrocodone 5–10 mg PO QID)

Pediatric: NSAID (e.g. ibuprofen 10 mg/kg PO q6–8 h)

Special cases:

■ *NSAID ineligibility or failure*: opioids such as oxycodone (5–10 mg PO q4–6 h)
■ *mild–moderate pain and wish to avoid strong opioids*: tramadol 50–75 mg PO q4–6 h in combination with acetaminophen (650–1000 mg PO QID) or an NSAID (e.g. ibuprofen 400–600 mg PO QID)
■ *high suspicion of inappropriate drug-seeking behavior*: local anesthetic injection
■ *infant teething, carious disease, or dental appliance pain*: benzocaine 10–20% topically, no more than four times daily as either monotherapy or adjunctive therapy

References

1. Dionne RA, Berthold CW. Therapeutic uses of non-steroidal anti-inflammatory drugs in dentistry. *Crit Rev Oral Biol Med*. 2001;**12**(4):315–330.
2. Forbes JA, Kehm CJ, Grodin CD, *et al*. Evaluation of ketorolac, ibuprofen, acetaminophen, and an acetaminophen–codeine combination in postoperative oral surgery pain. *Pharmacotherapy*. 1990;**10**(6 Pt 2):94S–105S.
3. Sadeghein A, Shahidi N, Dehpour AR. A comparison of ketorolac tromethamine and acetaminophen codeine in the management of acute apical periodontitis. *J Endod*. 1999;**25**(4):257–259.

4. Cooper SA, Engel J, Ladov M, *et al*. Analgesic efficacy of an ibuprofen-codeine combination. *Pharmacotherapy*. 1982;**2**(3):162–167.

5. Cooper SA. Five studies on ibuprofen for postsurgical dental pain. *Am J Med*. 1984;**77**(1A):70–77.

6. Curtis P, **Jr.,** Gartman LA, Green DB. Utilization of ketorolac tromethamine for control of severe odontogenic pain. *J Endod*. 1994;**20**(9):457–459.

7. Bartfield JM, Kern AM, Raccio-Robak N, *et al*. Ketorolac tromethamine use in a university-based emergency department. *Acad Emerg Med*. 1994;**1** (6):532–538.

8. Brown CR, Moodie JE, Wild VM, *et al*. Comparison of intravenous ketorolac tromethamine and morphine sulfate in the treatment of postoperative pain. *Pharmacotherapy*. 1990;**10**(6 Pt 2):116S–121S.

9. Mroszczak EJ, Jung D, Yee J, *et al*. Ketorolac tromethamine pharmacokinetics and metabolism after intravenous, intramuscular, and oral administration in humans and animals. *Pharmacotherapy*. 1990;**10**(6 Pt 2):33S–39S.

10. Penniston SG, Hargreaves KM. Evaluation of periapical injection of ketorolac for management of endodontic pain. *J Endod*. 1996;**22**(2):55–59.

11. Doyle G, Jayawardena S, Ashraf E, *et al*. Efficacy and tolerability of nonprescription ibuprofen versus celecoxib for dental pain. *J Clin Pharmacol*. 2002;**42**(8):912–919.

12. Huber MA, Terezhalmy GT. The use of COX-2 inhibitors for acute dental pain: A second look. *J Am Dent Assoc*. 2006;**137**(4):480–487.

13. Forbes JA, Beaver WT, Jones KF, *et al*. Effect of caffeine on ibuprofen analgesia in postoperative oral surgery pain. *Clin Pharmacol Ther*. 1991;**49**(6):674–684.

14. McQuay HJ, Carroll D, Watts PG, *et al*. Codeine 20 mg increases pain relief from ibuprofen 400 mg after third molar surgery. A repeat-dosing comparison of ibuprofen and an ibuprofen–codeine combination. *Pain*. 1989;**37**(1):7–13.

15. Nusstein JM, Beck M. Comparison of preoperative pain and medication use in emergency patients presenting with irreversible pulpitis or teeth with necrotic pulps. *Oral Surg Oral Med Oral Pathol Oral Radiol Endod*. 2003;**96** (2):207–214.

16. Haas DA. An update on analgesics for the management of acute postoperative dental pain. *J Can Dent Assoc*. 2002;**68**(8):476–482.

17. Hargreaves KM. Management of pain in endodontic patients. *Tex Dent J*. 1997;**114**(10):27–31.

18. Mickel AK, Wright AP, Chogle S, *et al*. An analysis of current analgesic preferences for endodontic pain management. *J Endod*. 2006;**32**(12):1146–1154.

19. Ma M, Lindsell CJ, Jauch EC, *et al.* Effect of education and guidelines for treatment of uncomplicated dental pain on patient and provider behavior. *Ann Emerg Med.* 2004;**44**(4):323–329.

20. Fricke JR, **Jr.,** Hewitt DJ, Jordan DM, *et al.* A double-blind placebo-controlled comparison of tramadol/acetaminophen and tramadol in patients with postoperative dental pain. *Pain.* 2004;**109**(3):250–257.

21. Doroschak AM, Bowles WR, Hargreaves KM. Evaluation of the combination of flurbiprofen and tramadol for management of endodontic pain. *J Endod.* 1999;**25**(10):660–663.

22. Halberstein RA, Abrahmsohn GM. Clinical management and control of alveolalgia ("dry socket") with vitamin C. *Am J Dent.* 2003;**16**(3):152–154.

23. Meechan JG, Kanaa MD, Corbett IP, *et al.* Pulpal anaesthesia for mandibular permanent first molar teeth: a double-blind randomized cross-over trial comparing buccal and buccal plus lingual infiltration injections in volunteers. *Int Endod J.* 2006;**39**(10):764–769.

24. Rood JP. Some anatomical and physiological causes of failure to achieve mandibular analgesia. *Br J Oral Surg.* 1977;**15**(1):75–82.

25. Vreeland DL, Reader A, Beck M, *et al.* An evaluation of volumes and concentrations of lidocaine in human inferior alveolar nerve block. *J Endod.* 1989;**15**(1):6–12.

26. McLean C, Reader A, Beck M, *et al.* An evaluation of 4% prilocaine and 3% mepivacaine compared with 2% lidocaine (1:100 000 epinephrine) for inferior alveolar nerve block. *J Endod.* 1993;**19**(3):146–150.

27. Dagher FB, Yared GM, Machtou P. An evaluation of 2% lidocaine with different concentrations of epinephrine for inferior alveolar nerve block. *J Endod.* 1997;**23**(3):178–180.

28. Dionne RA, Lepinski AM, Gordon SM, *et al.* Analgesic effects of peripherally administered opioids in clinical models of acute and chronic inflammation. *Clin Pharmacol Ther.* 2001;**70**(1):66–73.

29. Keenan JV, Farman AG, Fedorowicz Z, *et al.* A Cochrane Systematic Review finds no evidence to support the use of antibiotics for pain relief in irreversible pulpitis. *J Endod.* 2006;**32**(2):87–92.

30. Nagle D, Reader A, Beck M, *et al.* Effect of systemic penicillin on pain in untreated irreversible pulpitis. *Oral Surg Oral Med Oral Pathol Oral Radiol Endod.* 2000;**90**(5):636–640.

31. Garibaldi JA, Greenlaw J, Choi J, *et al.* Treatment of postoperative pain. *J Calif Dent Assoc.* 1995;**23**(4):71–72, 74.

32. Sveen OB, Yaekel M, Adair SM. Efficacy of using benzocaine for temporary relief of toothache. *Oral Surg Oral Med Oral Pathol.* 1982;**53**(6):574–576.

33. Jolley HM, Torneck CD, Siegel I. A topical choline salicylate gel for control of pain and inflammation in oral conditions: a controlled study. *J Can Dent Assoc (Toronto).* 1972;**38**(2):72–74.

Orthopedic extremity trauma – sprains, strains, and fractures

CATHERINE A. MARCO AND JASON B. LESTER

■ Agents

- Local anesthetics
- Acetaminophen
- NSAIDs
- Opioids

■ Evidence

While mechanical approaches (e.g. splinting) are important in managing sprain, strain, and fracture (SSF) pain, pharmacotherapy retains an important position for orthopedic analgesia. Systemic analgesics used for SSF include *acetaminophen (paracetamol)*, **NSAIDs**, and **opioids**. Although patients with severe pain or need for immediate relief should usually be given IV analgesia, other routes may be indicated in the acute care setting.[1]

This chapter focuses on systemically active analgesics. Pain relief for SSF can often be facilitated (or wholly provided) with local or regional injection of **local anesthetics**.[2–9] The high number of potential uses for **local anesthetics** in various SSF conditions precludes detailed discussion here, but ED physicians should always think first of this approach. Examples of high utility for **local anesthetic** injection include hip and radius fractures.[8–10] Evidence from RCTs of femur fractures suggests superiority of **local anesthetic** injection (for regional block) over *morphine* for managing pain in the ED.[10] The **local anesthetics** are also useful in management of rib fractures (discussed under chest wall trauma) and as adjuncts in ED procedural sedation and analgesia (outside this text's scope).

Acetaminophen (QID dose 650–1000 mg PO in adults, 15 mg/kg PO in children) can be effective in controlling mild-to-moderate pain. One RCT in patients with ankle sprains found *acetaminophen* (3900 mg daily) was not inferior to *ibuprofen*, but the **NSAID** dose was relatively low (1200 mg daily).[11] *Acetaminophen*'s main advantage is its relative safety in a broad range of patient populations. Evidence from a variety of study populations supports its employment as monotherapy (for mild pain) or as part of a combination regimen for myriad types of SSF pain.[12–17] It is the preferred initial agent for patients with pain that is not severe and who have contraindications for **NSAID** therapy.[18] In some countries, *acetaminophen* has an additional advantage of being available in an IV formulation (thus allowing patients to stay nil by mouth).

The **NSAIDs** (e.g. *ibuprofen* 400–600 mg or 10 mg/kg PO QID, *naproxen* 500 mg PO BID, *ketorolac* 15–30 mg IV) are traditional mainstays of SSF analgesia. This class is at least partly efficacious for SSF pain, and the **NSAIDs** are superior to *acetaminophen* (or *codeine*) for monotherapy of mild or moderate SSF pain.[19–21] The extensive clinical experience with **NSAIDs** and SSF pain relief is not to be discounted. However, review of evidence addressing **NSAIDs** for SSF indicates that the success of pain relief with **NSAIDs** is tempered by safety concerns.

The safety issues with **NSAIDs** are a combination of "generic" problems (i.e. those risks that are not related to SSF in particular) and SSF-specific problems. The generic problems of GI and renal complications are important owing to their relatively high likelihood in some SSF subgroups (e.g. elderly patients with hip fractures).

The first of two SSF-specific **NSAID** safety issues is related to the effects of this class on platelet function and hemostasis. Concerns about SSF-related bleeding exacerbation by **NSAIDs** are at this time largely theoretical. Nonetheless, absence of evidence addressing **NSAID**-associated SSF bleeding should not completely allay concerns about using these analgesics in patients with hematomas, or in those in whom operation may be necessary. Given the prevalence of hematoma and intraoperative bleeding in the setting of SSF, reports of *ketorolac*-induced operative bleeding in patients without SSF should give pause to clinicians considering **NSAID** administration to patients in whom bleeding could be problematic.[22]

A second SSF-specific **NSAID** problem, fracture healing and nonunion, has been addressed by studies, but the topic remains controversial as the data generated are not definitive. The available animal and human data suggest that **NSAIDs** should be used with caution in both the acute and chronic management of fractures because of the risk of delayed healing and nonunion.[23-27] The lack of definitive evidence for either safety or risk is a problem, especially in terms of managing these injuries prior to X-ray imaging (**local anesthetic** injection may be a partial solution).

To date, the use of **NSAIDs** for treatment of SSF pain is based upon decades of efficacy, and the existing evidence of their risk is insufficient for a sweeping proscription of their use in SSF. Both the general and SSF-specific risks of **NSAIDs** should be weighed against benefit from use of these drugs in any given patient. For the healthy young person with mild or moderate pain from a low-grade sprain or strain, the risk to-benefit ratio of **NSAIDs** favors use of this class. For other populations, pain relief alternatives (e.g. **opioids**, injection of **local anesthetics**) may be preferred and **NSAIDs** best avoided or delayed (e.g. until radiographs rule out fracture or need for operation). Until rigorous evidence demonstrates or refutes the case for **NSAIDs** in SSF, judgment should be exercised based on the anticipated risks and benefits of therapy.

Opioids have long been effectively used for severe SSF pain. Intravenous **opioids** (e.g. *morphine*) remain the most effective means for achieving both rapid analgesia and sustained relief (e.g. using patient-controlled analgesia) in most SSF conditions.[28] If the prototypical **opioid** *morphine* is to be avoided, *hydromorphone* is an alternative approach for potent analgesia.[29] *Fentanyl*'s demonstrated safety and efficacy in acute SSF pain (particularly in fractures) make this agent an attractive alternative for both children and adults in the acute phase. One study of fractures in children found that administration of IN *fentanyl* (150 µg/mL at a dose of 1.7 µg/kg) provided equivalent analgesia to that achieved with IV *morphine* (0.1 mg/kg).[30] Other acute care (prehospital) studies provide consistent evidence of *fentanyl*'s safety and efficacy for analgesia in acute trauma (including patients with extremity fractures).[31-34] Recent preliminary evidence in children with SSF suggests that oral transmucosal *fentanyl* (10–15 µg/kg) provides analgesia superior to that achieved with IV *morphine*; broad use of this approach must await further safety study.[35]

There is some evidence comparing various PO **opioid** approaches, although the studies directly comparing oral regimens are few. *Hydrocodone* (5–10 mg PO) and *oxycodone* (5–10 mg PO) are commonly used and efficacious.[36] *Hydrocodone* is preferable to *codeine* for SSF pain, based on a combination of efficacy and side effect profiles.[36] *Hydrocodone* and *oxycodone* (each in a 5 mg PO regimen, in combination with *acetaminophen*) are similarly safe and efficacious for ED fracture treatment.[37] There is no difference between the two agents at pain assessments at 30 or 60 min, and adverse effect profiles are similar (although there may be higher incidence of subsequent constipation after *hydrocodone*).[37]

When combined with *acetaminophen*, the mixed-mechanism **opioid** *tramadol* is found to be equally efficacious to *hydrocodone* for relieving SSF pain. A study of patients with ankle sprain and partial ligament tear found coadministered *tramadol* (75 mg PO) with *acetaminophen* (650 mg PO) was equal in terms of both efficacy and side effects to *hydrocodone* (7.5 mg PO) when the following endpoints were assessed: pain relief magnitude during the first 4 h after dosing, rate of 30% analgesic response, and rate of 50% analgesic response.[38]

Many combination products are available. Such products often include an **opioid** and a weaker analgesic such as *acetaminophen* or *aspirin*. There is no reason to suspect that these combination products lack efficacy, but few studies have rigorously evaluated their performance against alternative approaches such as **opioid** monotherapy.

■ Summary and recommendations

First line:
- consider local or regional anesthesia (e.g. using lidocaine)
- NSAID (e.g. ibuprofen 400–800 mg PO QID)
- opioid (e.g. morphine initial dose 4–6 mg IV, then titrate)

Reasonable: any NSAID or opioid

Pediatric:
- NSAID (e.g. ibuprofen 10 mg/kg PO QID)
- opioids (e.g. hydrocodone 2.5 mg PO q4–6 h)

Pregnancy:

■ acetaminophen (650–1000 mg PO QID)
■ opioids (e.g. oxycodone 5–10 mg PO q4–6 h)

Special cases:

■ *concern for hemodynamics or possibility of other (e.g. abdominal) injuries*: fentanyl (initial dose 50–100 μg IV, then titrate)
■ *mild-moderate pain and NSAIDs not tolerated*: acetaminophen (650–1000 mg PO QID)

References

1. Fosnocht D, Hollifield M, Swanson E. Patient preference for route of pain medication delivery. *J Emerg Med*. 2004;**26**(1):7–11.
2. Singelyn EJ. Continuous peripheral nerve blocks and postoperative pain management. *Acta Anaesthesiol Belg*. 2006;**57**(2):109–112.
3. Ilfeld BM, Morey TE, Enneking FK. Infraclavicular perineural local anesthetic infusion: a comparison of three dosing regimens for postoperative analgesia. *Anesthesiology*. 2004;**100**(2):395–402.
4. Miller SL, Cleeman E, Auerbach J, *et al*. Comparison of intra-articular lidocaine and intravenous sedation for reduction of shoulder dislocations: a randomized, prospective study. *J Bone Joint Surg Am*. 2002,**04A**(12):2135–2139.
5. Kieninger AN, Bair HA, Bendick PJ, *et al*. Epidural versus intravenous pain control in elderly patients with rib fractures. *Am J Surg* 2005;**189**(3):327–330.
6. Trincr W, Levine J, Lai SY, *et al*. Femoral nerve block for femur fractures. *Ann Emerg Med*. 2005;**45**(6):679.
7. Bulger EM, Edwards T, Klotz P, *et al*. Epidural analgesia improves outcome after multiple rib fractures. *Surgery*. 2004;**136**(2):426–430.
8. Parker MJ, Griffiths R, Appadu BN. Nerve blocks (subcostal, lateral cutaneous, femoral, triple, psoas) for hip fractures. *Cochrane Database Syst Rev*. 2000(2): CD001159.
9. Handoll HH, Madhok R, Dodds C. Anaesthesia for treating distal radial fracture in adults. *Cochrane Database Syst Rev*. 2002(3):CD003320.
10. Wathen J, Gao D, Merritt G, *et al*. A randomized controlled trial comparing a fascia iliaca compartment nerve block to a traditional systemic analgesic for

femur fractures in a pediatric emergency department. *Ann Emerg Med.* 2007;**50**(2):162–171.

11. Dalton JD, Jr., Schweinle JE. Randomized controlled noninferiority trial to compare extended release acetaminophen and ibuprofen for the treatment of ankle sprains. *Ann Emerg Med.* 2006;**48**(5):615–623.

12. Hiller A, Meretoja OA, Korpela R, *et al.* The analgesic efficacy of acetaminophen, ketoprofen, or their combination for pediatric surgical patients having soft tissue or orthopedic procedures. *Anesth Analg.* 2006;**102**(5):1365–1371.

13. Sinatra RS, Jahr JS, Reynolds LW, *et al.* Efficacy and safety of single and repeated administration of 1 gram intravenous acetaminophen injection (paracetamol) for pain management after major orthopedic surgery. *Anesthesiology.* 2005;**102**(4):822–831.

14. Drendel AL, Lyon R, Bergholte J, *et al.* Outpatient pediatric pain management practices for fractures. *Pediatr Emerg Care.* 2006;**22**(2):94–99.

15. Hynes D, McCarroll M, Hiesse-Provost O. Analgesic efficacy of parenteral paracetamol (propacetamol) and diclofenac in postoperative orthopaedic pain. *Acta Anaesthesiol Scand.* 2006;**50**(3):374–381.

16. Ripouteau C, Conort O, Lamas JP, *et al.* Effect of multifaceted intervention promoting early switch from intravenous to oral acetaminophen for postoperative pain: controlled, prospective, before and after study. *BMJ.* 2000;**321** (7274):1460–1463.

17. Peduto VA, Ballabio M, Stefanini S. Efficacy of propacetamol in the treatment of postoperative pain. Morphine-sparing effect in orthopedic surgery. Italian Collaborative Group on Propacetamol. *Acta Anaesthesiol Scand.* 1998;**42** (3):293–298.

18. Hyllested M, Jones S, Pedersen JL, *et al.* Comparative effect of paracetamol, NSAIDs or their combination in postoperative pain management: a qualitative review. *Br J Anaesth.* 2002;**88**(2):199–214.

19. Dahl V, Dybvik T, Steen T, *et al.* Ibuprofen vs. acetaminophen vs. ibuprofen and acetaminophen after arthroscopically assisted anterior cruciate ligament reconstruction. *Eur J Anaesthesiol.* 2004;**21**(6):471–475.

20. Graham GG, Graham RI, Day RO. Comparative analgesia, cardiovascular and renal effects of celecoxib, rofecoxib and acetaminophen (paracetamol). *Curr Pharm Des.* 2002;**8**(12):1063–1075.

21. Clark E, Plint AC, Correll R, *et al.* A randomized, controlled trial of acetaminophen, ibuprofen, and codeine for acute pain relief in children with musculoskeletal trauma. *Pediatrics.* 2007;**119**(3):460–467.

22. Vuilleumier H, Halkic N. Ruptured subcapsular hematoma after laparoscopic cholecystectomy attributed to ketorolac-induced coagulopathy. *Surg Endosc.* 2003;**17**(4):659.

23. Gerstenfeld LC, Thiede M, Seibert K, *et al.* Differential inhibition of fracture healing by non-selective and cyclooxygenase-2 selective non-steroidal anti-inflammatory drugs. *J Orthop Res.* 2003;**21**(4):670–675.

24. Giannoidis P, Furlong A, Macdonald D, *et al.* Non-union of the femoral diaphysis: the influence of reaming and non-steroidal anti-inflammatory drugs (NSAIDs). *J Bone Joint Surg.* 2000;**82B**:655–658.

25. Beck A, Salem K, Krischak G, *et al.* Nonsteroidal anti-inflammatory drugs (NSAIDs) in the perioperative phase in traumatology and orthopedics effects on bone healing. *Oper Orthop Traumatol.* 2005;**17**(6):569–578.

26. Dahners LE, Mullis BH. Effects of nonsteroidal anti-inflammatory drugs on bone formation and soft-tissue healing. *J Am Acad Orthop Surg.* 2004;**12**(3):139–143.

27. Allen HL, Wase A, Bear WT. Indomethacin and aspirin: effect of nonsteroidal anti-inflammatory agents on the rate of fracture repair in the rat. *Acta Orthop Scand.* 1980;**51**(4):595–600.

28. Capdevila X, Dadure C, Bringuier S, *et al.* Effect of patient-controlled perineural analgesia on rehabilitation and pain after ambulatory orthopedic surgery: a multicenter randomized trial. *Anesthesiology.* 2006;**105**(3):566–573.

29. Chang AK, Bijur PE, Meyer RH, *et al.* Safety and efficacy of hydromorphone as an analgesic alternative to morphine in acute pain: a randomized clinical trial. *Ann Emerg Med.* 2006;**48**(2):164–172.

30. Borland M, Jacobs I, King B, *et al.* A randomized controlled trial comparing intranasal fentanyl to intravenous morphine for managing acute pain in children in the emergency department. *Ann Emerg Med.* 2007;**49**(3):335–340.

31. DeVellis P, Thomas S, Wedel S, *et al.* Prehospital fentanyl analgesia in air-transported pediatric trauma patients. *Pediatr Emerg Care.* 1998;**14**(5):321–323.

32. DeVellis P, Thomas SH, Wedel SK. Prehospital and emergency department analgesia for air-transported patients with fractures. *Prehosp Emerg Care.* 1998;**2**(4):293–296.

33. Frakes MA, Lord WR, Kociszewski C, *et al.* Efficacy of fentanyl analgesia for trauma in critical care transport. *Am J Emerg Med.* 2006;**24**(3):286–289.

34. Galinski M, Dolveck F, Borron SW, *et al.* A randomized, double-blind study comparing morphine with fentanyl in prehospital analgesia. *Am J Emerg Med.* 2005;**23**(2):114–119.

35. Mahar PJ, Rana JA, Kennedy CS, *et al.* A randomized clinical trial of oral transmucosal fentanyl citrate versus intravenous morphine sulfate for initial control of pain in children with extremity injuries. *Pediatr Emerg Care.* 2007;**23**(8):544–548.

36. Turturro MA, Paris PM, Yealy DM, *et al.* Hydrocodone versus codeine in acute musculoskeletal pain. *Ann Emerg Med.* 1991;**20**(10):1100–1103.

37. Marco CA, Plewa MC, Buderer N, *et al.* Comparison of oxycodone and hydrocodone for the treatment of acute pain associated with fractures: a double-blind, randomized, controlled trial. *Acad Emerg Med.* 2005;**12**(4):282–288.

38. Hewitt DJ, Todd KH, Xiang J, *et al.* Tramadol/acetaminophen or hydrocodone/acetaminophen for the treatment of ankle sprain: a randomized, placebo-controlled trial. *Ann Emerg Med.* 2007;**49**(4):468–480, e461–e462.

Osteoporotic vertebral compression fracture

SUSAN R. WILCOX AND STEPHEN H. THOMAS

■ Agents

- Acetaminophen
- NSAIDs
- Opioids
- Calcitonin
- Pamidronate

■ Evidence

Treatment of osteoporotic vertebral compression fracture (OVCF) is multi-faceted, but most techniques (e.g. kyphoplasty, nerve blocks, jacket splints) require orthopedic consultation. For the acute care provider, OVCF pharmacotherapy begins with *acetaminophen (paracetamol)*.[1,2] Although **NSAIDs** are sometimes a second line choice, the increased risk of GI and renal complications in the elderly, the population at highest risk for OVCF, renders this class of analgesics less than ideal.[1,3] (Issues relevant to **NSAID** use and fracture-specific risks are discussed in the chapter on extremity fractures.)

Since the pain from OVCF is often too severe for adequate control with relatively weak analgesics such as *acetaminophen* and **NSAIDs**, **opioids** are commonly the next choice. The ability of **opioids** to alleviate OVCF pain is not doubted, although there is little high-level evidence addressing the subject. The problem, as discussed in the chapter on geriatric analgesia (p. 42), lies with the relatively high complication rates associated with **opioid** use in the (elderly) population with OVCF. In fact, the relative frequency of **opioid**-related side effects (e.g. falls, constipation) in OVCF is largely responsible for the exploration of alternative analgesic approaches that is the focus of this chapter.[1-3]

Once-daily *calcitonin*, either IM, PR, SC, or IN may be known to some providers as an outpatient preventative therapy for those at risk of OVCF.[4,5] In terms of its relief of bony pain, *calcitonin* has had disappointing results in some arenas (see the chapter on cancer and tumor pain, p. 151), but there is promise for its use in OVCF. Trials indicate that *calcitonin* is associated with better pain relief and earlier mobilization than achieved with *acetaminophen* monotherapy or placebo.[6–8]

The exact mechanism of *calcitonin's* analgesia provision is not known, but effects can be expected as early as 48 h after institution of therapy.[2,7–9] Meta-analysis of five RCTs evaluating *calcitonin* versus placebo for acute OVCF concluded that the drug significantly reduces pain, with an effect consistently identified within seven days of treatment.[2] The reduction in pain score over that associated with placebo is both long-lasting – persisting through four weeks of follow-up – and substantial (over 3 units on a 10-point pain scale).[2] *Calcitonin's* pain-relieving effects extend to reduction of discomfort associated with sitting, standing, and walking.[2]

Meta-analysis finds a potential trend toward faster pain relief with IM *calcitonin*, although there are too few studies for definitive conclusions.[2] Evidence shows equivalence between IN and SC routes for *calcitonin*, and data also demonstrate significant pain reductions with the PR formulation.[5,9] Therefore, there is little evidence base to recommend one administration route over another.

Where specified, the majority of the studies use salmon *calcitonin*. There are no studies comparing the effectiveness of salmon-derived versus synthetic forms of the hormone. If patients are not allergic to fish products, the salmon-derived formulation seems a reasonable choice.

There are no studies that specifically address the utility of *calcitonin* in the ED. There is also an absence of data addressing use of *calcitonin* for non-osteoporotic compression fractures. In our judgment, it is reasonable to extrapolate non-ED evidence of *calcitonin's* pain relief efficacy to the acute care setting for OVCF. We are less convinced about the appropriateness of extrapolating evidence of *calcitonin's* efficacy in osteoporotic fracture pain to compression fractures not related to osteoporosis.

Like *calcitonin*, the **bisphosphonates** have been studied for bony tumor and cancer-related pain (see the chapter on cancer and tumor pain, p. 151). There is less evidence addressing their use for OVCF. One placebo-controlled OVCF trial found *pamidronate* improved pain.[10] Another study found similar pain relief between *pamidronate* and *calcitonin*.[11] Given the relative strengths of evidence for *calcitonin* and the **bisphosphonates**, and the drugs' safety and side effect profiles, we recommend reserving *pamidronate* for situations where other approaches fail or are contraindicated.

■ Summary and recommendations

First line:

- acetaminophen (650–1000 mg PO QID) for mild–moderate pain
- opioids (e.g. oxycodone 2.5–5 mg PO q4–6h) for 2–3 days until calcitonin takes effect
- calcitonin (200 IU salmon-derived preparation IN QD)

Reasonable: NSAIDs (e.g. ibuprofen 600–800 mg PO q6–8h, maximum daily 2400 mg) if favorable risk profile

Special cases:

- *patient allergic to fish*: use synthetic calcitonin (200 IU IN QD)
- *intolerability or failure of other approaches*: pamidronate (in consultation with follow-up physicians)

References

1. Lyles KW. Management of patients with vertebral compression fractures. *Pharmacotherapy*. 1999;**19**(1 Pt 2):21S–24S.
2. Old JL, Calvert M. Vertebral compression fractures in the elderly. *Am Fam Physician*. 2004;**69**(1):111–116.
3. Kanis JA, McCloskey EV. Effect of calcitonin on vertebral and other fractures. *Q J Med*. 1999;**92**(3):143–149.
4. Knopp J, Diner B, Blitz M, *et al*. Calcitonin for treating acute pain of osteoporotic vertebral compression fractures: a systematic review of randomized, controlled trials. *Osteoporos Int*. 2005;**16**(10):1281–1290.
5. Lyritis G, Ioannidis G, Karachalios T, *et al*. Analgesic effect of salmon calcitonin suppositories in patients with acute pain due to recent osteoporotic vertebral crush fractures: a prospective, double-blind, randomized, placebo-controlled clinical study. *Clin J Pain*. 1999;**15**(4):284–289.

6. Combe B, Cohen C, Aubin F. Equivalence of nasal spray and subcutaneous formulations of salmon calcitonin. *Calcif Tissue Int.* 1997;**61**(1):10–15.

7. Lyritis G, Paspati I, Karachalios T, *et al.* Pain relief from nasal salmon calcitonin in osteoporotic vertebral crush fractures: a double-blind, placebo-controlled clinical study. *Acta Orthop Scand Suppl.* 1997;**275**:112–114.

8. Lyritis G, Tsakalakos N, Magiasis B, *et al.* Analgesic effect of salmon calcitonin suppositories in patients with acute pain due to recent osteoporotic vertebral crush fractures: a double-blind placebo-controlled clinical study. *Calcif Tissue Int.* 1991;**49**(6):369–372.

9. Chesnut C, Silverman S, Andriano K, *et al.* A randomized trial of nasal spray salmon calcitonin in postmenopausal women with established osteoporosis: the Prevent Recurrence of Osteoporotic Fractures (PROOF) Study. *Am J Med.* 2000;**109**(4):267–276.

10. Armingeat T, Brondino R, Pham T, *et al.* Intravenous pamidronate for pain relief in recent osteoporotic vertebral compression fracture: a randomized double-blind controlled study. *Osteoporos Int.* 2006;**17**(11):1659–1665.

11. Laroche M, Cantogrel S, Jamard B, *et al.* Comparison of the analgesic efficacy of pamidronate and synthetic human calcitonin in osteoporotic vertebral fractures: a double-blind controlled study. *Clin Rheumatol.* 2006;**25**(5):683–686.

Otitis media and externa

KELLY YOUNG

■ Agents

- NSAIDs
- Acetaminophen
- Topical local anesthetics
- Topical naturopathics
- Topical antihistamines
- Topical corticosteroids
- Opioids

■ Evidence

Given the frequency of otitis media (OM) and otitis externa (OE), there is surprisingly little evidence on treating pain associated with these conditions. For both conditions, there can be utility in mechanical interventions (myringotomy for OM, ear canal cleaning and drying for OE). An additional part of otalgia control is patient instruction. Patients with OM should avoid pressure changes (e.g. flying), and those with OE need to avoid further ear canal irritation (e.g. swimming). As for pharmacotherapy, guidelines emphasize the importance of pain management, but recommendations are based on expert panel consensus rather than methodologically rigorous comparative trials.[1,2]

The **NSAIDs** are typically recommended as first-line treatment, although evidence is sparse. One RCT in young children found that *ibuprofen* and *acetaminophen* (*paracetamol*) similarly outperformed placebo in terms of OM pain relief.[3] While the analgesic benefit of the **NSAID** (like that of *acetaminophen*) seems likely, the effect magnitude is probably small since two smaller trials failed to identify any benefit (compared with placebo) for *naproxen* use in painful OM.[4,5]

Topically applied **local anesthetics**, generally *benzocaine*, are widely used for otalgia. The evidence is limited, but available data from one study indicate benefit from this approach.[6,7] When compared with application of olive oil as a control, topical application of *benzocaine* (in a glycerin vehicle) is associated with lower pain scores assessed at 10, 20, and 30 min, although statistical significance is only found for the 30 min assessment.[7] In addition to the topical analgesia, all patients in the study received *acetaminophen* (15 mg/kg). As commonly used, *benzocaine* is combined with the anti-inflammatory *antipyrine*; the drugs are instilled as drops in the ear canal (or administered and plugged into place with cotton in children). Since little or no systemic absorption occurs, toxicity is not a concern.

At least one other **local anesthetic** approach is described for otic analgesia. A *eutectic mixture of local anesthetics* (*EMLA*), which contains *lidocaine* and *prilocaine*, is described as effective for relieving OE pain.[8] This preparation is also useful for anesthetizing the tympanic membrane prior to myringotomy.[9] However, no randomized trials have assessed *EMLA*'s efficacy for otalgia caused by OE or OM. Furthermore, there are concerns about middle ear toxicity from topical agents that are applied in patients with (known or unknown) tympanic membrane perforation.[10]

Naturopathic topical approaches for OM are found by one investigator to be more effective than the topical **local anesthetic** *amethocaine*.[11,12] The results of these studies are called into question because of problems related to non-blinding and statistical methodology.[13] A preliminary report of another study, also methodologically limited, assessed the endpoint of treatment failure and found no benefit (over placebo) to a homeopathic approach.[14]

Trial evidence and reviews find neither **antihistamines** nor **corticosteroids** are effective in reducing OM pain.[1,15] For OE, there are no data addressing **antihistamine** use but conclusions about **corticosteroids** parallel those for OM. An RCT in OE, comparing treatment with topical **antibiotic** solutions with and without **corticosteroids**, found no analgesic advantage to inclusion of the **corticosteroid** component (although pain relief was not the study's primary endpoint).[16]

There are no data assessing otalgia relief for systemically administered **opioids**. However, expert panel evidence supports use of oral agents such as *oxycodone* or *hydrocodone* (usually in combination with *acetaminophen* or *ibuprofen*) for severe otalgia from either OM or OE.[1,2]

■ Summary and recommendations

First line: NSAID (e.g. ibuprofen 600–800 q6–8 h, maximum 2400 mg/day)

Reasonable:

- acetaminophen 650–1000 mg PO QID (if pain is mild and NSAID contraindicated)
- topical benzocaine (3–4 drops 20% solution q1–4 h, with insertion of saturated cotton plug) if tympanic membrane is not perforated

Pregnancy:

- acetaminophen
- topical benzocaine (3–4 drops 20% solution q3–4 h, with insertion of saturated cotton plug) if tympanic membrane is not perforated

Pediatric:

- NSAID (e.g. ibuprofen 10 mg/kg PO QID)
- topical benzocaine (3–4 drops 20% solution q3–4 h, with insertion of saturated cotton plug) if tympanic membrane is not perforated

Special case:

- *severe pain*: opioid (e.g. oxycodone 5–10 mg PO q4–6 h)

References

1. American Academy of Pediatrics and American Academy of Family Physicians. Diagnosis and management of acute otitis media. *Pediatrics*. 2004;**113** (5):1451–1465.

2. Rosenfeld RM, Brown L, Cannon CR, *et al*. Clinical practice guideline: acute otitis externa. *Otolaryngol Head Neck Surg*. 2006;**134**(4 Suppl):S4–23.

3. Bertin L, Pons G, d'Athis P, *et al*. A randomized, double-blind, multicentre controlled trial of ibuprofen versus acetaminophen and placebo for symptoms of acute otitis media in children. *Fundam Clin Pharmacol*. 1996;**10** (4):387–392.

4. Abramovich S, O'Grady J, Fuller A, *et al*. Naproxen in otitis media with effusion. *J Laryngol Otol*. 1986;**100**(3):263–266.

5. Varsano IB, Volovitz BM, Grossman JE. Effect of naproxen, a prostaglandin inhibitor, on acute otitis media and persistence of middle ear effusion in children. *Ann Otol Rhinol Laryngol.* 1989;**98**(5, Pt 1):389–392.

6. Foxlee R, Johansson A, Wejfalk J, *et al.* Topical analgesia for acute otitis media. *Cochrane Database Syst Rev.* 2006(3):CD005657.

7. Hoberman A, Paradise JL, Reynolds EA, *et al.* Efficacy of Auralgan for treating ear pain in children with acute otitis media. *Arch Pediatr Adolesc Med.* 1997;**151**(7):675–678.

8. Premachandra DJ. Use of EMLA cream as an analgesic in the management of painful otitis externa. *J Laryngol Otol.* 1990;**104**(11):887–888.

9. Roberts C, Carlin WV. A comparison of topical EMLA cream and prilocaine injection for anaesthesia of the tympanic membrane in adults. *Acta Otolaryngol.* 1989;**108**(5–6):431–433.

10. Woldman S. Treating ear pain in children with acute otitis media. *Arch Pediatr Adolesc Med.* 1998;**152**(1):102.

11. Sarrell EM, Cohen HA, Kahan E. Naturopathic treatment for ear pain in children. *Pediatrics.* 2003;**111**(5, Pt 1):e574–e579.

12. Sarrell EM, Mandelberg A, Cohen HA. Efficacy of naturopathic extracts in the management of ear pain associated with acute otitis media. *Arch Pediatr Adolesc Med.* 2001;**155**(7):796–799.

13. Kemper AR, Krysan DJ. Reevaluating the efficacy of naturopathic ear drops. *Arch Pediatr Adolesc Med.* 2002;**156**(1):88–89.

14. Jacobs J, Springer DA, Crothers D. Homeopathic treatment of acute otitis media in children: a preliminary randomized placebo-controlled trial. *Pediatr Infect Dis J.* 2001;**20**(2):177–183.

15. Chonmaitree T, Saeed K, Uchida T, *et al.* A randomized, placebo-controlled trial of the effect of antihistamine or corticosteroid treatment in acute otitis media. *J Pediatr.* 2003;**143**(3):377–385.

16. Schwartz RH. Once-daily ofloxacin otic solution versus neomycin sulfate/polymyxin B sulfate/hydrocortisone otic suspension four times a day: a multi-center, randomized, evaluator-blinded trial to compare the efficacy, safety, and pain relief in pediatric patients with otitis externa. *Curr Med Res Opin.* 2006;**22**(9):1725–1736.

Pancreatitis

STEPHEN H. THOMAS AND JONATHAN S. ILGEN

■ Agents

- Opioids
- NSAIDs
- Cholecystokinin receptor agents
- Octreotide
- Glucagon

■ Evidence

Opioids remain the most commonly used, and most commonly recommended, treatment for acute (and acute-on-chronic) pancreatitis [1] Evidence addressing **opioids'** effect on the sphincter of Oddi and biliary tract pain (see the chapter on biliary tract pain) may also be applicable in pancreatitis.

The data show little difference in efficacy between various **opioids**. Authors criticizing the widespread practice of using *meperidine* (*pethidine*) for pancreatitis pain have noted that there is no contraindication to routine use of *morphine*.[2,3]

While most **opioids** are acceptable, there are reasons to select the mixed agonist–antagonist *buprenorphine*. *Buprenorphine* appears to have advantages related to a paucity of effect on Oddi's sphincter. Perhaps related to this property are reports of *buprenorphine* success when pure-agonist **opioids** fail to control pancreatitis pain.[4,5] For instance, a trial has found that *buprenorphine* achieves better analgesia than *meperidine*.[6] Use of an agent with limited effects on the sphincter of Oddi can reduce confusion about the etiology of the pancreatitis, by eliminating the **opioid** as a possible cause.[7] (In the rare instance in which mu receptor agonists cause pancreatitis, *naloxone* is the indicated therapy.)

There may be situations in which oral agents may be appropriate for ED therapy (e.g. chronic or less-severe pancreatitis). In these cases, PO *tramadol* (which lacks effects on the sphincter of Oddi) is more efficacious and causes fewer GI motility side effects than PO *morphine*.[4,8]

There is conflicting information as to the role of **NSAIDs** in treating pancreatitis pain. One expert consensus panel included **NSAIDs** as a first-line treatment for flares of chronic pancreatitis.[9] In a study with potential relevance to the ED setting, an RCT in outpatients with chronic pancreatitis found that *indomethacin* (50 mg PR every 12 h) provided effective analgesia and had an **opioid**-sparing effect.[10] However, the human-subjects literature on pancreatitis and **NSAIDs** (including those agents with COX-2 selectivity) consists primarily of sporadic reports of **NSAID**-induced pancreatitis.[11] Risk of this rare but concerning complication tempers enthusiasm for ED use of **NSAIDs** for pancreatitis. The **COX-2 selective NSAID** *misoprostol* has been described as useful in chronic pancreatitis, but comprehensive reviews of available evidence find insufficient data to support ED use of **COX-2 selective NSAIDs**.[12,13]

The **cholecystokinin (CCK)-receptor antagonists** *proglumide* and *loxiglumide* appear to be effective in ameliorating pain from acute exacerbations of pancreatitis. One study demonstrated improvement in both subjective and objective (laboratory) parameters.[14] Another trial found that multiple oral regimens of *loxiglumide* improved acute pancreatitis symptoms; a 600 mg/day dosage improved pain in over half of the patients.[15] There may be an occasional ED role for **CCK-receptor antagonists** for pancreatitis pain that is refractory to **opioids**. The ED physician's lack of familiarity with **CCK-receptor antagonists** will usually mean *proglumide* or *loxiglumide* are reserved for use after consultation with physicians more accustomed to these agents.

Other drugs for which any pancreatitis analgesia role lies outside the ED include the viscosity-lowering agent *bromhexine*, the platelet-activating factor receptor antagonist *lexipafant*, and the protease inhibitors *aprotinin* or *gabexate*.[16,17] There are varying degrees of evidentiary support for these agents' efficacies, but none of the applicable data supports their early use in the acute care setting.

Given potent inhibitory effects on pancreatic secretion, *somatostatin* and its analog *octreotide* have been studied for use in pancreatitis. Prophylactic *somatostatin* may reduce the rate of pancreatitis after endoscopic retrograde cholangiopancreatography.[18] The acute care indications for this drug class are less clear. While some trial data suggests that *octreotide* (250 µg SC, followed by IV infusion of 0.5 µg/kg per h) useful for acute pancreatitis, meta-analysis of available evidence suggests minimal overall benefit.[19,20]

Several RCTs with analgesia as an endpoint failed to identify a pancreatitis treatment role for *glucagon*, *procaine*, or *cimetidine*.[21–23]

■ Summary and recommendations

First line: buprenorphine (initial dose 0.3 mg IV, then titrate)

Reasonable: other opioids (e.g. morphine initial dose 4–6 mg IV, then titrate)

Pregnancy: buprenorphine (initial dose 0.3 mg IV, then titrate)

Pediatric: buprenorphine (initial dose 2–6 µg/kg, then titrate)

Special cases:

- *opioid ingestion prior to, and suspected of causing, pancreatitis*: naloxone (0.4 mg IV)
- *known or suspected involvement of biliary tract*: buprenorphine (initial dose 0.3 mg IV, then titrate)
- *oral therapy appropriate*: tramadol (25–50 mg PO q4–6 h)

References

1. Mayerle J, Hlouschek V, Lerch MM. Current management of acute pancreatitis. *Nat Clin Pract Gastroenterol Hepatol*. 2005;**2**(10):473–483.
2. Thompson DR. Narcotic analgesic effects on the sphincter of Oddi: a review of the data and therapeutic implications in treating pancreatitis. *Am J Gastroenterol*. 2001;**96**(4):1266–1272.
3. Beckwith MC, Fox ER, Chandramouli J. Removing meperidine from the health-system formulary: frequently asked questions. *J Pain Palliat Care Pharmacother*. 2002;**16**(3):45–59.
4. Staritz M, Poralla T, Manns M, *et al*. Effect of modern analgesic drugs (tramadol, pentazocine, and buprenorphine) on the bile duct sphincter in man. *Gut*. 1986;**27**(5):567–569.

5. Hubbard GP, Wolfe KR. Meperidine misuse in a patient with sphincter of Oddi dysfunction. *Ann Pharmacother.* 2003;**37**(4):534–537.

6. Blamey SL, Finlay IG, Carter DC, *et al.* Analgesia in acute pancreatitis: comparison of buprenorphine and pethidine. *BMJ Clin Res Ed.* 1984;**288** (6429):1494–1495.

7. Moreno Escobosa MC, Amat Lopez J, Cruz Granados S, *et al.* Pancreatitis due to codeine. *Allergol Immunopathol (Madrid).* 2005;**33**(3):175–177.

8. Wilder-Smith CH, Hill L, Osler W, *et al.* Effect of tramadol and morphine on pain and gastrointestinal motor function in patients with chronic pancreatitis. *Dig Dis Sci.* 1999;**44**(6):1107–1116.

9. Ihse I, Andersson R, Albiin N, *et al.* [Guidelines for management of patients with chronic pancreatitis. Report from a consensus conference.] *Lakartidningen.* 2003;**100**(32–33):2518–2525.

10. Ebbehoj N, Friis J, Svendsen LB, *et al.* Indomethacin treatment of acute pancreatitis. A controlled double-blind trial. *Scand J Gastroenterol.* 1985;**20** (7):798–800.

11. Famularo G, Bizzarri C, Nicotra GC. Acute pancreatitis caused by ketorolac tromethamine. *J Clin Gastroenterol.* 2002;**34**(3):283–284.

12. Grover JK, Yadav S, Vats V, *et al.* Cyclo-oxygenase 2 inhibitors: emerging roles in the gut. *Int J Colorectal Dis.* 2003;**18**(4):279–291.

13. Davies NM, Longstreth J, Jamali F. Misoprostol therapeutics revisited. *Pharmacotherapy.* 2001;**21**(1):60–73.

14. McCleane GJ. The cholecystokinin antagonist proglumide has an analgesic effect in chronic pancreatitis. *Pancreas.* 2000;**21**(3):324–325.

15. Shiratori K, Takeuchi T, Satake K, *et al.* Clinical evaluation of oral administration of a cholecystokinin-A receptor antagonist (loxiglumide) to patients with acute, painful attacks of chronic pancreatitis: a multicenter dose-response study in Japan. *Pancreas.* 2002;**25**(1):e1–e5.

16. Tsujimoto T, Tsuruzono T, Hoppo K, *et al.* Effect of bromhexine hydrochloride therapy for alcoholic chronic pancreatitis. *Alcohol Clin Exp Res.* 2005;**29** (12 Suppl):272S–276S.

17. Valderrama R, Perez-Mateo M, Navarro S, *et al.* Multicenter double-blind trial of gabexate mesylate (FOY) in unselected patients with acute pancreatitis. *Digestion.* 1992;**51**(2):65–70.

18. Poon RT, Yeung C, Lo CM, *et al.* Prophylactic effect of somatostatin on post-ERCP pancreatitis: a randomized controlled trial. *Gastrointest Endosc.* 1999;**49** (5):593–598.

19. Heinrich S, Schafer M, Rousson V, *et al.* Evidence-based treatment of acute pancreatitis: a look at established paradigms. *Ann Surg.* 2006;**243**(2):154–168.

20. Beechey-Newman N. Controlled trial of high-dose octreotide in treatment of acute pancreatitis. Evidence of improvement in disease severity. *Dig Dis Sci.* 1993;**38**(4):644–647.

21. Broe PJ, Zinner MJ, Cameron JL. A clinical trial of cimetidine in acute pancreatitis. *Surg Gynecol Obstet.* 1982;**154**(1):13–16.

22. Olazabal A, Fuller R. Failure of glucagon in the treatment of alcoholic pancreatitis. *Gastroenterology.* 1978;**74**(3):489–491.

23. Kahl S, Zimmermann S, Pross M, *et al.* Procaine hydrochloride fails to relieve pain in patients with acute pancreatitis. *Digestion.* 2004;**69**(1):5–9.

Pharyngitis

KELLY YOUNG

■ Agents

- NSAIDs
- Aspirin
- Acetaminophen
- Corticosteroids
- Ambroxol mucolytic lozenges
- Local anesthetics
- Herbal preparations
- Antibiotics

■ Evidence

This chapter focuses on sore throat caused by viral or bacterial infection, and it assumes that clinicians exercise appropriate precautions about airway management and possible complicating diagnoses (e.g. retropharyngeal abscess). It is acknowledged that noninfectious causes of pharyngeal pain are important, and that these etiologies of sore throat have specific therapies. Examples are **proton pump inhibitors** for gastroesophageal reflux pain and *sucralfate* for postoperative pain (e.g. after uvulopalatopharyngoplasty).[1,2]

The **NSAIDs**, most commonly *ibuprofen*, are usually recommended for pain treatment of mild-to-moderate viral or bacterial pharyngitis (PG) in both adults and children.[3,4] The most commonly used initial dose is *ibuprofen* 400 mg PO (10 mg/kg in children), although doses up to 600–800 mg (maximum 2400 mg/day) are commonly prescribed. Other **NSAIDs** are likely similarly effective.[5,6]

Although there is no reason to suspect that IV administration (e.g. *ketorolac* 15 mg) relieves pain better than orally administered **NSAIDs**, avoiding the PO route may be advantageous. An alternative method of **NSAID** delivery that does not require swallowing (which can be painful or even impossible in

PG) is the lozenge; RCT data from the UK found *flurbiprofen* lozenges (8.75 or 15 mg) to be effective for infectious throat pain.[7-9]

Benzydamine, a topical **NSAID** (administered as a mouth rinse or spray), was found in trials in the 1980s to be effective for relieving PG pain, but there is no clear advantage to its use and the preparation is not available in the USA.[10,11] Other **NSAIDs**, including a mouthwash of *ketoprofen*, are superior in providing lasting pain relief in PG.[12]

Aspirin, commonly dosed at 400–800 mg orally, is also an effective PG pain reliever and is associated with symptomatic improvement as assessed at 2, 4, and 6 h post-administration.[13] *Aspirin* should not be given to children with PG because of the risk of Reye's syndrome. In adults, the addition of *caffeine* (64 mg) improves PG pain relief from *aspirin*.[14] Since *aspirin* causes more adverse events than *ibuprofen* or *acetaminophen* (*paracetamol*), there seems little reason to recommend its first-line use in the ED.[15]

Acetaminophen is also an effective reliever of mild pain, providing better PG relief than placebo within as little as 15 min.[16] The typical dose is 1000 mg (15 mg/kg in children). Even at (PO) doses of 1000 mg, *acetaminophen* is less effective than *ibuprofen* 400 mg PO.[3,17] In the (usually healthy) population with PG, *acetaminophen* and *ibuprofen* have similar tolerability and adverse event rates.[15]

Corticosteroids, administered IM or PO in single or multiple doses, hasten onset of both partial and complete pain relief in adults. In adults with exudative pharyngitis, *dexamethasone* (10 mg IM or PO) speeds onset of pain relief by 4 to 6 h, and speeds complete pain relief by 20 h.[18,19] *Prednisone* (60 mg PO) has similar effects.[15,20] The longer half-life of *dexamethasone* renders this **corticosteroid** preferable. There is no advantage in administering the (painful) IM injection, and the PO route should be used in patients who can tolerate it.[21]

In children, the utility of *dexamethasone* probably mirrors that of use of **corticosteroids** in adults with PG. Data from RCTs of children with moderate-to-severe PG demonstrate that PO *dexamethasone* (0.6 mg/kg to maximum of 10 mg) quickened onset of pain relief by 6–9 h.[22,23] In one of the pediatric studies, onset of pain relief was only hastened in the subset of patients with a positive rapid test for *Streptococcus*.[22] In terms of its effect on time to reach complete pain relief in children, *dexamethasone* was found of no benefit in one study but useful in another (which found it speeds time to pain resolution by 13 h).[22,23] In children, a multiple-dose approach (comprising three doses of *dexamethasone*) may bring complete pain relief more effectively than a single dose.[24] *Dexamethasone* has also been shown effective in treating pediatric PG presumed to be caused by mononucleosis.[25]

Although not commonly used in most ED settings, lozenges that deliver 20 mg *ambroxol* (a metabolite of the **mucolytic** *bromhexine*) may be of utility. Placebo-controlled trials have found these agents, administered up to six times daily, to have some benefit at relieving PG pain.[26,27]

Benzocaine (delivered by lozenges or spray) is commonly used for PG pain, but there are little applicable data for this indication. The lack of data for *benzocaine* use in PG, the demonstrated failure of this approach for some related throat conditions (e.g. post-tonsillectomy pain), and the potential risks of methemoglobinemia combine to render *benzocaine* an unlikely choice for acute care PG relief.[28–30]

Although there is little supporting evidence, the common practice of **opioid** prescription for some patients with PG pain appears to be for refractory or severe cases. A mild **opioid** such as *hydrocodone* (in combination with *acetaminophen*) is a reasonable, if not solidly evidence-based, approach.

Although occasional studies indicate possible benefit from some herbal preparations (e.g. herbal tea, sage spray), a 2007 Cochrane review concluded that there was insufficient evidence to recommend herbal preparations for relief of PG.[31–33] Another Cochrane review found that **antibiotics** probably confer some benefit in terms of pain relief, but the magnitude of the effect is small and other approaches will better serve the interests of the patient.[34,35] Recent evidence suggests that patients who request **antibiotics** for PG are really more interested in getting pain relief.[36]

■ Summary and recommendations

First line:

- NSAID (e.g. ibuprofen 400–800 mg PO QID; maximum daily dose 2400 mg)
- single-dose dexamethasone (0.6 mg/kg PO, maximum 10 mg)

Reasonable:

- acetaminophen (1000 mg PO QID)
- ambroxol 20 mg lozenge (up to six lozenges daily)

Pregnancy:

- acetaminophen (1000 mg PO)
- opioids for severe pain

Pediatric:

- NSAID (e.g. ibuprofen 10 mg/kg PO QID)
- single-dose dexamethasone 0.6 mg/kg PO (maximum of 10 mg)

Special cases:

- *inability to take oral medications*: single-dose IM dexamethasone (0.6 mg/kg to maximum dose of 10 mg)
- *severe pain*: opioids (e.g. oxycodone 5–10 mg PO q4-6 h)

References

1. Dore MP, Pedroni A, Pes GM, *et al*. Effect of antisecretory therapy on atypical symptoms in gastroesophageal reflux disease. *Dig Dis Sci*. 2007;**52**(2):463–468.
2. Zodpe P, Cho JG, Kang HJ, *et al*. Efficacy of sucralfate in the postoperative management of uvulopalatopharyngoplasty: a double-blind, randomized, controlled study. *Arch Otolaryngol Head Neck Surg*. 2006;**132**(10):1082–1085.
3. Schachtel BP, Fillingim JM, Thoden WR, *et al*. Sore throat pain in the evaluation of mild analgesics. *Clin Pharmacol Ther*. 1988; **44**(6):704–711.
4. Schachtel BP, Thoden WR. A placebo-controlled model for assaying systemic analgesics in children. *Clin Pharmacol Ther*. 1993; **53**(5):593–601.
5. Conti M. [Comparative, randomized, parallel clinical study of the effectiveness and safety of aceclofenac vs. paracetamol in the treatment of viral pharyngoamygdalitis.] *Acta Otorrinolaringol Esp*. 1997; **48**(2):133–137.
6. Weckx LL, Ruiz JE, Duperly J, *et al*. Efficacy of celecoxib in treating symptoms of viral pharyngitis: a double-blind, randomized study of celecoxib versus diclofenac. *J Int Med Res*. 2002;**30**(2):185–194.

7. Blagden M, Christian J, Miller K, *et al.* Multidose flurbiprofen 8.75 mg lozenges in the treatment of sore throat: a randomised, double-blind, placebo-controlled study in UK general practice centres. *Int J Clin Pract.* 2002;**56**(2):95–100.

8. Watson N, Nimmo WS, Christian J, *et al.* Relief of sore throat with the anti-inflammatory throat lozenge flurbiprofen 8.75 mg: a randomised, double-blind, placebo-controlled study of efficacy and safety. *Int J Clin Pract.* 2000; **54**(8):490–496.

9. Schachtel BP, Homan HD, Gibb IA, *et al.* Demonstration of dose response of flurbiprofen lozenges with the sore throat pain model. *Clin Pharmacol Ther.* 2002;**71**(5):375–380.

10. Wethington JF. Double-blind study of benzydamine hydrochloride, a new treatment for sore throat. *Clin Ther.* 1985;**7**(5):641–646.

11. Whiteside MW. A controlled study of benzydamine oral rinse ("Difflam") in general practice. *Curr Med Res Opin.* 1982;**8**(3):188–190.

12. Passali D, Volonte M, Passali GC, *et al.* Efficacy and safety of ketoprofen lysine salt mouthwash versus benzydamine hydrochloride mouthwash in acute pharyngeal inflammation: a randomized, single-blind study. *Clin Ther.* 2001;**23**(9):1508–1518.

13. Eccles R, Loose I, Jawad M, *et al.* Effects of acetylsalicylic acid on sore throat pain and other pain symptoms associated with acute upper respiratory tract infection. *Pain Med.* 2003;**4**(2):118–124.

14. Schachtel BP, Fillingim JM, Lane AC, *et al.* Caffeine as an analgesic adjuvant. A double-blind study comparing aspirin with caffeine to aspirin and placebo in patients with sore throat. *Arch Intern Med.* 1991;**151**(4):733–737.

15. Moore N, Le Parc JM, van Ganse E, *et al.* Tolerability of ibuprofen, aspirin and paracetamol for the treatment of cold and flu symptoms and sore throat pain. *Int J Clin Pract.* 2002;**56**(10):732–734.

16. Burnett I, Schachtel B, Sanner K, *et al.* Onset of analgesia of a paracetamol tablet containing sodium bicarbonate: a double-blind, placebo-controlled study in adult patients with acute sore throat. *Clin Ther.* 2006;**28**(9):1273–1278.

17. Lala I, Leech P, Montgomery L, *et al.* Use of a simple pain model to evaluate analgesic activity of ibuprofen versus paracetamol. *East Afr Med J.* 2000;**77**(9):504–507.

18. O'Brien JF, Meade JL, Falk JL. Dexamethasone as adjuvant therapy for severe acute pharyngitis. *Ann Emerg Med.* 1993;**22**(2):212–215.

19. Wei JL, Kasperbauer JL, Weaver AL, *et al.* Efficacy of single-dose dexamethasone as adjuvant therapy for acute pharyngitis. *Laryngoscope.* 2002;**112**(1):87–93.

20. Kiderman A, Yaphe J, Bregman J, *et al.* Adjuvant prednisone therapy in pharyngitis: a randomised controlled trial from general practice. *Br J Gen Pract.* 2005;**55**(512):218–221.

21. Marvez-Valls EG, Stuckey A, Ernst AA. A randomized clinical trial of oral versus intramuscular delivery of steroids in acute exudative pharyngitis. *Acad Emerg Med.* 2002;**9**(1):9–14.

22. Bulloch B, Kabani A, Tenenbein M. Oral dexamethasone for the treatment of pain in children with acute pharyngitis: a randomized, double-blind, placebo-controlled trial. *Ann Emerg Med.* 2003;**41**(5):601–608.

23. Olympia RP, Khine H, Avner JR. Effectiveness of oral dexamethasone in the treatment of moderate to severe pharyngitis in children. *Arch Pediatr Adolesc Med.* 2005;**159**(3):278–282.

24. Niland ML, Bonsu BK, Nuss KE, *et al.* A pilot study of 1 versus 3 days of dexamethasone as add-on therapy in children with streptococcal pharyngitis. *Pediatr Infect Dis J.* 2006;**25**(6):477–481.

25. Roy M, Bailey B, Amre DK, *et al.* Dexamethasone for the treatment of sore throat in children with suspected infectious mononucleosis: a randomized, double blind, placebo-controlled, clinical trial. *Arch Pediatr Adolesc Med.* 2004;**158**(3):250–254.

26. Fischer J, Pschorn U, Vix JM, *et al.* Efficacy and tolerability of ambroxol hydrochloride lozenges in sore throat. Randomised, double-blind, placebo-controlled trials regarding the local anaesthetic properties. *Arzneimittelforschung.* 2002;**52**(4):256–263.

27. Schutz A, Gund HJ, Pschorn U, *et al.* Local anaesthetic properties of ambroxol hydrochloride lozenges in view of sore throat. Clinical proof of concept. *Arzneimittelforschung.* 2002;**52**(3):194–199.

28. Dempster JH. Post-tonsillectomy analgesia: the use of benzocaine lozenges. *J Laryngol Otol.* 1988;**102**(9):813–814.

29. Becker K, Becker C, Frieling T, *et al.* Topical benzocaine anaesthesia lacks analgesic effects in painful non-acid oesophagitis. *Aliment Pharmacol Ther.* 1997;**11**(5):953–957.

30. Dahshan A, Donovan GK. Severe methemoglobinemia complicating topical benzocaine use during endoscopy in a toddler: a case report and review of the literature. *Pediatrics.* 2006;**117**(4):e806–e809.

31. Shi Y, Gu R, Liu C, *et al.* Chinese medicinal herbs for sore throat. *Cochrane Database Syst Rev.* 2007(3):CD004877.

32. Hubbert M, Sievers H, Lehnfeld R, *et al.* Efficacy and tolerability of a spray with *Salvia officinalis* in the treatment of acute pharyngitis: a randomised, double-blind, placebo-controlled study with adaptive design and interim analysis. *Eur J Med Res.* 2006;**11**(1):20–26.

33. Brinckmann J, Sigwart H, van Houten Taylor L. Safety and efficacy of a traditional herbal medicine (Throat Coat) in symptomatic temporary relief of pain in patients with acute pharyngitis: a multicenter, prospective, randomized, double-blinded, placebo-controlled study. *J Altern Complement Med.* 2003;**9**(2):285–298.

34. Del Mar CB, Glasziou PP, Spinks AB. Antibiotics for sore throat. *Cochrane Database Syst Rev.* 2006(4):CD000023.

35. Danchin MH, Curtis N, Nolan TM, *et al.* Treatment of sore throat in light of the Cochrane verdict: is the jury still out? *Med J Aust.* 2002;**177**(9):512–515.

36. van Driel ML, De Sutter A, Deveugele M, *et al.* Are sore throat patients who hope for antibiotics actually asking for pain relief? *Ann Fam Med.* 2006;**4**(6):494–499.

Postdural puncture headache

SOHAN PAREKH AND ANDY JAGODA

■ Agents

- Caffeine
- Gabapentin
- Epidural blood patch

■ Evidence

Postdural puncture headache (PDPH) complicates up to 5% of spinal taps and is also frequently seen postpartum (from anesthesia-related dural puncture). The best "treatment" for PDPH is prevention (e.g. use of small-caliber 22- or 24-gauge spinal needles, avoidance of multiple dural penetrations, replacement of stylet prior to withdrawing needle). Given PDPH's frequency, and the usual failure (as shown by meta-analysis) of nondrug interventions (i.e. bedrest), pharmacotherapy remains an important consideration.[1]

Case series data outline some utility of *acetaminophen* (*paracetamol*) for PDPH in postpartum patients.[2] Usually, more potent analgesia is required in patients presenting to the ED.

Although a variety of approaches to PDPH have been mentioned in reviews, the drug therapy with the most supporting evidence is *caffeine*. Oral formulations of *caffeine* (300 mg per dose) are more effective than placebo for PDPH.[3] Intravenous administration of *caffeine* (250–500 mg every 8 h) has been studied in a placebo-controlled fashion, but many of the supporting data includes co-administration of other drugs. Although the potential confounding effects of co-administered agents cannot be quantified, there is consistent indication that IV *caffeine* is at least partially effective for PDPH.[4]

Thrice-daily *gabapentin* is reported in case series to have efficacy in PDPH.[5] The evidence is preliminary, but administration of this **anticonvulsant** is of potential utility when *caffeine* fails or is not an option, and patients are not candidates for (or refuse) *epidural blood patch*.

Case report evidence also suggests efficacy of *corticotropin* (*adrenocorticotropic hormone*), but the data are insufficient to support a recommendation for its ED use in PDPH.[6,7]

Myriad types of epidural injections (e.g. *saline*, *dextran*) have been used in treating postdural puncture headaches.[8] By far the most common technique is the *epidural blood patch*, which entails injecting 10–25 mL of the patient's own blood into the epidural space. The *blood patch* should not be placed in the first 24 h after dural puncture, because of limitations in efficacy.[9,10] Furthermore, the technical requirements and training required to safely perform an *epidural blood patch* are beyond most acute care providers' scope of practice. When the *blood patch* is used, trial evidence and expert reviews suggest it is more efficacious than pharmacotherapy with either *caffeine* or **NSAIDs**.[10] For instance, one large series finds that the *epidural blood patch* completely alleviates pain in 75% of patients; 18% of patients have partial relief, and 7% have no symptomatic improvement.[11] The responsibility of the acute care provider to the patient with PDPH is often administration of temporizing pharmacotherapy pending availability of an *epidural blood patch*.

■ Summary and recommendations

First line: caffeine (300 mg PO, may be repeated in 4 h)

Reasonable: caffeine (500 mg IV, diluted in 1 L of IV fluid and administered over 1 h; may be repeated in 4 h)

Pregnancy:
- acetaminophen (1000 mg PO q6 h)
- caffeine (300 mg PO or 500 mg IV, diluted in 1 L of IV fluid and administered over 1 h; may be repeated in 4 h)

Pediatric: caffeine if age at least 12 years; IV dose of 250 mg diluted in 1 L of IV fluid and administered over 1 h; may be repeated in 4 h)

Special cases:
- *refractory pain and at least 24 h after dural puncture*: epidural blood patch
- *need for alternative to caffeine*: gabapentin 300 mg PO QD on day 1, 300 mg PO BID on day 2, then 300 mg PO TID

References

1. Thoennissen J, Herkner H, Lang W, *et al*. Does bed rest after cervical or lumbar puncture prevent headache? A systematic review and meta-analysis. *CMAJ*. 2001;**165**(10):1311–1316.

2. Imarengiaye C, Ekwere I. Postdural puncture headache: a cross-sectional study of incidence and severity in a new obstetric anaesthesia unit. *Afr J Med Sci*. 2006;**35**(1):47–51.

3. Camann WR, Murray RS, Mushlin PS, *et al*. Effects of oral caffeine on post-dural puncture headache. A double-blind, placebo-controlled trial. *Anesth Analg*. 1990;**70**(2):181–184.

4. Turnbull DK, Shepherd DB. Post-dural puncture headache: pathogenesis, prevention and treatment. *Br J Anaesth*. 2003;**91**(5):718–729.

5. Lin YT, Sheen MJ, Huang ST, *et al*. Gabapentin relieves post-dural puncture headache: a report of two cases. *Acta Anaesthesiol Taiwan*. 2007;**45**(1):47–51.

6. Ghai A, Wadhera R. Adrenocorticotrophic hormone: is a single dose sufficient for post-dural puncture headache? *Acta Anaesthesiol Scand*. 2007;**51**(2):266.

7. Kshatri AM, Foster PA. Adrenocorticotropic hormone infusion as a novel treatment for postdural puncture headache. *Reg Anesth*. 1997;**22**(5):432–434.

8. Choi A, Laurito CE, Cunningham FE. Pharmacologic management of post-dural puncture headache. *Ann Pharmacother*. 1996;**30**(7–8):831–839.

9. Gaiser R. Postdural puncture headache. *Curr Opin Anaesthesiol*. 2006;**19**(3):249–253.

10. Sandesc D, Lupei MI, Sirbu C, *et al*. Conventional treatment or epidural blood patch for the treatment of different etiologies of post dural puncture headache. *Acta Anaesthesiol Belg*. 2005;**56**(3):265–269.

11. Safa Tisseront V, Thormann F, Malassine P, *et al*. Effectiveness of epidural blood patch in the management of post-dural puncture headache. *Anesthesiology*. 2001;**95**(2):334–339.

Post-herpetic neuralgia

JEREMY ACKERMAN AND ADAM J. SINGER

■ Agents

- ■ Tricyclic antidepressants
- ■ Anticonvulsants
- ■ Opioids
- ■ Local anesthetics
- ■ Capsaicin
- ■ Ketamine

■ Evidence

Post-herpetic neuralgia (PHN) is one of the more commonly encountered manifestations of neuropathic pain. Pharmacotherapy remains the mainstay of PHN treatment, although other interventions (e.g. nerve stimulation, biofeedback) may have utility outside the acute care environment.[1,2] It should be emphasized that prompt treatment of acute herpes zoster decreases the risk of PHN development (and reduces the severity of PHN that does occur).[3]

Post-herpetic neuralgia is one of the many neuropathies for which **tricyclic antidepressants** (**TCAs**) are useful. At least three RCTs compare PHN pain relief between placebo and **TCAs** (*amitriptyline* in two studies and *desipramine* in the other).[4] Only two PHN patients need to be treated at least to achieve 50% pain relief in at least one study. Though the clinical difference is probably marginal, there is evidence to support selection of *nortriptyline* over *amitriptyline* based on the former agent achieving equal efficacy with fewer adverse effects.[5]

A placebo-controlled trial testing the **anticonvulsant** *gabapentin* found that one patient in three achieved significant pain relief.[6] Studies comparing **antidepressants** with **anticonvulsants** demonstrate similar efficacies (i.e. overlapping confidence intervals for pain relief measures). However, the incidence of adverse events leading to drug withdrawal is greater for the **TCAs**.[7] Consequently, based on the combination of efficacy with a favorable side effect profile, *gabapentin* is arguably the PO drug of first choice for PHN (*pregabalin* is another first-line choice, as noted below). The starting daily dose for *gabapentin* is 300 mg PO HS on day one, then 300 mg PO BID day two, and 300 mg PO TID thereafter (with up-titration as needed to 1800 mg/day maximum).

A multicenter trial of *pregabalin* found this agent to be useful for PHN, with a response rate of approximately one in three patients.[8] Another well-designed trial confirmed the utility of *pregabalin* as a means to control both pain and associated symptoms in PHN.[9]

Double-blind, randomized, crossover trials comparing the analgesic effects of **TCAs** and **opioids** have demonstrated that both approaches provide a similar degree of superiority over placebo.[10,11] Multiple **opioids** have been evaluated for PHN management, but other than data showing a lack of efficacy for *dextromethorphan*, no solid evidence exists to demonstrate superiority of one particular member of this class.[11-13]

Topical agents can also be used to treat PHN, and this can minimize systemic drug side effects. Pain and allodynia associated with PHN is reduced by various formulations of local anesthetics (e.g. 2% *lidocaine* gel, *eutectic mixture of local anesthetics* [*EMLA*] cream, 5% *lidocaine* impregnated patches).[14-16] The good quality of available evidence supporting topical *lidocaine* use for PHN has been highlighted by expert reviews of neuropathy treatment.[2] A useful approach allows for application of up to three 5% *lidocaine* impregnated patches to the painful area, for up to 12 h. Other approaches (e.g. for diabetic neuropathy treatment) have also been described. The *lidocaine* patch can be cut to fit the skin area over the involved dermatone; this serves to protect allodynic skin as well as providing a depot for the continuous release of the drug. Any topical preparation should only be applied to intact healed skin.

In addition to use by topical application, **local anesthetics** such as *lidocaine* may be efficacious when used for peripheral nerve blockade. There is little methodologically rigorous evidence addressing use of nerve blocks (e.g. of intercostal nerves). However, a large noncontrolled study found that virtually all patients with PHN in the study (96%) achieved pain relief after local SC 2% *lidocaine*, 0.5% *bupivacaine*, and 4 mg/mL *dexamethasone*.[17]

Administration of IV boluses of *lidocaine* (5 mg/kg) may be effective for PHN, but the potential dangers of this route rule out suggestion of its routine use.[18]

While its exact mechanism is unknown, topical *capsaicin* cream (0.025% to 0.075%) may reduce PHN pain in some patients. Clinical trials reveal a modest salutary effect of this chili pepper derivative, but its use is limited by the significant burning sensation many patients feel upon drug application.[12,19] Even trials suggesting *capsaicin*'s utility (e.g. studies finding it relieves pain in up to half of patients who can tolerate it) report that a third of those in whom the cream is tried find its application-associated burning "unbearable."[20]

Meta-analysis has been conducted to assess and compare some of the many treatments for PHN. Available data from RCT data for PHN show that roughly half of patients respond to **TCAs** or *oxycodone*, one in three improves with *gabapentin*, and approximately one in five achieves significant relief with *capsaicin*; *dextromethorphan* has no efficacy.[12]

Ketamine, commonly used in the ED as an adjunct for procedural sedation, has antagonistic effects at N-methyl-D-aspartic acid receptors. This activity is known to reduce pain and allodynia associated with PHN, but the overall side effect profile of *ketamine* does not allow its endorsement for regular use in PHN.[21]

■ Summary and recommendations

First line: 5% lidocaine patch (1–3 patches, applied up to 12 h/day)

Reasonable:
- gabapentin (300 mg PO HS day 1, 300 mg BID day 2, 300 mg TID thereafter)
- pregabalin (50 mg PO TID)

Pregnancy:
- 5% lidocaine patch (1–3 patches, applied up to 12 h/day)
- capsaicin cream (0.025% applied 4–5 times daily)

Pediatrics:

- 5% lidocaine patch (1–3 patches, applied up to 12 h/day)
- capsaicin cream (0.025% applied 4–5 times daily)

Special case:

- *patient failing above approaches*: nortriptyline (10–25 mg PO QHS), opioids (e.g. extended-release oxycodone 10 mg PO BID)

References

1. Kanazi GE, Johnson RW, Dworkin RH. Treatment of postherpetic neuralgia: an update. *Drugs*. 2000;**59**(5):1113–1126.
2. Attal N, Cruccu G, Haanpaa M, *et al*. EFNS guidelines on pharmacological treatment of neuropathic pain. *Eur J Neurol*. 2006;**13**(11):1153–1169.
3. Kost RG, Straus SE. Postherpetic neuralgia: pathogenesis, treatment, and prevention. *N Engl J Med*. 1996;**335**(1):32–42.
4. Collins SL, Moore RA, McQuay HJ, *et al*. Antidepressants and anticonvulsants for diabetic neuropathy and postherpetic neuralgia: a quantitative systematic review. *J Pain Symptom Manage*. 2000;**20**(6):449–458.
5. Watson CP, Vernich L, Chipman M, *et al*. Nortriptyline versus amitriptyline in postherpetic neuralgia: a randomized trial. *Neurology*. 1998;**51**(4):1166–1171.
6. Rice AS, Maton S. Gabapentin in postherpetic neuralgia: a randomised, double blind, placebo controlled study. *Pain*. 2001;**94**(2):215–224.
7. Chandra K, Shafiq N, Pandhi P, *et al*. Gabapentin versus nortriptyline in post herpetic neuralgia patients: a randomized, double-blind clinical trial – the GONIP Trial. *Int J Clin Pharmacol Ther*. 2006;**44**(8):358–363.
8. Dworkin RH, Corbin AE, Young JP, Jr., *et al*. Pregabalin for the treatment of postherpetic neuralgia: a randomized, placebo-controlled trial. *Neurology*. 2003;**60**(8):1274–1283.
9. Sabatowski R, Galvez R, Cherry DA, *et al*. Pregabalin reduces pain and improves sleep and mood disturbances in patients with post-herpetic neuralgia: results of a randomised, placebo-controlled clinical trial. *Pain*. 2004;**109**(1–2):26–35.
10. Watson CP, Babul N. Efficacy of oxycodone in neuropathic pain: a randomized trial in postherpetic neuralgia. *Neurology*. 1998;**50**(6):1837–1841.

11. Raja SN, Haythornthwaite JA, Pappagallo M, *et al.* Opioids versus antidepressants in postherpetic neuralgia: a randomized, placebo-controlled trial. *Neurology.* 2002;**59**(7):1015–1021.

12. Sindrup SH, Jensen TS. Efficacy of pharmacological treatments of neuropathic pain: an update and effect related to mechanism of drug action. *Pain.* 1999;**83**(3):389–400.

13. Rowbotham MC, Twilling L, Davies PS, *et al.* Oral opioid therapy for chronic peripheral and central neuropathic pain. *N Engl J Med.* 2003;**348**(13):1223–1232.

14. Galer BS, Rowbotham MC, Perander J, *et al.* Topical lidocaine patch relieves postherpetic neuralgia more effectively than a vehicle topical patch: results of an enriched enrollment study. *Pain.* 1999;**80**(3):533–538.

15. Rowbotham MC, Davies PS, Fields HL. Topical lidocaine gel relieves postherpetic neuralgia. *Ann Neurol.* 1995;**37**(2):246–253.

16. Attal N, Brasseur L, Chauvin M, *et al.* Effects of single and repeated applications of a eutectic mixture of local anaesthetics (EMLA) cream on spontaneous and evoked pain in post-herpetic neuralgia. *Pain.* 1999;**81**(1–2):203–209.

17. Bhargava R, Bhargava S, Haldia KN, *et al.* Jaipur block in postherpetic neuralgia. *Int J Dermatol.* 1998;**37**(6):465–468.

18. Kastrup J, Petersen P, Dejgard A, *et al.* Intravenous lidocaine infusion: a new treatment of chronic painful diabetic neuropathy? *Pain.* 1987;**28**(1):69–75.

19. Watson CP, Tyler KL, Bickers DR, *et al.* A randomized vehicle-controlled trial of topical capsaicin in the treatment of postherpetic neuralgia. *Clin Ther.* 1993;**15**(3):510–526.

20. Watson CP, Evans RJ, Watt VR. Post-herpetic neuralgia and topical capsaicin. *Pain.* 1988;**33**(3):333–340.

21. Eide PK, Jorum E, Stubhaug A, *et al.* Relief of post-herpetic neuralgia with the *N*-methyl-D-aspartic acid receptor antagonist ketamine: a double-blind, cross-over comparison with morphine and placebo. *Pain.* 1994;**58**(3):347–354.

Renal colic

ANDREW WORSTER

■ Agents studied

- Opioids
- NSAIDs
- Antispasmodics
- Diuretics

■ Evidence

Opioids have long served as the first-line analgesics for patients suffering from acute renal colic (RC). The two most-studied and most commonly used **opioids** for the ED treatment of RC are *morphine* and *meperidine* (*pethidine*). *Meperidine* is a synthetic **opioid** with higher lipid solubility than *morphine*; this means that *meperidine* has faster onset and a shorter duration of action. *Meperidine*'s pharmacologic characteristics, which increase its abuse potential, combine with risks from accumulation of a toxic metabolite (normeperidine) to render the drug theoretically less attractive than *morphine* for RC (or any other) analgesia. An ED-based RCT of patients with RC demonstrated equal analgesia between *morphine* (10 mg) and *meperidine* (100 mg).[1] Based on equianalgesia and the overall characteristics of the two most commonly used **opioids** for RC, we recommend *morphine* over *meperidine*.

If there is need for an **opioid** alternative to *morphine*, *hydromorphone* is recommended. The only RCT evaluating *hydromorphone* for ED treatment of RC compares fixed IV doses of either *hydromorphone* (1 mg) or *meperidine* (50 mg).[2] The authors reported that *hydromorphone* is more effective than *meperidine* in all patient-important outcomes.

The **NSAIDs** are believed to reduce RC-associated pain by inhibiting prostaglandin synthesis and release. Cochrane review of RCTs of RC comparing any **opioid** with any **NSAID** concluded that both reduce patient-reported pain scores.[3] The Cochrane review also reported that those receiving **NSAIDs** are less likely to require rescue medication and less likely to vomit than those receiving opioids. However, the review did not address GI bleeding or renal impairment, which constitute the two most serious **NSAID**-associated adverse events. Furthermore, since *meperidine* was the **opioid** used in most of the reviewed studies, it is possible that some of the effects attributed to **opioids** might, in fact, be less likely in patients receiving *morphine* or *hydromorphone*.

An RCT published after that Cochrane review adds important data to the consideration of RC treatment in the ED. A comparison of *morphine* (5 mg IV, repeated after 20 min), *ketorolac* (15 mg IV, repeated after 20 min), and a combination of both, found that dual therapy provides significantly better pain relief than either drug alone. The combination of *morphine* plus *ketorolac* was also associated with a decreased requirement for rescue analgesia.[4] In North America, the major advantage of *ketorolac* is its availability for parenteral delivery. This advantage is important, since many patients with RC have associated nausea and vomiting and cannot tolerate oral medication. There is also a role for *ketorolac* monotherapy for patients in whom **opioids** are contraindicated. The **NSAID** *metamizole* is found in Cochrane review to be effective when given IV, but this agent's association with blood dyscrasias renders it unavailable in some countries (e.g. USA, UK) and its use is not recommended.[5]

Currently developing evidence suggests that the most effective pain medications for RC might prove to be neither **NSAIDs** nor **opioids**. Instead, the optimal approach to RC relief may entail administration of medications that relieve symptoms by inducing rapid stone passage. A systematic review of RCTs evaluating **calcium channel blockers** or **alpha-adrenergic blockers** for RC found both effectively relieved pain and facilitated stone passage in patients amenable to conservative management.[6] Although the results are promising for ED patients, acute care use of this therapeutic approach requires tailoring therapy to stone size and location. In the future, ED provider understanding of this information may broaden acute care therapeutic options for RC.

The fact that ureteral smooth muscle spasm is a primary mediator of RC pain has prompted investigations of **antispasmodic** (**antimuscarinic**) agents for analgesia. Unfortunately, available data fail to demonstrate utility for this approach. In patients receiving primary RC analgesia with *ketorolac*, addition of sublingual *hyoscyamine sulfate* (0.125 mg) offers no advantage over placebo.[7] Another well-designed RCT revealed that there was no benefit in adding *hyoscine butylbromide* for patients receiving *morphine*; the lack of benefit was consistent regardless of *indomethacin* co-administration.[8] The use of **antimuscarinic** agents for the treatment of RC pain, while theoretically attractive, has no basis in clinical evidence.

Given the fact that most ureteral stones are small enough to pass spontaneously, it is thought that **diuretics** (with or without IV fluid therapy) might relieve RC pain by facilitating movement of the stone into the bladder. The evidence does not support diuresis as a means for pain relief. A Cochrane systematic review evaluating the benefits and harms of **diuretics** (with or without above-maintenance IV fluid administration) found no data supporting efficacy.[9] Furthermore, the review cautioned that attempting to "flush stones through" risks ureteral rupture or renal damage secondary to rapid increases in collecting system pressure.[9] Adequate fluid replacement is important, since dehydration is often contributory to ureteral stone formation. However, there is no role for aggressive administration of IV fluids.

■ Summary and recommendations

First line: combination therapy with morphine (initial dose 4–6 mg IV, then titrate) plus ketorolac (15–30 mg IV QID)

Reasonable: hydromorphone (initial dose 1 mg IV, then titrate) plus an NSAID (e.g. ibuprofen 600–800 mg PO QID, maximum daily dose 2400 mg)

Pregnancy: morphine (initial dose 4–6 mg IV, then titrate)

Pediatric: combination therapy with morphine (initial dose 0.05–0.1 mg/kg IV, then titrate) plus ketorolac (0.5 mg/kg IV QID)

Special case:
■ *patients in whom opioids are to be avoided*: ketorolac 15–30 mg IV QID

References

1. O'Connor A, Schug SA, Cardwell H. A comparison of the efficacy and safety of morphine and pethidine as analgesia for suspected renal colic in the emergency setting. *J Accid Emerg Med.* 2000;**17**(4):261–264.

2. Jasani NB, O'Conner RE, Bouzoukis JK. Comparison of hydromorphone and meperidine for ureteral colic. *Acad Emerg Med.* 1994;**1**(6):539–543.

3. Holdgate A, Pollock T. Nonsteroidal anti-inflammatory drugs (NSAIDs) versus opioids for acute renal colic. *Cochrane Database Syst Rev.* 2005(2):CD004137.

4. Safdar B, Degutis L, Landry K, *et al.* Intravenous morphine plus ketorolac is superior to either drug alone for treatment of acute renal colic. *Ann Emerg Med.* 2006;**48**:173–181.

5. Edwards JE, Meseguer F, Faura C, *et al.* Single dose dipyrone for acute renal colic pain. *Cochrane Database Syst Rev.* 2002(4):CD003867.

6. Hollingsworth JM, Rogers MA, Kaufman SR, *et al.* Medical therapy to facilitate urinary stone passage: a meta-analysis. *Lancet.* 2006;**368**(9542):1171–1179.

7. Jones JB, Giles BK, Brizendine EJ, *et al.* Sublingual hyoscyamine sulfate in combination with ketorolac tromethamine for ureteral colic: a randomized, double-blind, controlled trial. *Ann Emerg Med.* 2001;**37**(2):141–146.

8. Holdgate A, Oh CM. Is there a role for antimuscarinics in renal colic? A randomized controlled trial. *J Urol.* 2005;**174**(2):572–575; discussion 575.

9. Worster A, Richards C. Fluids and diuretics for acute ureteric colic. *Cochrane Database Syst Rev.* 2005(3):CD004926.

Sialolithiasis

SAMUEL KIM AND JOHN H. BURTON

■ Agents

- ■ NSAIDs
- ■ Opioids
- ■ Sialogogues

■ Evidence

Conservative treatment of sialolithiasis pain consists of **sialagogues** (e.g. lemon drops), mild analgesics (e.g. *acetaminophen [paracetamol]*, **NSAIDs**), **opioids**, mechanical stimulation, and warm compresses.[1] A variety of nonpharmacological treatment modalities may be necessary if, as is often the case, pharmacotherapy fails.[2,3] The goal of drug therapy is to temporize until, and hopefully facilitate (in the case of **sialogogues**), passage of the stone.[4]

Unfortunately, in many cases, the stone moves into the salivary gland (e.g. parotid) rather than passing externally. Surgical intervention is frequently needed and analgesic approaches in acute care do not obviate the need for ENT evaluation.

Given the importance of surgical intervention to relieve salivary tract stone disease (and symptoms), it is not surprising that no clinical trials assess the comparative efficacy of drug treatment options for treating sialolithiasis pain. Textbooks recommend traditional analgesics, separately or in combination. **NSAIDs**, *acetaminophen*, and various **opioids** (e.g. *hydrocodone*, *oxycodone*) are usually recommended. Given the inflammatory component to parotitis and sialolithiasis, **NSAIDs** are the most reasonable initial choice, but it must be acknowledged that there is little evidence basis for treatment decisions in this population.

■ Summary and recommendations

First line:

■ sialogogues (e.g. tart candies such as lemon drops)
■ NSAIDs (e.g. ibuprofen 400–600 mg PO QID)

Reasonable: acetaminophen (650–1000 mg PO QID)

Pregnancy: tart candies and acetaminophen (650–1000 mg PO QID)

Pediatric: tart candies, NSAIDs (e.g. ibuprofen 400–600 mg PO QID)

Special case:

■ *severe or refractory pain*: opioids (e.g. oxycodone 5–10 mg PO q4–6 h)

References

1. Pollack CV, Jr., Severance HW, Jr. Sialolithiasis: case studies and review. *J Emerg Med*. 1990;**8**(5):561–565.
2. Knight J. Diagnosis and treatment of sialolithiasis. *Ir Med J*. 2004;**97**(10):314–315.
3. McGurk M, Escudier MP, Brown JE. Modern management of salivary calculi. *Br J Surg*. 2005;**92**(1):107–112.
4. Williams MF. Sialolithiasis. *Otolaryngol Clin North Am*. 1999;**32**(5):819–834.

Sickle cell crisis

HANS BRADSHAW AND DALE WOOLRIDGE

■ Agents

- Oxygen
- Opioids
- NSAIDs
- Ribonuclease reductase inhibitor
- Corticosteroids
- Nitric oxide
- Poloxamer 188

■ Evidence

The analgesic approach to sickle cell vaso-occlusive crisis (VOC) depends on the episode's severity, which can vary between patients and even within an individual's successive presentations. Therapy may be further complicated by the fact that patients with VOC represent a population with recurring pain and frequent ED visits. Frustration on the part of patients and providers can result, putting VOC patients at risk for oligoanalgesia even in current times of focus on appropriate pain medication administration.[1,2]

In VOC, the directive to "trust the patient" is of paramount importance: patients' self-reports of pain should be heeded and acted upon, even if patients are sometimes demanding (as would be expected, given the frequent undertreatment of their symptoms). Sickle cell crisis remains a manifestation of a disease process that is ultimately fatal. Acute care providers should keep this eventuality in mind when dealing with these patients.

An improving understanding of VOC pathophysiology is outlined by a broad and informative literature. Clinicians are well aware of the imperative to seek and correct any underlying causes of VOC (e.g. renal failure, sepsis, pulmonary dysfunction). However, there are surprisingly few data directly comparing one therapy with another. In fact, a recent Cochrane review concluded that there is insufficient evidence to allow for definitive assessments across different regimens.[3] Consequently, consensus guidelines play an important role in differentiating from the available analgesic approaches.

SUPPORTIVE MEASURES: OXYGEN AND INTRAVENOUS FLUIDS

The first interventions in managing VOC pain are supportive therapies. Recommendations to decrease VOC duration by administration of *oxygen* and *IV fluids* are physiologically well grounded, and such interventions form part of nearly all VOC care protocols.[4] Given the plausibility of benefit and implausibility of harm, we concur with this recommendation.[5] Nonetheless, it is noteworthy that the evidence supporting utility of *oxygen* and *IV fluids* is not robust. Furthermore, there are very few data guiding decisions as to how *oxygen* or *IV fluids* should be given.

An example placebo-controlled pediatric study assessed administration of 50% *oxygen* as adjunctive therapy to continuously administered *morphine*. The investigators could show no further analgesic effect with *oxygen*; it reduced neither pain severity nor number of pain sites.[6] Another RCT, while finding *oxygen* reduced the number of reversibly sickled cells, failed to demonstrate *oxygen*-mediated effects on pain severity, need for **opioids**, or hospitalization rate.[7] Clinical trials have also failed to demonstrate any VOC pain endpoint advantages to adding *oxygen* to non-opioid therapy (e.g. *hydroxyurea*).[8]

Most studies assess use of 50% *oxygen*, but there are no data to demonstrate superiority for this concentration. Some data indicate potential VOC utility for *hyperbaric oxygen*, which effectively improves oxygenation and can reverse local sickling.[9,10] Since there are no methodologically rigorous data demonstrating the utility of *hyperbaric oxygen* in VOC, and since its induction of vasoconstriction has been theorized to be deleterious in sickle cell patients, we do not recommend emergent *hyperbaric oxygen* for VOC.[11]

The theory underlying *IV fluid* administration is that, like supplemental *oxygen*, hydration reduces the duration of the VOC episode. Many experienced clinicians use hypotonic *IV fluids*. Recommendations from an NIH panel are typical: $D_5\frac{1}{2}NS$ (plus 20 mEq/L potassium), with total fluid infusion equal to 1.5 times maintenance.[12] While such a choice is not based upon definitive evidence, it is physiologically reasonable: intravascular sludging and low-flow states undoubtedly contribute to sickling and VOC pain. Despite the rational underpinning to *IV fluid* therapy in VOC, a 2007 Cochrane review failed to find studies addressing types, quantities, or administration routes for fluid replacement in acute sickle disease.[4] Therefore, recommendations for adjunctive *IV fluids* in VOC are accompanied by acknowledgment of the need for further studies assessing relative values of differing approaches.

Supportive therapy with *oxygen* and *IV fluids* constitute adjunctive measures only. They must be complemented by a stepwise pain medication regimen that, for ED purposes, currently consists of occasional *acetaminophen* (*paracetamol*) and **NSAIDs**, with **opioids** forming the mainstay of therapy.

ACETAMINOPHEN AND NSAIDs

Mild VOC pain can be treated with oral *acetaminophen* or **NSAIDs**.[12–14] Other oral **NSAIDs** are probably equally acceptable for nonsevere VOC pain; among those recommended are *naproxen* and *diclofenac*.[13] In VOC patients who present to the ED, the most likely role for PO *acetaminophen* or **NSAID** therapy will be in situations where VOC pain is mild, or when **opioid** use is to be avoided or minimized.[12]

Although there is some role for PO **NSAIDs** in mild VOC, the place of parenteral **NSAIDs** is not as clear. Relevant lessons from the available literature follow. First, there are no trials demonstrating superiority of IV or IM **NSAIDs** over the same or similar medications administered orally. Second, there is a divergence between nontrial evidence (e.g. clinical reviews), which often includes mention of *ketorolac*'s utility, and evidence from clinical trials, which suggest only limited efficacy of parenteral **NSAID**.[15–20] Third, *ketorolac* monotherapy provides adequate pain relief in only half of unselected VOC patients.[19] Monotherapy with the injectable **NSAID** appears most likely to succeed where pain is not severe (i.e. pain score is less than 7 on a 10-point scale), and when there is VOC pain in three or fewer body sites.[19,20]

One potentially useful advantage to *ketorolac* (or any other **NSAID**) would be if its administration had an **opioid**-sparing effect. The question has been assessed in studies, which gave mixed results. A pediatric RCT of *ketorolac* (0.9 mg/kg IV) versus placebo for adjunctive analgesia (to *morphine*) found no *ketorolac*-associated benefit in total **opioid** dose, reduction in pain severity, rate of hospitalization, or (for discharged patients) rate of return to the ED.[21] Two studies in adults report opposite findings. A trial with limited applicability to current ED practice suggested that *ketorolac* may provide clinical synergism with IM *meperidine* (*pethidine*).[22] A more methodologically rigorous ED RCT found no **opioid**-sparing effect associated with IM *ketorolac*.[23] Consensus reviews tend to conclude that there is some **opioid**-sparing effect from *ketorolac*, and that the injectable **NSAIDs** have a role in the initial therapy of VOC.[13,14] The reviews are consistent in their recommendations that *ketorolac* be used for no more than three to five days in a given episode of VOC.[13]

Like other **NSAIDs**, *ketorolac* is not without risk in VOC. The patient may be at increased risk for **NSAID**-associated effects on renal blood flow and platelet function.[12] Close attention to renal function should accompany *ketorolac* use in VOC patients, but the **NSAID** side effects do not preclude occasional utility of this class in VOC – especially when therapy is limited to a few initial doses to help to get pain under control.[24]

OPIOIDS

Although the **NSAIDs** may be occasionally used as monotherapy, and may have some efficacy as adjuvant therapy, the cornerstone of VOC treatment in the ED is **opioids**. Administered by a variety of methods, **opioids** can safely and effectively relieve VOC pain. As is the case with many chronic disease states, there are inevitable issues with respect to **opioid** dependency. The role of the acute care provider is to act within the patient's longitudinal care plan, coordinating **opioid** care with outpatient providers where possible. However, the prime goal of the ED provider remains relief of the patient's pain using whatever means are possible; physicians should err on the side of **opioid** administration when other choices are unavailable.

The first route to consider for **opioids** in VOC is the PO route. Although most VOC patients in the ED will have IV access, and the IV route remains preferred for severe pain, clinical experience and Cochrane review concur that there is a role for PO **opioids**.[3] One of the most common indications for PO **opioids** is use in a patient who has had adequate relief with IV **opioids** and who will be discharged from the ED. In such cases a predischarge trial of an orally administered agent such as *morphine* is recommended.

Orally administered controlled-release preparations of *morphine* have been used with success in VOC, as long as they are supplemented with additional medication (oral or parenteral) as needed. Recommended dosages for controlled-release *morphine* are 30–60 mg every 8–12 h for adults (maximum 180 mg daily), and for children 1.9 mg/kg every 12 h, with doses rounded off to the nearest strength of 15, 30, or 60 mg.[25] Physicians in ED lacking experience prescribing these controlled-release **opioid** preparations are well advised to discuss the care with the physician who will be providing follow-up.

Although the PO and (for patients with no IV access) SC routes of **opioid** administration may be useful in acute care management of VOC, most patients in the ED setting should be treated with IV **opioids**.[2,12] The benchmark **opioid** for parenteral therapy of VOC is *morphine*, which for acute sickle cell pain is best administered by scheduled around-the-clock dosing, or via PCA (see discussion below).[13,14] The usual level of VOC pain severity warrants aggressive *morphine* dosing: doses of 5–10 mg in adults (0.10–0.15 mg/kg in children) should be repeated as needed, with literature supporting frequent administration (as often as every 5 min initially, with appropriate monitoring).[12,13,25–27] *Hydromorphone* (1.5 mg in adults, or 0.015–0.020 mg/kg in children) is also recommended.[12]

As a (non-PCA) continuous infusion, *morphine* can be administered in adults at a starting dose of 0.8 mg/h. Higher starting doses will often be necessary since VOC patients are not **opioid** naïve, and the infusion rate can be titrated up to 10 mg/h. For children, a starting dose of 0.04 mg/kg per hour can be titrated to relief (in increments of 0.02 mg/kg per hour) to a maximum of 0.1 mg/kg per hour.[13] Continuous *hydromorphone* infusions can also be administered for adults, at a starting dose of 0.25 mg/h (titrate to a maximum of 0.5 mg/h), and in children (starting dose of 0.004 mg/kg per hour, titrated in increments of 0.002 mg/kg per hour to a maximum of 0.01 mg/kg per hour).[13,25,27,28]

There is evidence suggesting that *morphine* and its metabolite, morphine 6-glucuronide, may play a role in development of acute chest crisis (by respiratory depression, histamine release, or via an unknown mechanism). However, these data appear to apply to chronic use of oral *morphine*.[29] The acute care clinician should not allow these concerns to prevent appropriate dosing of *morphine*.

Other **opioid** agonists and agonist–antagonists have been investigated for IV use in VOC. Alternatives include *fentanyl*, which is particularly useful for patients who cannot tolerate *morphine* owing to excessive pruritis and nausea.[13] *Methadone*'s long half-life and associated titration difficulty render it a poor choice for VOC pain.[13,14]

The role of *meperidine* in VOC is a subject of dispute. The weight of expert opinion is such that it simply cannot be recommended for routine use.[12] However, *meperidine* has an extensive history of efficacy, and patients in whom it has safely relieved pain for years are understandably suspicious when they are informed that the drug is "unsafe." Even critics of *meperidine*'s use in VOC acknowledge its role for brief treatment courses in patients who have responded well to it in the past, and who may not tolerate other agents.[13] Accumulation of *meperidine*'s metabolite, normeperidine, does indeed incur risks of irritability, CNS stimulation, seizures, and poor pain control – but such accumulation is highly unlikely in the initial hours of an ED stay.[13,14,25,26,30,31] If patients in pain insist upon *meperidine*, the acute care clinician should exercise judgment rather than categorically refuse to administer the drug. *Meperidine* should be an **opioid** of choice in patients with documented intolerance (e.g. anaphylaxis) to *morphine* and *hydromorphone*.[13,14] *Meperidine* use should be limited to less than 48 h, at doses less than 600 mg per day, and use of the drug should be avoided in patients with renal compromise or in those taking monoamine oxidase inhibitors. *Meperidine* is also a poor choice for use in PCA devices, since its repeat administration poses particular seizure risks in VOC patients.[32]

Nalbuphine, a synthetic **opioid** with agonist–antagonist activity, may be useful in children and adults who require infrequent pain treatment. The benefits of *nalbuphine* (adult dosage, 0.3 mg/kg up to 20 mg, with maximum dose 160 mg/day) include an excellent adverse effect profile. *Nalbuphine* is associated with relatively less nausea, sedation, and respiratory depression compared with pure **opioid** agonists. A retrospective analysis of children receiving *nalbuphine* for VOC found this agonist–antagonist at least as effective as *morphine*, with some endpoints (e.g. development of acute chest syndrome) favoring *nalbuphine*.[33] The authors concluded that prospective study is necessary to delineate any advantages of *nalbuphine*.[33] More study is required before widespread adoption of *nalbuphine*, since the agent's antagonist properties have disadvantages. The most important issue with *nalbuphine* is its ceiling dose of 20 mg every 3 h, which is necessitated by the agent's antagonist activity. Therefore, if pain is not controlled after titration to 20 mg every 3 h, *nalbuphine* should be stopped and the patient should be given a pure **opioid** agonist. Also, *nalbuphine*'s antagonist properties preclude its use in patients who have frequent or regular need for pure-agonist **opioids** (owing to the risk of acute withdrawal symptoms).[13,14,28]

Transdermal *fentanyl* (25–50 µg/h) has been administered to children in an open-label trial assessing its use as adjunctive therapy to *morphine* PCA.[34] The trial's authors concluded that further study is necessary to elucidate the pharmacology of transdermal *fentanyl* in children. While acute care recommendation of this approach must await further data, the finding of subjective improvement in pain relief in 70% of patients indicates promise for transdermal *fentanyl*. At this time, the role of transdermal *fentanyl* appears limited to chronic-care use.[12]

Opioids comprise the mainstay of therapy of VOC in pregnancy, although *acetaminophen* may also be useful in gravida with mild pain.[35]

PATIENT-CONTROLLED ANALGESIA

The PCA technology is of high potential utility in the ED management of VOC. Pumps can be set for basal (i.e. constant) infusion rate and bolus doses; a "lockout" interval after each bolus dose prevents stacking of analgesic doses and reduces chances of toxicity. The PCA is a valuable tool for ED clinicians, but acute care providers who are unfamiliar with the device should execute PCA orders in consultation with experienced users.

Before discussion of particular regimens, some initial points are important to make. First, PCA pumps are not universally available in EDs, and intermittent IV **opioids** remain a reasonable therapeutic choice. Second, even if PCA devices are to be used, adequate pain relief should be obtained before institution of PCA therapy.[13,36] Third, although PCA therapy for VOC offers the ability to achieve and maintain optimal analgesia with minimal sedation and few side effects, pharmacokinetic data demonstrate the critical import of an individualized approach.[36-39] Finally, it is necessary to monitor pain, since some patients (particularly children who do not properly understand PCA) fail to self-administer analgesia despite ongoing pain.[17]

For those acute care providers who do have access to PCA, VOC offers an excellent opportunity to take full advantage of the technology. Trials demonstrate safety and efficacy of PCA administration of constant and demand low-dose *morphine* or *hydromorphone* in patients as young as eight years of age.[13,40-44] A small nonrandomized, nonblinded trial of PCA **opioid** treatment for pediatric VOC found that patients, families, and hospital staff preferred PCA to traditional IV bolus therapy.[40] As assessed by a variety of physiological and psychological endpoints, most patients and families were satisfied with PCA use.[41-43]

The PCA regimen appears to be related to therapeutic success for VOC. A nonrandomized review of 26 children, hospitalized with PCA therapy on 60 occasions, compared the alternative regimens of high bolus dose with low basal infusion, and low bolus dose with high basal infusion. The high bolus/low basal regimen was preferable; children receiving this regimen used significantly less **opioid**, had shorter hospital stays, and reported lower pain scores by the second day of therapy.[44]

Specific regimens for PCA use in VOC have been investigated. *Morphine* is often used and is both safe and effective.[13,14,26] The PCA parameters for *morphine* include bolus doses of 0.01 to 0.05 mg/kg, with a lockout interval of 6–15 min. Basal infusion can be provided either around the clock or at nighttime, in doses ranging between 0.01 to 0.07 mg/kg per hour.[13] For patients with an established bolus dosing pattern, the basal infusion can be instituted at 25% of the hourly bolus dose that has been required to control pain.

For *hydromorphone* use in PCA pumps, adults should receive bolus doses between 0.05 and 0.5 mg IV, with a lockout interval of 5–15 min. The supplemental basal infusion should be titrated up to 0.2 mg/h. For children, *hydromorphone* bolus doses should be 0.003 to 0.005 mg/kg, with the same lockout interval as adults (5–15 min), and a basal infusion of 0.001 mg/kg per hour.

OTHER AGENTS

The role of **corticosteroids** in treating VOC continues to evolve. Data of primarily historical interest suggest potential utility of *hydrocortisone* monotherapy (with *IV fluids*).[45] More recently, a 2006 Cochrane review provides supporting evidence for use of **corticosteroids** in VOC. The review concluded that acute care use of this class incurs little risk, and that such use shortens both the the time period over which **opioids** are required and also the length of hospital stay.[3] One of the review's cited studies is a trial of high-dose *methylprednisolone* (15 mg/kg IV upon presentation and 24 h later) that found **corticosteroid** administration reduced the duration of VOC episodes.[46] Patients receiving acute **corticosteroids** do not have significant side effects, but those receiving *methylprednisolone* are significantly more likely to have recurrent VOC soon after hospital discharge than those receiving placebo.[46] Others consider that **corticosteroid** use in VOC is controversial and have identified poor tolerance of longer courses of **corticosteroids**.[47] Given the lack of definitive evidence supporting use in the ED, the need for high-dose therapy, and the fact that supporting evidence requires a **corticosteroid** regimen that must be given during hospitalization, the ED physician is advised to consult with admitting physicians before instituting **corticosteroid** therapy for VOC.

Preliminary data demonstrate potential utility for *nitric oxide* (80 ppm administered with 21% oxygen) for VOC. An RCT of children receiving **opioid** analgesia found that *nitric oxide* administration was associated with a decrease in **opioid** requirement over 6 h (but not over 4 h) compared with placebo.[48] When pain score changes (on a 10 cm scale) over the study treatment time were considered, patients receiving *nitric oxide* had a 1 cm/h greater reduction in pain over the course of the treatment.[48] The failure of the study's endpoints results to demonstrate consistent benefit from *nitric oxide* mean that there is no current indication for *nitric oxide* in ED therapy of VOC, but that further data may identify a future role.

Of the novel therapies for treating VOC, *hydroxyurea*, a **ribonuclease reductase inhibitor** that increases amounts of fetal hemoglobin (which does not sickle), appears to have the most promise. *Hydroxyurea* can decrease the incidence and severity of pain episodes by as much as 50%, but the existing studies primarily address its utility in management settings outside the ED.[49-52] There is suggestion that short-term use of *hydroxyurea* may someday have a role in acute management, but there is no current indication for its use as ED therapy.[51,53]

Adults receiving *hydroxyurea*, as well as children under 15 years of age, appear to be potential beneficiaries from administration of IV *poloxamer 188* (a rheologic compound that is theorized to improve tissue oxygenation).[54] One trial found that administration of *poloxamer 188* (100 mg/kg for 1 h followed by 30 mg/kg per hour for 47 h) reduced the duration of VOC and increased the proportion of patients achieving crisis resolution.[55] A more recent pooled analysis sheds light on patients most likely to benefit from *poloxamer 188*, identifying children under 15 as a potentially high-yield group for rheologic therapy.[54] For undifferentiated patients with VOC, the pooled analysis indicates there is safety, but little efficacy, for *poloxamer 188*.[54] *Poloxamer 188* may have a role in the acute care setting, particularly for patients who are expected to be in the ED for an extended duration of time. However, since the infusion is a prolonged one, and since there is a paucity of supporting data, the ED physician considering *poloxamer 188* is advised to discuss use of the drug with the physician who will be admitting the patient.

SUMMARY AND RECOMMENDATIONS

First line:

- oxygen (50%)
- above-maintenance IV fluids (e.g. $D_5\frac{1}{2}NS$)

- morphine bolus dosing (initial dose 4–6 mg IV, then titrate) followed if possible by PCA (0.01–0.04 mg/kg per hour basal rate, 0.01–0.05 mg/kg bolus dose with lockout 6–15 min)

Reasonable: other opioid (e.g. hydromorphone initial dose 1 mg IV, then titrate)

Pregnancy:
- acetaminophen (650–1000 mg PO QID)
- morphine bolus dosing (initial dose 4–6 mg IV, then titrate) followed if possible by PCA (0.01–0.04 mg/kg per hour basal rate, 0.01–0.05 mg/kg bolus dose with lockout 6–15 min)

Pediatric: morphine bolus dosing (initial dose 0.05–0.1 mg IV, then titrate) followed if possible by PCA (0.01–0.04 mg/kg per hour basal rate, 0.01–0.05 mg/kg bolus dose with lockout 6–15 min)

Special cases:
- *mild VOC pain*: acetaminophen PO (1 g in adults, 10–15 mg/kg in children) or ibuprofen (600–800 mg in adults, 10 mg/kg in children); other NSAIDs are also acceptable
- *if renal function normal*: consider NSAID (e.g. ketorolac 15–30 mg IV QID)
- *transitioning to oral morphine*:
  - initial PO dose of regular-release morphine 0.3 mg/kg (or 10–30 mg), q3–4 h
  - initial PO dose of controlled-release morphine 1.9 mg/kg, rounded off to nearest available strength (15, 30, 60 mg), q12 h
- *if patient is being admitted and has refractory pain*: consider corticosteroids, hydroxyurea, or poloxamer 188 in consultation with admitting team

References

1. Linklater DR, Pemberton L, Taylor S, *et al*. Painful dilemmas: an evidence-based look at challenging clinical scenarios. *Emerg Med Clin North Am*. 2005;**23** (2):367–392.
2. Tanabe P, Myers R, Zosel A, *et al*. Emergency department management of acute pain episodes in sickle cell disease. *Acad Emerg Med*. 2007;**14**(5):419–425.

3. Dunlop RJ, Bennett KC. Pain management for sickle cell disease. *Cochrane Database Syst Rev.* 2006(2):CD003350.

4. Okomo U, Meremikwu MM. Fluid replacement therapy for acute episodes of pain in people with sickle cell disease. *Cochrane Database Syst Rev.* 2007(2):CD005406.

5. Hargrave DR, Wade A, Evans JP, *et al.* Nocturnal oxygen saturation and painful sickle cell crises in children. *Blood.* 2003;**101**(3):846–848.

6. Robieux IC, Kellner JD, Coppes MJ, *et al.* Analgesia in children with sickle cell crisis: comparison of intermittent opioids vs. continuous intravenous infusion of morphine and placebo-controlled study of oxygen inhalation. *Pediatr Hematol Oncol.* 1992;**9**(4):317–326.

7. Zipursky A, Robieux IC, Brown EJ, *et al.* Oxygen therapy in sickle cell disease. *Am J Pediatr Hematol Oncol.* 1992;**14**(3):222–228.

8. Tavakkoli F, Nahavandi M, Wyche MQ, *et al.* Effects of hydroxyurea treatment on cerebral oxygenation in adult patients with sickle cell disease: an open-label pilot study. *Clin Ther.* 2005;**27**(7):1083–1088.

9. Reynolds JD. Painful sickle cell crisis. Successful treatment with hyperbaric oxygen therapy. *JAMA.* 1971;**216**(12):1977–1978.

10. Wallyn CR, Jampol LM, Goldberg MF, *et al.* The use of hyperbaric oxygen therapy in the treatment of sickle cell hyphema. *Invest Ophthalmol Vis Sci.* 1985;**26**(8):1155–1158.

11. Petrini M, Galimberti S, DeIaco G. Hyperbaric oxygen therapy in a case of combined sickle cell and hemoglobin Lepore disease. *Transfus. Altern Transfus Med.* 2006;**8**(4):210–212.

12. NIH Division of Blood Diseases and Resources. *Publication 02-2117: The Management of Sickle Cell Disease*, 4th edn. Bethesda, MD: National Heart, Lung, and Blood Institute, 2002.

13. Stinson J, Naser B. Pain management in children with sickle cell disease. *Paediatr Drugs.* 2003;**5**(4):229–241.

14. Benjamin LJ, Dampier CD, Jacox A. *Guideline for the Management of Acute and Chronic Pain in Sickle Cell Disease*, Vol 1. Glenview, IL: American Pain Society, 1999.

15. Jacob E, Miaskowski C, Savedra M, *et al.* Quantification of analgesic use in children with sickle cell disease. *Clin J Pain.* 2007;**23**(1):8–14.

16. de Franceschi L, Finco G, Vassanelli A, *et al.* A pilot study on the efficacy of ketorolac plus tramadol infusion combined with erythrocytapheresis in the management of acute severe vaso-occlusive crises and sickle cell pain. *Haematologica.* 2004;**89**(11):1389–1391.

17. Jacob E, Miaskowski C, Savedra M, *et al.* Management of vaso-occlusive pain in children with sickle cell disease. *J Pediatr Hematol Oncol.* 2003;**25**(4):307–311.

18. Gillis JC, Brogden RN. Ketorolac. A reappraisal of its pharmacodynamic and pharmacokinetic properties and therapeutic use in pain management. *Drugs.* 1997;**53**(1):139–188.

19. Beiter JL, Jr., Simon HK, Chambliss CR, *et al.* Intravenous ketorolac in the emergency department management of sickle cell pain and predictors of its effectiveness. *Arch Pediatr Adolesc Med.* 2001;**155**(4):496–500.

20. Cordner S, De Ceulaer K. Musculoskeletal manifestations of hemoglobinopathies. *Curr Opin Rheumatol.* 2003;**15**(1):44–47.

21. Hardwick WE, Jr., Givens TG, Monroe KW, *et al.* Effect of ketorolac in pediatric sickle cell vaso-occlusive pain crisis. *Pediatr Emerg Care.* 1999;**15** (3):179–182.

22. Perlin E, Finke H, Castro O, *et al.* Enhancement of pain control with ketorolac tromethamine in patients with sickle cell vaso-occlusive crisis. *Am J Hematol.* 1994;**46**(1):43–47.

23. Wright SW, Norris RL, Mitchell TR. Ketorolac for sickle cell vaso-occlusive crisis pain in the emergency department: lack of a narcotic-sparing effect. *Ann Emerg Med.* 1992;**21**(8):925–928.

24. Simckes AM, Chen SS, Osorio AV, *et al.* Ketorolac-induced irreversible renal failure in sickle cell disease: a case report. *Pediatr Nephrol.* 1999; **13**(1):63–67.

25. Hick JL, Nelson SC, Hick K, *et al.* Emergency management of sickle cell disease complications: review and practice guidelines. *Minn Med.* 2006; **89** (2):42–44, 47.

26. Platt A, Eckman JR, Beasley J, *et al.* Treating sickle cell pain: an update from the Georgia comprehensive sickle cell center. *J Emerg Nurs.* 2002;**28**(4):297–303.

27. Koumoukelis H. *Paediatric Pain Management Dosing Guideline.* Toronto, ON: Department of Anaesthesia, Toronto Hospital for Sick Children, 2002.

28. Platt OS, Thorington BD, Brambilla DJ, *et al.* Pain in sickle cell disease. Rates and risk factors. *N Engl J Med.* 1991;**325**(1):11–16.

29. Kopecky EA, Jacobson S, Joshi P, *et al.* Systemic exposure to morphine and the risk of acute chest syndrome in sickle cell disease. *Clin Pharmacol Ther.* 2004;**75**(3):140–146.

30. Nadvi SZ, Sarnaik S, Ravindranath Y. Low frequency of meperidine-associated seizures in sickle cell disease. *Clin Pediatr (Philadelphia).* 1999; **38**(8):459–462.

31. Turner E, Shapiro B. Pharmacological management of pain. In Shapiro B, Schechter NL, Ohene-Frempong K (eds.) *The Genetic Resource for Sickle Cell*

Disease-related Pain: Assessment and Management. Mt. Desert, ME: New England Regional Genetics Group, 1994:27–38.

32. Hagmeyer KO, Mauro LS, Mauro VF. Meperidine-related seizures associated with patient-controlled analgesia pumps. *Ann Pharmacother.* 1993;**27**(1):29–32.

33. Buchanan ID, Woodward M, Reed GW. Opioid selection during sickle cell pain crisis and its impact on the development of acute chest syndrome. *Pediatr Blood Cancer.* 2005;**45**(5):716–724.

34. Christensen ML, Wang WC, Harris S, *et al.* Transdermal fentanyl administration in children and adolescents with sickle cell pain crisis. *J Pediatr Hematol Oncol.* 1996;**18**(4):372–376.

35. Alam M, Saqib M. Management of painful sickle cell crisis in pregnancy. *J Coll Physicians Surg Pak.* 2004;**14**(2):115–116.

36. Melzer-Lange MD, Walsh-Kelly CM, Lea G, *et al.* Patient-controlled analgesia for sickle cell pain crisis in a pediatric emergency department. *Pediatr Emerg Care.* 2004;**20**(1):2–4.

37. Dampier CD, Setty BN, Logan J, *et al.* Intravenous morphine pharmacokinetics in pediatric patients with sickle cell disease. *J Pediatr.*Mar 1995;**126**(3):461–467.

38. White PF. Use of patient-controlled analgesia for management of acute pain. *JAMA.* 1988;**259**(2):243–247.

39. Yaster M, Kost-Byerly S, Maxwell LG. The management of pain in sickle cell disease. *Pediatr Clin North Am.* 2000;**47**(3):699–710.

40. Holbrook CT. Patient-controlled analgesia pain management for children with sickle cell disease. *J Assoc Acad Minor Phys.* 1990;**1**(3):93–96.

41. Shapiro BS, Cohen DE, Howe CJ. Patient-controlled analgesia for sickle-cell-related pain. *J Pain Symptom Manage.* 1993;**8**(1):22–28.

42. Schechter NL, Berrien FB, Katz SM. The use of patient-controlled analgesia in adolescents with sickle cell pain crisis: a preliminary report. *J Pain Symptom Manage.* 1988;**3**(2):109–113.

43. Stinson J, Naser B. Analgesie autocontrolee chez les enfants atteints d'anemie falciforme: L'experience d'un centre canadien. *Doul Analg.* 2000;**1**(1):21–26.

44. Trentadue NO, Kachoyeanos MK, Lea G. A comparison of two regimens of patient-controlled analgesia for children with sickle cell disease. *J Pediatr Nurs.* 1998;**13**(1):15–19.

45. de Araujo JT, Comerlatti LK, de Araujo RA, *et al.* [Treatment of sickle cell anemia crisis with dipyrone, hydrocortisone, and fluid therapy.] *Rev Hosp Clin Fac Med Sao Paulo.* 1994;**49**(1):13–16.

46. Griffin TC, McIntire D, Buchanan GR. High-dose intravenous methylprednis-olone therapy for pain in children and adolescents with sickle cell disease. *N Engl J Med*. 1994;**330**(11):733–737.

47. Couillard S, Benkerrou M, Girot R, *et al.* Steroid treatment in children with sickle-cell disease. *Haematologica*. 2007;**92**(3):425–426.

48. Weiner DL, Hibberd PL, Betit P, *et al.* Preliminary assessment of inhaled nitric oxide for acute vaso-occlusive crisis in pediatric patients with sickle cell disease. *JAMA*. 2003;**289**(9):1136–1142.

49. Steinberg MH. Management of sickle cell disease. *N Engl J Med*. 1999;**340**(13):1021–1030.

50. Ohene-Frempong K. Indications for red cell transfusion in sickle cell disease. *Semin Hematol*. 2001;**38**(1 Suppl 1):5–13.

51. Claster S, Vichinsky EP. Managing sickle cell disease. *BMJ*. 2003;**327**(7424):1151–1155.

52. Davies S, Olujohungbe A. Hydroxyurea for sickle cell disease. *Cochrane Database Syst Rev*. 2001(2):CD002202.

53. Ferster A, Tahriri P, Vermylen C, *et al.* Five years of experience with hydroxy-urea in children and young adults with sickle cell disease. *Blood*. 2001;**97**(11):3628–3632.

54. Gibbs WJ, Hagemann TM. Purified poloxamer 188 for sickle cell vaso-occlusive crisis. *Ann Pharmacother*. 2004;**38**(2):320–324.

55. Orringer EP, Casella JF, Ataga KI, *et al.* Purified poloxamer 188 for treatment of acute vaso-occlusive crisis of sickle cell disease: a randomized controlled trial. *JAMA*. 2001;**286**(17):2099–2106.

Temporomandibular disorders

NATHANAEL WOOD AND JOHN H. BURTON

■ Agents

- NSAIDs
- Opioids
- Amitriptyline
- Glucosamine sulfate
- Benzodiazepines
- Muscle relaxants

■ Evidence

Tricyclic antidepressants (TCAs), **NSAIDs**, **anxiolytic agents**, and **muscle relaxants** are the most common agents used to treat temporomandibular disorder (TMD) and its most common manifestation, temporomandibular joint (TMJ) pain. A National Institutes of Health conference on TMD, as well as recent literature reviews, conclude that the current body of evidence does not support any one drug as superior in the management of TMD.[1-3] Acute care analgesic regimens are typically combined with soft diet and habit reversal (e.g. gum-chewing cessation).

Although **NSAIDs** are the analgesic mainstay for acute TMD, trial evidence supporting use of this class is mixed. Two RCTs demonstrate no therapeutic advantage of oral **NSAIDs** over placebo for treatment of TMD. The first of these RCTs found therapeutic equivalence between *ibuprofen* (2400 mg PO daily) and placebo after four weeks of treatment for myofacial pain.[4] The second trial also found no benefit for **NSAIDs**, showing no advantage of *piroxicam* (20 mg PO daily) over placebo for TMD.[5] Another study, focusing on patients with chronic TMD (over 90 days in duration), found that **NSAIDs** added no pain relief over that achieved by **benzodiazepines** (see below).[4]

An RCT in patients with clinical TMD (and lacking radiographic evidence of osteoarthritis) demonstrated that *ampiroxicam* (27 mg PO daily), combined with TID jaw-opening exercises, was associated with symptomatic improvement in 60% of patients after a month's therapy (compared with a placebo response rate of 30%).[6] Another recent study found no difference between patients treated with *ibuprofen* (400 mg PO TID) and those receiving *glucosamine sulfate* (500 mg PO TID); each group showed a 60–70% improvement in pain after three months of therapy.[7] *Naproxen* (500 mg PO BID) outperformed placebo in a 2004 RCT of TMD patients; the same trial showed no benefit (over placebo) from use of the **COX-2 selective NSAID** *celecoxib* (100 mg PO BID).[8]

The role of **opioids** in the treatment of TMD remains controversial. Traditionally, authors have recommended avoiding **opioids** (owing to concerns about chronic use and abuse), and there is no published evidence supporting use of this class. **Opioids** are typically employed when pain is severe or refractory.

Although low-dose **TCAs** have been studied for the treatment of various chronic pain states, the literature addressing their use in TMD is sparse. Two small placebo-controlled RCTs of low-dose *amitriptyline* demonstrated reduced symptoms in patients with chronic TMD and facial pain. A Brazilian study of women with TMD found 75% improvement (nearly three times better than placebo) after two weeks of treatment with *amitriptyline* (25 mg PO daily).[9] Another study, assessing 28 patients with chronic orofacial pain, demonstrated improvement with *amitriptyline* (10 mg PO qHS) after four weeks of treatment.[10] In addition to its nonspecific analgesic effects, *amitriptyline* is thought to reduce the nighttime bruxism that is often a predisposing or exacerbating factor in TMD.[11]

Benzodiazepines are commonly used for TMD, particularly when symptoms are thought to include a muscular component. Available evidence suggests a role for this drug class, but supporting data are not definitive. A placebo-controlled pilot study demonstrated improvement for TMD patients treated for 30 days with *clonazepam* (10 mg PO qHS), but the study's size ($n = 10$) limits conclusions that can be drawn.[12] *Diazepam* (2.5–5 mg PO qHS) reduces nocturnal bruxism and alleviates pain from chronic TMD conditions (i.e. those lasting longer than three months).[4,13]

Other **muscle relaxants**, such as *cyclobenzaprine* or *metaxalone*, are occasionally used in TMD with a significant myofacial component. There is no evidence in the medical literature to support or refute this practice.

■ Summary and recommendations

First line: NSAID (e.g. ibuprofen 400–600 mg PO QID; naproxen 500 mg PO BID)

Reasonable:

- amitriptyline 10–25 mg PO qHS
- clonazepam 10 mg PO qHS *or* diazepam 2.5–5 mg PO qHS

Pregnancy:

- acetaminophen (650–1000 mg PO QID)
- opioids (e.g. oxycodone 5–10 mg PO q4–6 h)

Pediatric: ibuprofen (10 mg/kg PO QID)

Special cases:

- *TMD caused by anxiety*: clonazepam 10 mg PO qHS *or* diazepam 2.5–5 mg PO qHS
- *nighttime bruxism*: amitriptyline 10–25 mg PO qHS *or* clonazepam 10 mg PO qHS *or* diazepam 2.5–5 mg PO qHS
- *chronic TMD*: diazepam 2.5–5 mg PO qHS

References

1. National Institutes of Health. *Technology Assessment Conference on Management of Temporomandibular Disorders*. Bethesda, MD: National Institutes of Health, 1996.
2. List T, Axelsson S, Leijon G. Pharmacologic interventions in the treatment of temporomandibular disorders, atypical facial pain, and burning mouth syndrome. A qualitative systematic review. *J Orofac Pain*. 2003;**17**(4):301–310.
3. Dionne RA. Pharmacologic treatments for temporomandibular disorders. *Oral Surg Oral Med Oral Pathol Oral Radiol Endod*. 1997;**83**(1):134–142.
4. Singer E, Dionne R. A controlled evaluation of ibuprofen and diazepam for chronic orofacial muscle pain. *J Orofac Pain*. 1997;**11**(2):139–146.
5. Gordon S. Comparative efficacy of piroxicam versus placebo for temporomandibular pain. *J Dent Res*. 1990;**69**:S83.

6. Yuasa H, Kurita K. Randomized clinical trial of primary treatment for temporomandibular joint disk displacement without reduction and without osseous changes: a combination of NSAIDs and mouth-opening exercise versus no treatment. *Oral Surg Oral Med Oral Pathol Oral Radiol Endod.* 2001;**91** (6):671–675.

7. Thie NM, Prasad NG, Major PW. Evaluation of glucosamine sulfate compared to ibuprofen for the treatment of temporomandibular joint osteoarthritis: a randomized double blind controlled 3 month clinical trial. *J Rheumatol.* 2001;**28**(6):1347–1355.

8. Ta LE, Dionne RA. Treatment of painful temporomandibular joints with a cyclooxygenase 2 inhibitor: a randomized placebo-controlled comparison of celecoxib to naproxen. *Pain.* 2004;**111**(1–2):13–21.

9. Rizzatti Barbosa CM, Nogueira MT, de Andrade ED, *et al.* Clinical evaluation of amitriptyline for the control of chronic pain caused by temporomandibular joint disorders. *Cranio.* 2003;**21**(3):221–225.

10. Sharav Y, Singer E, Schmidt E, *et al.* The analgesic effect of amitriptyline on chronic facial pain. *Pain.* 1987;**31**(2):199–209.

11. Ware JC. Tricyclic antidepressants in the treatment of insomnia. *J Clin Psychiatry.* 1983;**44**(9 Pt 2):25–28.

12. Harkins S, Linford J, Cohen I, *et al.* Administration of clonazepam in the treatment of TMD and associated myofascial pain: a double-blind pilot study. *J Craniomandib Disord.* 1991;**5**(3):179–186.

13. Montgomery M. Effect of diazepam on nocturnal masticatory muscle activity. *J Dent Res.* 1986;**65**(3):180.

Tension-type headache

SOHAN PAREKH AND ANDY JAGODA

■ Agents

- Triptans
- Antiemetics
- NSAIDs
- Acetaminophen

■ Evidence

In the ED, diagnostic differentiation between migrainous pain and tension headache (TH) can be difficult. Fortunately, the best ED migraine therapies (the **triptans** and the **antiemetics** *metoclopromide* and *prochlorperazine*) are also efficacious for tension-type cephalalgia.[1–4] At a minimum, the "anti-migraine" agents may be used as second-line therapy for TH. In actual practice, given the often-encountered situation in which **NSAIDs** have either failed or are best avoided, the **triptans** or **antiemetics** constitute preferred pharmacotherapy for TH.

For many years, traditional employment of **NSAIDs** as the ED therapy of choice for TH was based upon a paucity of supporting data. Recently, the state of the evidence has improved, with trials assessing **NSAIDs**' perform-ance both against placebo and in comparison with each other. The placebo-controlled trials find TH benefit from myriad agents (e.g. *aspirin*, *ibuprofen*, *diclofenac*, *naproxen*, *ketoprofen*, *lumaricoxib*), and similar performance across different **NSAIDs**.[5–9] Some representative studies are presented here.

Pain relief in TH is similar for *ibuprofen* (400 mg PO) and *diclofenac* (12.5 mg PO).[10] Low-dose *ibuprofen* (200 mg PO) relieves TH better than placebo, but not as well as *ketoprofen* (25 mg PO).[11] Some of *aspirin*'s unique pharmacologic effects (i.e. compared with other **NSAIDs**) may make it relatively more useful in TH, but there are no data demonstrating *aspirin* superiority for this diagnosis.[6] **COX-2 selective NSAIDs** have also been found superior to placebo for TH relief, although there appears little reason to use these drugs for single-dose therapy in the ED.[5]

Compared with migraine headache, TH is less likely associated with nausea and an inability to tolerate oral analgesia. Therefore, the need to provide injectable **NSAIDs** is less important, but parenteral agents such as *ketorolac* and *metamizol* (not available in the USA because of potential bone marrow suppression) have been found to outperform placebo.[7,12]

There are conflicting data on the question of whether **NSAIDs** or *acetaminophen* (*paracetamol*) provide better TH relief. Two trials have found equivalence between *acetaminophen* (1000 mg PO) and *aspirin* (1000 mg PO) or *naproxen* (375 mg PO).[9,13] Other studies report mixed results from comparison of *acetaminophen* (1000 mg PO) with *ketoprofen* (25 mg PO); in one trial, the agents performed equally and in the other the **NSAID** was superior.[8,14] Some of the inconsistency in the results may reflect the time of assessment of the pain relief endpoint. There is suggestion that **NSAIDs** such as *ibuprofen* (400 mg PO) provide faster (although not necessarily more profound) TH relief than *acetaminophen*.[15,16]

Overall, it appears unlikely that there are clinically important efficacy differences between individual **NSAIDs**, or between the **NSAIDs** and *acetaminophen*. These agents should be tried on a case-by-case basis, with the clinician maintaining therapeutic flexibility (an individual patient may respond differently to different agents in the same class).

The "tension"-type pain of TH is sometimes treated with **benzodiazepines**. However, a multicenter RCT of TH patients could detect no overall benefit from adding a **benzodiazepine** (*etizolam*, 0.5 mg PO) to **NSAID** monotherapy (*mefenamic acid*, 250 mg PO).[17]

Muscle relaxants such as *cyclobenzaprine*, *chlormezanone*, and *tizanidine* have been investigated for TH, but the existing evidence does not support their use in the ED.[18-20]

The anti-dopaminergic effects of *chlorpromazine* (0.1 mg/kg IV) probably mediate this agent's reported effectiveness in relieving TH pain, but side effects limit broad use of this agent.[21]

Some drugs, such as *mirtazapine*, have promise for prophylaxis of chronic TH but there is no ED role for these agents.[22,23] Other drugs reportedly useful for TH, but lacking evidence basis for current recommendations in acute care, include *niacin* and *botulinum toxin*.[24,25]

Although **opioids** may have some role for refractory TH, evidence support for their use is limited. Anecdotal reports endorse use of PO *tramadol* for TH.[26] One of the few existing comparisons between an **opioid** and an **antiemetic** found *meperidine* less reliable for TH relief than *metoclopramide*.[4] Nevertheless, some patients with suspected TH will fail to respond to standard therapy. The clinician should not assume these patients are drug seekers; it may well be the case that the diagnosis of TH is in error. Assuming the pain is real, and providing appropriate rescue analgesia (which will often be best achieved with **opioids**), is the best course for TH or any other headache syndrome.

■ Summary and recommendations

First line: NSAID (e.g. ibuprofen 400–600 mg PO q6–8 h)

Reasonable: acetaminophen (1000 mg PO q6 h)

Pregnancy: acetaminophen (1000 mg PO q6 h)

Pediatric: NSAID (e.g. ibuprofen 10 mg/kg PO q6–8 h)

Special case:

■ *pain unresponsive to NSAIDs or acetaminophen*: triptans (e.g. sumatriptan 6 mg SC) or antiemetic (e.g. prochlorperazine 10 mg IV)

References

1. Miner JR, Smith SW, Moore J, *et al.* Sumatriptan for the treatment of undifferentiated primary headaches in the ED. *Am J Emerg Med.* 2007;**25**:60–64.

2. Thomas S, Stone C, Ray V, *et al.* Intravenous vs. rectal prochlorperazine for the treatment of benign vascular or tension headache. *Ann Emerg Med.* 1994;**23**:923–927.

3. Jones J, Sklar D, Dougherty J, *et al.* Randomized double-blind trial of intravenous prochlorperazine for the treatment of acute headache. *JAMA.* 1989;**261**:1174–1176.

4. Cicek M, Karcioglu O, Parlak I, *et al*. Prospective, randomised, double blind, controlled comparison of metoclopramide and pethidine in the emergency treatment of acute primary vascular and tension type headache episodes. *Emerg Med J*. 2004;**21**:323–326.

5. Packman E, Packman B, Thurston H, *et al*. Lumiracoxib is effective in the treatment of episodic tension-type headache. *Headache*. 2005;**45**:1163–1170.

6. Farinelli I, Martelletti P. Aspirin and tension-type headache. *J Headache Pain*. 2007;**8**:49–55.

7. Harden R, Rogers D, Fink K, *et al*. Controlled trial of ketorolac in tension-type headache. *Neurology*. 1998;**50**:507–509.

8. Steiner T, Lange R. Ketoprofen (25 mg) in the symptomatic treatment of episodic tension-type headache: double-blind placebo-controlled comparison with acetaminophen (1000 mg). *Cephalalgia*. 1998;**18**:38–43.

9. Steiner T, Lange R, Voelker M. Aspirin in episodic tension-type headache: placebo-controlled dose-ranging comparison with paracetamol. *Cephalalgia*. 2003;**23**:59–66.

10. Kubitzek F, Ziegler G, Gold M, *et al*. Low-dose diclofenac potassium in the treatment of episodic tension-type headache. *Eur J Pain*. 2003;**7**:155–162.

11. van Gerven J. Self-medication of a single headache episode with ketoprofen, ibuprofen or placebo, home-monitored with an electronic patient diary. *Eur J Pain*. 1996;**7**:155–162.

12. Bigal ME, Bordini CA, Speciali JG. Intravenous metamizol (Dipyrone) in acute migraine treatment and in episodic tension-type headache: a placebo-controlled study. *Cephalalgia*. 2001;**21**:90–95.

13. Prior M, Cooper K, May L, *et al*. Efficacy and safety of acetaminophen and naproxen in the treatment of tension-type headache: a randomized, double-blind, placebo-controlled trial. *Cephalalgia*. 2002;**22**:740–748.

14. Mehlisch D, Weaver M, Fladung B. Ketoprofen, acetaminophen, and placebo in the treatment of tension headache. *Headache*. 1998;**38**:579–589.

15. Packman B. Solubilized ibuprofen: evaluation of onset, relief, and safety of a novel formulation in the treatment of episodic tension-type headache. *Headache*. 2000;**40**:561–567.

16. Schachtel B, Furey S, Thoden W. Nonprescription ibuprofen and acetaminophen in the treatment of tension-type headache. *J Clin Pharmacol*. 1996;**36**:1120–1125.

17. Hirata K, Tatsumoto M, Araki N, *et al*. Multi-center randomized control trial of etizolam plus NSAID combination for tension-type headache. *Intern Med*. 2007;**46**:467–472.

18. Lance JW, Anthony M. Cyclobenzaprine in the treatment of chronic tension headache. *Med J Aust.* 1972;**2**:1409–1411.

19. Larsson B, Melin L, Doberl A. Recurrent tension headache in adolescents treated with self-help relaxation training and a muscle relaxant drug. *Headache.* 1990;**30**:665–671.

20. Saper JR, Winner PK, Lake AE, 3rd. An open-label dose-titration study of the efficacy and tolerability of tizanidine hydrochloride tablets in the prophylaxis of chronic daily headache. *Headache.* 2001;**41**:357–368.

21. Bigal ME, Bordini CA, Speciali JG. Intravenous chlorpromazine in the acute treatment of episodic tension-type headache: a randomized, placebo controlled, double-blind study. *Arq Neuropsiquiatr.* 2002;**60**:537–541.

22. Bendtsen L, Buchgreitz L, Ashina S, *et al.* Combination of low-dose mirtazapine and ibuprofen for prophylaxis of chronic tension-type headache. *Eur J Neurol.* 2007;**14**:187–193.

23. Tajti J, Almasi J. [Effects of mirtazapine in patients with chronic tension-type headache. Literature review.] *Neuropsychopharmacol Hung.* 2006;**8**:67–72.

24. Evers S, Frese A. Recent advances in the treatment of headaches. *Curr Opin Anaesthesiol.* 2005;**18**:563–568.

25. Prousky J, Seely D. The treatment of migraines and tension-type headaches with intravenous and oral niacin (nicotinic acid): systematic review of the literature. *Nutr J.* 2005;**4**:3.

26. Robbins L. Tramadol for tension-type headache. *Headache.* 2004;**44**:192–193.

Trigeminal neuralgia

SOHAN PAREKH AND ANDY JAGODA

■ Agents

- Anticonvulsants
- Baclofen

■ Evidence

The **anticonvulsants** constitute the major drug therapy for trigeminal neuralgia (TN). Cochrane review has shown that, of the older agents, the treatment of choice is *carbamazepine* (200–400 mg PO BID, titrated up to 1200 mg daily maximum dose).[1] *Carbamazepine*'s keto-analog *oxcarbazepine* (300–600 mg PO BID) is equally effective.

Most of the evidence for *carbamazepine*'s efficacy in TN comes from the outpatient setting. However, given the drug's decades of usefulness, it is a reasonable first-line choice for ED therapy of TN.[1,2] In addition to its utility in the general population of patients with TN, *carbamazepine* is recommended for treatment of TN in the elderly.[3]

Phenytoin and *valproic acid* can be of some use in TN. *Phenytoin* is likely a good second-choice agent, but *carbamazepine*'s "number needed to treat for 50% pain relief" of 1.8 reflects its superiority over the other older **anticonvulsants**.[1,4,5]

Just as *carbamazepine* incurs certain risks (e.g. blood cell counts and liver function tests must be monitored), *phenytoin*'s use in TN is associated with some chance of side effects such as psychosis.[6] A preliminary case series found that *fosphenytoin* helps in acute refractory TN, but the evidence for this approach remains limited.[7]

There are data to suggest utility of new-generation **anticonvulsants** for TN. Currently, the main ED role for these agents in TN is for patients who fail to respond to, or cannot tolerate, single-drug therapy with *carbamazepine*. In the near future, though, the newer **anticonvulsants** may replace *carbamazepine* as the initial drug of choice for TN. An emerging body of RCT evidence supports first-line TN treatment with *lamotrigine* (400 mg PO QD).[8–10] Case series data for TN patients with multiple sclerosis found *gabapentin* (300 mg PO daily) and *topiramate* (25 mg PO BID) particularly useful.[11,12]

Baclofen, a gamma-aminobutyric acid (GABA) agonist usually used as an antispasticity agent, is an effective, though second-line, therapy for TN.[10,13,14] Animal models of TN suggest that *baclofen* mediates pain relief via a mechanism (attenuation of allodynia-type response) that differs from that of *carbamaze-pine*.[15] This is clinically relevant, because the complementary pain relief mechanisms of the two drugs may be responsible for the observation that pain relief is improved with dual therapy (i.e. *baclofen* 10–20 mg PO q6–8 h, plus *carbama-zepine*).[14] Although there is promise for *baclofen*'s use in TN, the overall level of evidence is insufficient to recommend its first-line use in the ED setting.[16,17]

■ Summary and recommendations

First line: carbamazapine (200 mg PO BID)

Reasonable: gabapentin (300 mg PO QD)

Pregnancy: there is insufficient evidence to recommend therapy without consultation; baclofen and gabapentin (both Category C) may be options, but carbamazepine and phenytoin are Category D and should not be prescribed by the ED provider for TN

Pediatric: carbamazepine 100 mg PO BID for age at least 6 years (gabapentin 5 mg/kg PO TID may also be used with monitoring for CNS side effects)

Special case:

■ *multiple sclerosis with trigeminal neuralgia*: gabapentin (300 mg PO daily)

References

1. Wiffen PJ, McQuay HJ, Moore RA. Carbamazepine for acute and chronic pain. *Cochrane Database Syst Rev*. 2005(3):CD005451.
2. Nicol CF. A four year double-blind study of tegretol in facial pain. *Headache*. 1969;**9**(1):54–57.

3. Kaminski HJ, Ruff RL. Treatment of the elderly patient with headache or trigeminal neuralgia. *Drugs Aging*. 1991;**1**(1):48–56.

4. McCleane GJ. Intravenous infusion of phenytoin relieves neuropathic pain: a randomized, double-blinded, placebo-controlled, crossover study. *Anesth Analg*. 1999;**89**(4):985–988.

5. Wiffen P, Collins S, McQuay H, *et al.* Anticonvulsant drugs for acute and chronic pain. *Cochrane Database Syst Rev*. 2005(3):CD001133.

6. Gatzonis SD, Angelopoulos E, Sarigiannis P, *et al.* Acute psychosis due to treatment with phenytoin in a nonepileptic patient. *Epilepsy Behav*. 2003;**4** (6):771–772.

7. Cheshire WP. Fosphenytoin: an intravenous option for the management of acute trigeminal neuralgia crisis. *J Pain Symptom Manage*. 2001;**21**(6): 506–510.

8. Zakrzewska JM, Chaudhry Z, Nurmikko TJ, *et al.* Lamotrigine (lamictal) in refractory trigeminal neuralgia: results from a double-blind placebo controlled crossover trial. *Pain*. 1997;**73**(2):223–230.

9. Lunardi G, Leandri M, Albano C, *et al.* Clinical effectiveness of lamotrigine and plasma levels in essential and symptomatic trigeminal neuralgia. *Neurology*. 1997;**48**(6):1714–1717.

10. Canavero S, Bonicalzi V. Drug therapy of trigeminal neuralgia. *Expert Rev Neurother*. 2006;**6**(3):429–440.

11. Khan OA. Gabapentin relieves trigeminal neuralgia in multiple sclerosis patients. *Neurology*. 1998;**51**(2):611–614.

12. Zvartau-Hind M, Din MU, Gilani A, *et al.* Topiramate relieves refractory trigeminal neuralgia in MS patients. *Neurology*. 28 2000;**55**(10): 1587–1588.

13. Fromm GH. Baclofen as an adjuvant analgesic. *J Pain Symptom Manage*. 1994;**9**(8):500–509.

14. Baker KA, Taylor JW, Lilly GE. Treatment of trigeminal neuralgia: use of baclofen in combination with carbamazepine. *Clin Pharm*. 1985;**4**(1):93–96.

15. Idanpaan-Heikkila JJ, Guilbaud G. Pharmacological studies on a rat model of trigeminal neuropathic pain: baclofen, but not carbamazepine, morphine or tricyclic antidepressants, attenuates the allodynia-like behaviour. *Pain*. 1999;**79**(2–3):281–290.

16. Fromm GH, Terrence CF. Comparison of L-baclofen and racemic baclofen in trigeminal neuralgia. *Neurology*. 1987;**37**(11):1725–1728.

17. Parmar BS, Shah KH, Gandhi IC. Baclofen in trigeminal neuralgia: a clinical trial. *Indian J Dent Res*. 1989;**1**(4):109–113.

Undifferentiated abdominal pain

FRANK LOVECCHIO AND STEPHEN H. THOMAS

■ Agents

- Opioids
- NSAIDs

■ Evidence

This chapter is intended to address one of the broadest topics in acute care pain management: abdominal pain of uncertain etiology. Although some patients present to the ED with known diagnoses (e.g. recurrent kidney stone), the acute care provider is usually in a position in which analgesia decisions must be made in the setting of diagnostic imprecision. In truth, diagnostic certainty after an initial ED evalaution is often elusive. There will always be need for some degree of judgment as to appropriate analgesia, given patients' conditions, levels of pain, and relative likelihood of varying diagnoses (e.g. leaking aortic aneurysm versus renal colic). With that caveat, the reader is referred to other chapters of this text for cases in which the cause of abdominal pain is known. This chapter's discussion is intended to serve two functions. First, the chapter is intended to address treatment for patients where the cause of pain is unclear. Second, the chapter is intended to provide general guidance for treatment of abdominal (including pelvic) pain, serving as a reference for conditions (e.g. salpingitis, bowel obstruction) lacking sufficient analgesia data to warrant a separate chapter.

Perhaps the most important, and certainly the most historically controversial, issue with respect to treatment of undifferentiated abdominal pain (UAP) is whether *any* analgesia should be given. Based on physical examination concerns that have inertia from nearly a century of clinical application, some authors still write that relief of pain can dangerously obfuscate the diagnostic process.[1] Those concerns are mentioned here for the express purpose of categorically disagreeing with the practice of withholding analgesia in patients with UAP. Expert opinion, based upon a wealth of available evidence and anecdotal experience, and published in the world's leading journals in general medicine, surgery, and emergency medicine, is near unanimous: it is inappropriate to allow patient suffering on the pretext of preserving the physical examination.[2–5] The literature clearly demonstrates that neither proximal endpoints (e.g. specific examination findings such as Murphy's sign) nor downstream outcomes are significantly adversely impacted by administration of analgesics.[3,6–8] Rather than being caused by relief of pain, errors in diagnosis of UAP are more likely to be caused by premature cessation of the diagnostic process, or even from poor history owing to pain-clouded consciousness (particularly in the elderly). This issue's level of certainty has progressed to the point where it would be unethical to randomize to placebo the necessary number of UAP patients (i.e. thousands) needed to detect any outcomes detriment.[2]

Opioids remain the most commonly used, and most commonly recommended, treatment for acute UAP (including that which may be a result of surgical disease).[2,3,8] Other than the abovementioned issues with respect to **opioids**' effect on the physical examination, there have been questions about the effects of mu receptor agonists on the Oddi sphincter. The relevant evidence is addressed in detail in the biliary colic chapter (p. 111); the conclusions are that there is no relevant difference between the pure opioid agonists, and that if Oddi sphincter tone is a particular concern *buprenorphine* (0.3 mg IV) is a good choice. In the setting of UAP, there is no evidence supporting clinical practice of administering *meperidine* (*pethidine*) (over *morphine*) in case the pain is related to biliary tract spasm.[9–11]

There are a number of RCTs (with placebo controls) addressing *morphine* use for UAP, including pain suspected to be from appendicitis. The evidence clearly and consistently demonstrates safety and efficacy from *morphine* use in the UAP population.[3,6,8,12–16] Other **opioids** have also been studied and found effective, although evidence for other agents is generally less rigorous than that supporting *morphine* use.[3,6,12,15–24]

The use of *fentanyl* is theoretically attractive, since this agent has a short duration of action and is therefore easier to titrate. One study assessing IV *fentanyl* use for UAP found this approach safe and effective, but the data have only been reported in abstract form.[17] Another study compared IV *fentanyl* with a nebulized inhaled formulation of the same drug, and suggested similar efficacy between the two administration routes.[25] Based upon the limited data for *fentanyl* use in nontraumatic UAP, and the consistent demonstrations of *fentanyl*'s safety and efficacy in adults and children with undifferentiated trauma (many having abdominal injuries), we recommend the use of IV *fentanyl* when hemodynamic concerns or need for close titration are paramount.[26–29]

Both *morphine* and *oxycodone* (PO) have been specifically studied in children with UAP.[12,20,24] Either approach appears safe and efficacious in RCTs, but *morphine* offers the substantial advantage of keeping patients nil by mouth.

Whether *morphine* or any other **opioid** is administered, the need for *naloxone* reversal has been rare and the serious adverse event rates have been very low (and similar to placebo rates).[3,4] It is advisable to avoid having to use the reversal agent, because reversal complicates patient evaluation and renders subsequent analgesia difficult.

The mixed-mechanism agent *tramadol*, administered IV, has been found efficacious for UAP in one clinical trial.[21] Based upon the paucity of current evidence, and the efficacy of other agents with overlapping mechanisms of action, there is no basis for recommending *tramadol* as a preferred agent for UAP.

The use of **NSAIDs** in UAP has not been well studied. Use of **NSAIDs** is likely to help to alleviate any pain from stone movement. There is also evidence basis for COX-2 inhibition as a means to moderate pain from pelvic inflammatory disease.[30] Additionally, administration of parenteral *ketorolac* offers the advantage of preserving the nil by mouth status of a patient who may need surgery. However, there are problems with giving **NSAIDs** to patients with potential need for operative intervention. The issue of **NSAID**-associated operative bleeding is discussed in the chapter on biliary colic, but the message for UAP is that there is no reason to withhold **opioids** and run even a small (but preventable) risk of bleeding complications.[31,32]

■ Summary and recommendations

First line: morphine (initial dose 4–6 mg IV, then titrate)

Reasonable: any opioid (no advantage to use of meperidine)

Pregnancy: morphine (initial dose 4–6 mg IV, then titrate)

Pediatric: morphine (initial dose 0.05–0.1 mg/kg IV, then titrate)

Special cases:

- *Oral therapy appropriate*: oxycodone or hydrocodone (5–10 mg PO q4–6 h)
- *Opioids to be avoided, low likelihood of operative intervention*: ketorolac (15–30 mg IV q6 h)
- *Concern for hemodynamics or need for close titration*: fentanyl (initial dose 50–100 μg IV, then titrate)
- *Suspected biliary tract pain with Oddi sphincter concern*: buprenorphine (initial dose 0.3 mg IV, then titrate)

References

1. Nissman SA, Kaplan LJ, Mann BD. Critically reappraising the literature-driven practice of analgesia administration for acute abdominal pain in the emergency room prior to surgical evaluation. *Am J Surg*. 2003;**185**:291–296.
2. Ranji SR, Goldman LE, Simel DL, *et al*. Do opiates affect the clinical evaluation of patients with acute abdominal pain? *JAMA*. 2006;**296**:1764–1774.
3. Gallagher EJ, Esses D, Lee C, *et al*. Randomized clinical trial of morphine in acute abdominal pain. *Ann Emerg Med*. 2006;**48**:150–160.
4. Thomas SH, Silen W. Effect on diagnostic efficiency of analgesia for undifferentiated abdominal pain. *Br J Surg*. 2003;**90**:5–9.
5. Klein-Kremer A, Goldman RD. Opioid administration for acute abdominal pain in the pediatric emergency department. *J Opioid Manag*. 2007;**3**:11–14.
6. Thomas S, Silen W, Cheema F. Effects of morphine analgesia on diagnostic accuracy in emergency department patients with abdominal pain: a prospective, randomized trial. *J Am Coll Surg*. 2003;**196**:18–31.
7. Nelson B, Senecal E, Hong C, *et al*. Opioid analgesia and assessment of the sonographic Murphy's sign. *J Emerg Med*. 2005;**28**:409–413.
8. Bailey B, Bergeron S, Gravel J, *et al*. Efficacy and impact of intravenous morphine before surgical consultation in children with right lower quadrant pain suggestive of appendicitis: a randomized controlled trial. *Ann Emerg Med*. 2007;**50**:371–378.

9. Thompson DR. Narcotic analgesic effects on the sphincter of Oddi: a review of the data and therapeutic implications in treating pancreatitis. *Am J Gastroenterol.* 2001;**96**:1266–1272.

10. Beckwith MC, Fox ER, Chandramouli J. Removing meperidine from the health-system formulary: frequently asked questions. *J Pain Palliat Care Pharmacother.* 2002;**16**:45–59.

11. Latta KS, Ginsberg B, Barkin RL. Meperidine: a critical review. *Am J Ther.* 2002;**9**:53–68.

12. Green R, Bulloch B, Kabani A, *et al.* Early analgesia for children with acute abdominal pain. *Pediatrics.* 2005;**116**:978–983.

13. Kim MK, Strait RT, Sato TT, *et al.* A randomized clinical trial of analgesia in children with acute abdominal pain. *Acad Emerg Med.* 2002;**9**:281–287.

14. LoVecchio F, Oster N, Sturmann K, *et al.* The use of analgesics in patients with acute abdominal pain. *J Emerg Med.* 1997;**15**:775–779.

15. Pace S, Burke T. Intravenous morphine for early pain relief in patients with acute abdominal pain. *Acad Emerg Med.* 1996;**3**:1086–1092.

16. Vermeulen B, Morabia A, Unger PF, *et al.* Acute appendicitis: influence of early pain relief on the accuracy of clinical and US findings in the decision to operate – a randomized trial. *Radiology.* 1999;**210**:639–643.

17. Garyfallou G, Grillo A, Fulda ROCG, *et al.* A controlled trial of fentanyl analgesia in emergency department patients with abdominal pain: can treatment obscure the diagnosis? *Acad Emerg Med.* 1997;**4**:405.

18. Zoltie N, Cust MP. Analgesia in the acute abdomen. *Ann R Coll Surg Engl.* 1986;**68**:209–210.

19. LoVecchio F, Oster N, Sturmann K. The use of analgesics in patients with acute abdominal pain. *J Emerg Med.* 1997;**15**:775–779.

20. Kim M, Strait R, Sato T, *et al.* A randomized clinical trial of analgesia in children with acute abdominal pain. *Acad Emerg Med.* 2002;**9**:281–287.

21. Mahadevan M, Graff L. Prospective randomized study of analgesic use for ED patients with right lower quadrant abdominal pain. *Am J Emerg Med.* 2000;**18**:753–756.

22. Attard A, Kidner JCN, Leslie A, *et al.* Safety of early pain relief for acute abdominal pain. *BMJ.* 1992;**305**:554–556.

23. Zoltie N, Cust M. Analgesia in the acute abdomen. *Ann Royal Coll Surg.* 1986;**68**:209–210.

24. Kokki H, Lintula H, Vanamo K, *et al.* Oxycodone vs placebo in children with undifferentiated abdominal pain: a randomized, double-blind clinical trial of

the effect of analgesia on diagnostic accuracy. *Arch Pediatr Adolesc Med.* 2005;**159**:320–325.

25. Bartfield JM, Flint RD, McErlean M, *et al.* Nebulized fentanyl for relief of abdominal pain. *Acad Emerg Med.* 2003;**10**:215–218.

26. DeVellis P, Thomas S, Wedel S, *et al.* Prehospital fentanyl analgesia in air-transported pediatric trauma patients. *Pediatr Emerg Care.* 1998;**14**:321–323.

27. Galinski M, Dolveck F, Borron SW, *et al.* A randomized, double blind study comparing morphine with fentanyl in prehospital analgesia. *Am J Emerg Med.* 2005;**23**:114–119.

28. Kanowitz A, Dunn TM, Kanowitz EM, *et al.* Safety and effectiveness of fentanyl administration for prehospital pain management. *Prehosp Emerg Care.* 2006;**10**:1–7.

29. Thomas S. Fentanyl in the prehospital setting. *Am J Emerg Med.* 2007;**25** (7):842–843.

30. Chiantera A, Tesauro R, Di Leo S, *et al.* Nimesulide in the treatment of pelvic inflammatory diseases. A multicentre clinical trial conducted in Campania and Sicily. *Drugs.* 1993;**46**(Suppl 1):134–136.

31. Vuilleumier H, Halkic N. Ruptured subcapsular hematoma after laparoscopic cholecystectomy attributed to ketorolac-induced coagulopathy. *Surg Endosc.* 2003;**17**:659.

32. Varrassi G, Panella L, Piroli A, *et al.* The effects of perioperative ketorolac infusion on postoperative pain and endocrine-metabolic response. *Anesth Analg.* 1994;**78**:514–519.

Tables

Selected nonsteroidal anti-inflammatory drugs (NSAIDs)

Medication	Example tradename	Route^a	Initial adult dose^b	Initial pediatric dose	Maintenance adult dose^c	Maintenance pediatric dose
Salicylates						
Aspirin	Ecotrin	PO	650–1000 mg	10–15 mg/kg	325–1000 mg q6 h	10–15 mg/kg q4–6 h
Diflunisal	Dolobid	PO	1000 mg		500 mg q12 h	
Salsalate	Disalcid, Salflex	PO	1500 mg		1500 mg q12 h	
Acetic acids						
Diclofenac	Cataflam, Voltaren	PO^b	50–75 mg		50 mg q8–12 h	
	Solaraze	topical	3% (11.6 mg/g) gel, 50 mg diclofenac component		50 mg diclofenac component TID	
Etodolac	Lodine	PO	200–400 mg	400 mg q0 for age > 6 yr	200–400 mg q6–8 h	400–1000 mg QD
Indomethacin	Indocin	PO	50 mg	0.5–1 mg/kg for age > 2 yr	25–50 mg q8–12 h	1–2 mg/kg daily, divided BID–QID
		Spray	0.25% spray		0.25% spray q4–6 h	
Ketorolac	Toradol	PO	20 mg		10 mg q4–6 h	
	Toradol	IV	30 mg	0.5–1.0 mg/ kg for age >6 mth	30 mg q6 h	0.5 mg/kg q6 h

Selected nonsteroidal anti-inflammatory drugs (NSAIDs) (cont.)

Medication	Example tradename	Route[a]	Initial adult dose[b]	Initial pediatric dose	Maintenance adult dose[c]	Maintenance pediatric dose
	Toradol	IM	60 mg	1 mg/kg for age >6 mth	30 mg q6 h	1 mg/kg q6 h
	Acular	Ocular drops	1 drop (0.25 mg)	1 drop (0.25 mg) for age >3 yr	1 drop q6 h	1 drop q6 h
Sulindac	Clinoril	PO	150–200 mg	1–2 mg/kg	150–200 mg BID	1–2 mg/kg BID
Tolmetin	Tolectin	PO	400 mg	10 mg/kg for age >2 yr	400–600 mg TID	10 mg/kg TID
Enolic acids						
Meloxicam	Mobic	PO	7.5–15 mg	0.125 mg/kg for age >2 yr	7.5–15 mg QD	0.125 mg/kg QD
Piroxicam	Feldene	PO	20 mg		20 mg QD	
Propionic acids						
Fenoprofen	Nalfon	PO	200–800 mg		200–800 mg QID	
Flurbiprofen	Ansaid	PO	50–100 mg		100 mg BID–TID	
Ibuprofen	Advil, Motrin, Rufen	PO	200–800 mg	5–10 mg/kg for age > 6 mth	200–800 mg q6–8 h	5–10 mg/kg q6–8 h
Ketoprofen	Orudis, Oruvail	PO	50–75 mg		25–75 mg q6–8 h	

Naproxen	Naprosyn	PO	250–750 mg	5–10 mg/kg for age >2 yr	250–500 mg BID	10–20 mg/kg daily, divided BID–TID
	Aleve				220 mg BID–TID	
Oxaprozin	Daypro	PO	1200 mg	600 mg for age >6 yr	1200 mg QD	600 mg QD
Fenamates						
Meclofenamate	Meclomen	PO	100 mg	100 mg for age >14 yr	100 mg TID	100 mg TID
Mefenamic acid	Ponstel	PO	500 mg	500 mg for age >14 yr	250 mg QID	250 mg QID
Cyclooxygenase 2 selective						
Celecoxib	Celebrex	PO	400 mg	50 mg for age >2 yr	200 mg BID	50–100 mg BID
Lumiracoxib	Prexige	PO	200 mg		200 mg BID	
Nabumetone[d]	Relafen	PO	1000 mg		1000 mg BID	

[a] Rectal forms of many NSAIDs are available (doses are similar to PO); ketorolac is the only parenteral NSAID available in the USA.

[b] Adjustment of dose or interval should be considered when prescribing NSAIDs to patients with renal compromise

[c] Maintenance doses prescribed from the ED are intended for approximately one week of therapy only.

[d] COX2 selectivity is diminished at higher doses.

Selected opioids

Medication	Example tradename	Route[a]	Initial adult dose[b]	Initial pediatric dose	Maintenance adult dose[c]	Maintenance pediatric dose
Pure agonists						
Codeine	Tylenol[d]	PO	30 mg	0.5–1 mg/kg for age >1 yr	15–60 mg q4–6 h	0.5–1 mg/kg q 4–6 h
Fentanyl	Sublimaze	IV	50–100 µg	1–2 µg/kg	50–100 µg q1–2 h	0.5–2 µg/kg q1–4 h
		IN	1–2 µg/kg	1–2 µg/kg	1–2 µg/kg q1–2 h	
		Nebulized	1–3 µg/kg	1–3 µg/kg	1–3 µg/kg q1–2 h	1–3 µg/kg q1–2 h
	Actiq	Lozenge	200 µg	10–15 µg/kg	>30 min interval between doses	>30 min interval between doses
	Fentora	Buccal tablet	100 µg		> 4 h interval between doses	
Hydrocodone	Vicodin[d]	PO	5–10 mg	2.5 mg for age > 6 yr	5–10 mg q4–6 h	2.5 mg q4–6 h
Hydromorphone	Dilaudid	PO	1–2 mg	0.03 mg/kg for age >6 mth	2–8 mg q3–4 h	0.03–0.08 mg/kg q4–6 h
		IV	1 mg	0.015 mg/kg for age >6 mth	1–4 mg q 4–6 h	0.015 mg/kg q4–6 h
Meperidine (pethidine)	Demerol	IV	50 mg	1.1–1.8 mg/kg	50–150 mg q3–4 h	1.1–1.8 mg/kg q3–4 h
Morphine	MSContin	PO	10–30 mg	0.2–0.5 mg/kg for age >6 mth	10–30 mg q3–4 h	0.2–0.5 mg/kg q4–6 h
		Oral rinse	15 mL 2:1000 solution		15 mL 2:1000 solution q2–4 h	

		IV	4-6 mg	0.1-0.2 mg/kg for age >6 mth	2.5-10 mg q2-6 h	0.1-0.2 mg/kg q2-4 h
		Nebulized	10-20 mg			
Oxycodone	Percocet[d]	PO	5-10 mg	0.05-0.15 mg/kg	5-30 mg q4 h	0.05-0.15 mg/kg q4-6 h
Tramadol	Ultram	PO	50-100 mg	25-50 mg for age >16 yr	50-100 mg q4-6 h	25-50 mg q4-6 h
		IV	50-100 mg	0.7 mg/kg	50-100 mg q4-6 h	0.7 mg/kg q4-6 h
Agonist-antagonists						
Buprenorphine	Buprenex	IV	0.3 mg	2-6 µg/kg for age 2-12 yr	0.3 mg q6-8 h	2-6 µg/kg q 4-6 h
Butorphanol	Stadol	IV	0.5-2 mg		0.5-2 mg q3-4 h	
	Stadol NS	IN	1 mg (1 spray)		2nd spray in other nostril in 1 h	
Nalbuphine	Nubain	IV	10 mg	0.1 mg/kg	10-20 mg q3-6 h	0.1 mg/kg q2-6 h

[a] The IV opioid dosage may also be used for IM or SC administration; IV administration is preferred in most cases.

[b] Initial doses may be higher for opioid-tolerant patients; opioid dosages and intervals should be adjusted in setting of significant liver or renal disease (creatinine clearance < 50 mL/min).

[c] Initial IV titration schedule can be more aggressive (e.g. every 15-30 min).

[d] This brand also contains acetaminophen.

Other analgesic drugs

Medication	Trade name	Route	Initial adult dose	Initial pediatric dose	Maintenance adult dose	Maintenance pediatric dose	Pregnancy Category	Lactation	Dosage adjustment in renal disease
Acetaminophen (paracetamol)	Tylenol	PO	650 mg	10–15 mg/kg	325–1000 mg q4–6 h	10–15 mg/kg q4–8 h	B	Safe	if CrCl < 60 ml/min
Anticonvulsants									
Gabapentin	Neurontin	PO	300 mg	5 mg/kg for age > 3 yrs (limited data)	300 mg BID day 2, then 300 mg TID (further titration to 600 mg TID)	5 mg/kg TID (limited data)	C	Unknown	If CrCl < 60 ml/min
Pregabalin	Lyrica	PO	75–100 mg		100–300 mg divided BID–TID		C	Unknown	If CrCl < 60 ml/min
Carbamazepine	Tegretol	PO	100 mg	100 mg for age > 6 yrs (limited data)	200–400 mg QD–BID	100 mg BID	D	Probably safe	None
Antidepressants									
Duloxetine	Cymbalta	PO	60 mg		60 mg QD or BID		C	Possibly unsafe	If CrCl < 25 ml/min
Nortriptyline	Pamelor	PO	50 mg	1 mg/kg for age > 5yrs	50 mg qHS	1 mg/kg qHS	D	Probably safe	None

									If CrCl < 70 ml/min
Venlafaxine	Effexor	PO	75 mg		75 mg QD-BID		C	Possibly unsafe	
Hormones									
Calcitonin	Fortical	IN	200 IU	200 IU (limited data)	200 IU QD (limited data)		C	Possibly unsafe	Undefined
	Miacalcin	IV	200 IU over 20 min	200 IU (limited data)	May repeat 200 IU dose once		C	Possibly unsafe	Undefined
Corticotropin (ACTH)	Acthar	IM	40–80 units		40–80 units q8–12 h to total of 2–3 doses		C	Possibly unsafe	None
Muscle relaxants									
Cyclobenzaprine	Flexeril	PO	5 mg	5 mg for age > 14 yrs	5–10 mg TID	5 mg TID	B	Unknown	None
Diazepam	Valium	PO	2–10 mg	0.12–0.8 mg/kg per day divided QID	2–10 mg TID	0.12–0.8 mg/kg per day div q6h	D	Possibly unsafe	None
Cardiovascular agents									
Nitroglycerin (glyceryl trinitrate)	Nitrostat	SL	0.4 mg q5 mins x3		Not applicable to ED		C	Unknown	None
	Tridil	IV	5 µg/min titrated	0.25–0.5 µg/kg per min titrated	Titrate to maximum usual dose of 100 µg/kg per min	Titrate to maximum usual dose of 5 µg/kg per min	C	Unknown	None
Metoprolol	Lopressor	PO	25–50 mg		50–200 mg BID		C	Probably safe	None
		IV	5 mg IV				C	Probably safe	None

Other analgesic drugs (cont.)

Medication	Trade name	Route	Initial adult dose	Initial pediatric dose	Maintenance adult dose	Maintenance pediatric dose	Pregnancy Category	Lactation	Dosage adjustment in renal disease
Agents used for GI pain									
Aluminum/ magnesium salts (antacids)	Maalox	PO	20 mL suspension	5–15 mL for age > 5 yrs	10–20 mL between meals and HS	5–15 mL QID	C	Probably safe	If CrCl < 50 ml/min
Nifedipine	Procardia	PO	10 mg	0.2 mg/kg (maximum dose 10 mg)	10 mg PO TID	0.2–0.5 mg/kg (max 10 mg) TID	C	Possibly unsafe	None
Omeprazole	Prilosec	PO	20–40 mg	10–20 mg for age > 2 yrs	20–40 mg QD	10–20 mg QD	C	Probably safe	None
Pantoprazole	Protonix	PO	40 mg		40 mg QD–BID		B	Probably safe	None
		IV	40 mg		40 mg QD–BID		B	Probably safe	None
Ranitidine	Zantac	PO	150 mg	2 mg/kg	150 mg BID	1–2 mg/kg BID	B	Probably safe	If CrCl < 50 ml/min
		IV	50 mg	2 mg/kg	50 mg q6–8 h	2–4 mg/kg per day divided TID	B	Probably safe	If CrCl < 50 ml/min
Sucralfate	Carafate	PO	1000 mg	10–20 mg/kg	1000 mg QID (before meals and HS)	10–20 mg/kg (before meals and HS)	B	Safe	None

		Oral rinse	5–10 mL (500–1000 mg)	5 mL (500 mg)	5–10 mL (500–1000 mg) QID	5 mL (500 mg) QID	B	Safe	None
Headache therapy									
Caffeine	Cafcit	PO	300–400 mg		250–500 mg q8 h		C	Probably safe	None
Caffeine	Cafcit	IV	500 mg (in 1 L IV fluid over 1 h)		500 mg q4–8 h		C	Probably safe	None
Sumatriptan	Imitrex	IN	20 mg	5 mg IN if < 25 kg, 10 mg if 25–50 kg, 20 mg if > 50 kg	One repeat dose 2 h after first dose	One repeat dose 2 h after first dose	C	Safe	None
		PO	25 mg		25–100 mg QD		C	Safe	Undefined
		SC	6 mg		Used for episodic pain		C	Safe	Undefined
Zolmitriptan	Zomig	PO	2.5 mg		One repeat dose 2 h after first dose		C	Probably safe	If CrCl < 25 ml/min
		IN	5 mg		One repeat dose 2 h after first spray		C	Probably safe	If CrCl < 25 ml/min
Prochlorperazine	Compazine	PO	10 mg		5–10 mg q6–8 h		C	Unknown	None
		IV	10 mg		5–10 mg q6–8 h		C	Unknown	None
Topical agents									
Amlexanox	Aphthasol	Mucosal surfaces	1/4 inch (0.6 cm) 5% oral paste		1/4 inch (0.6 cm) QID		B	Probably safe	None
Benzocaine	Orajel	Oral surfaces	Apply with cotton-tipped swab		Apply QID		C	Probably safe	None

Other analgesic drugs (cont.)

Medication	Trade name	Route	Initial adult dose	Initial pediatric dose	Maintenance adult dose	Maintenance pediatric dose	Pregnancy Category	Lactation	Dosage adjustment in renal disease
Benzocaine +antipyrine	Auralgan	Otic	3–4 drops into ear then insert saturated cotton plug	3–4 drops into ear then insert saturated cotton plug	3–4 drops into ear q1–2 h as needed	3–4 drops into ear q1–2 h as needed	C	Probably safe	None
Diltiazem	Cardizem	Perianal region	700 mg 2% gel		Apply BID		C	Safe	None
Doxepin		Oral rinse (for mucositis)	5 mg/mL		5 mg/mL rinse q4–6 h		C	Possibly unsafe	None
Lidocaine	Lidoderm	Skin	5% patch		1–3 patches BID		B	Probably safe	None
Phenazopyridine	Pyridium	PO (for urinary tract)	200 mg	4 mg/kg	200 mg PO TID	4 mg/kg PO TID	B	Probably safe	If CrCl < 80 ml/min
Witch hazel	Tucks	Medicated pads	Gently pat pad on affected area	Gently pat pad on affected area	Repeat after each bowel movement or up to six times per day	Repeat after each bowel movement or up to six times per day	Unknown	Probably safe	None

CrCL, creatine clearance.